Acta Neurochirurgica
Supplements

Cerebral Vasospasm

Edited by
R. W. Seiler and H.-J. Steiger

Acta Neurochirurgica
Supplement 77

Prof. Dr. R. W. Seiler
Neurochirurgische Univ.-Klinik, Inselspital, Bern, Switzerland

Univ.-Prof. Dr. H.-J. Steiger
Neurochirurgische Univ.-Klinik, Klinikum Großhadern, München, Germany

Printed in Austria

Typesetting: Asco Typesetters, Hong Kong
Printing: A. Holzhausen, A-1140 Wien
Binding: Fa. Papyrus, A-1100 Wien
Printed on acid-free and chlorine-free bleached paper
SPIN: 10832807

With 90 partly coloured Figures

Library of Congress Cataloging-in-Publication Data

Cerebral vasospasm / edited by R. W. Seiler and H.-J. Steiger.
p.; cm. — (Acta neurochirurgica. Supplement ; 77)
Includes bibliographical references and index.
ISBN 3211836500 (alk. paper)
1. Cerebrovascular spasm—Congresses. I. Seiler, Rolf W. II. Steiger, Hans-Jakob, 1953– III. International Conference on Cerebral Vasospasm (7th : 2000 Interlaken, Switzerland) IV. Series.
[DNLM: 1. Vasospasm, Intracranial—Congresses. WL 355 C41306 2001]
RC388.5 .C39782 2001
616.8′1—dc21

2001020800

ISSN 0065-1419
ISBN 3-211-83650-0 Springer-Verlag Wien New York

Preface

This book contains the proceedings of the 7th International Conference on Cerebral Vasospasm, held in Interlaken, Switzerland, June 2000. Previous meetings devoted to cerebral vasospasm were held in Jackson, Mississippi (1972), Amsterdam, Netherlands (1979), Charlottesville, Virginia (1987), Tokyo (1990), Edmonton, Canada (1993) and Sydney, Australia (1997). The book gives the state of the art in reviews of the major aspects of cerebral vasospasm by invited authors, and selected articles of the conference presenting important results of the most recent research in basic sciences and clinical management of cerebral vasospasm.

Prof. Helge Nornes from Oslo, Norway, was the honored guest of the conference. Prof. Nornes has made major contributions to the evaluation and clinical management of cerebral vasospasm. A tribute to his life and his clinical and scientific work was published recently in *Supplement 72* of *Acta Neurochirurgica* (1999).

The editors gratefully acknowledge the help of the staff of the Department of Neurosurgery of the University Hospital Berne, and especially of Mrs. Nicole Reinert-Flückiger, in the organization and running of the 7th International Conference on Cerebral Vasospasm. The editors extend their gratitude to the many participants of this most recent vasospasm symposium, who were also the contributors to this book. Special thanks belong also to Mrs. Ilona Anders for editing the manuscripts.

This book is dedicated to our families whose patient support is so important for our professional and scientific activities.

R. W. Seiler and *H.-J. Steiger*

Contents

Listed in Current Contents

Acta Neurochir (2001) [Suppl] 77: 1–4

Is Cerebral Vasospasm still a Clinical Problem?

R. W. Seiler and **R. Binggeli**

Department of Neurosurgery, University Hospital, Berne, Switzerland

The first International Conference on Cerebral Vasospasm (ICCV) took place in Jackson (Mississippi) in 1972, and the second meeting in Amsterdam in 1979. At that time, ischemic deficits due to cerebral vasospasm (VSP) were a major clinical problem. The International Cooperative Study on the Timing of Aneurysm Surgery evaluated the results of surgical and medical management in 3521 patients treated between 1980 and 1983. The results showed that 42,3% of all patients were dead or disabled, and the leading cause of death and disability was VSP which had been present in 33% of those patients [10], (Fig. 1).

Around 1980, the antifibrinolytic drug tranexamic acid was used for prevention of rebleedings. In a randomized study, it was found to be effective in reducing the number of rebleedings, but with a proportionally equal increase of ischemic deficits. The conclusion was that until some method can be found to minimize ischemic complications, tranexamic acid is of no benefit in patients with subarachnoid hemorrhage [24].

In 1967, Farhat and Schneider published their observation on the improvement of ischemic neurological deficits with increased systemic blood pressure [5]. In clinical vasospasm, regional cerebral blood flow (rCBF) is depressed and pressure autoregulation is impaired. Under these circumstances, rCBF is directly dependent on perfusion pressure. Despite this rationale, clinicians have been reluctant to use hypervolemia and vasopressors for fear of precipitating hemorrhagic infarction or rupture of unclipped aneurysms. In 1976, Kosnik and Hunt reported the reversal of delayed ischemic symptoms in 6 of 7 patients by the use of vasopressors and hypervolemia [12]. A larger series, published by Kassel *et al.* in 1982, reported on the response of 58 patients with ischemic deficits due to vasospasm who were treated with intravascular volume expansion and induced arterial hypertension [11]. After these reports, hemodynamic therapy with careful fluid management to avoid hypovolemia and strict blood pressure limits to ensure adequate perfusion pressure became standard for the management of patients with subarachnoid hemorrhage. When the patients, despite these measures, become symptomatic, induced hypertension is now routinely used to try to reverse the ischemic deficit.

In the 1980's, the calcium antagonist nimodipine was evaluated in several randomized studies, and its neuroprotective effect to reduce ischemic deficits after subarachnoid hemorrhage (SAH) was proven [1, 3, 15, 17, 18, 19] (Table 1). Combining hemodynamic therapy, nimodipine and early aneurysm operation, we were able to reduce the frequency of permanent ischemic deficits due to vasospasm to about 5% of all

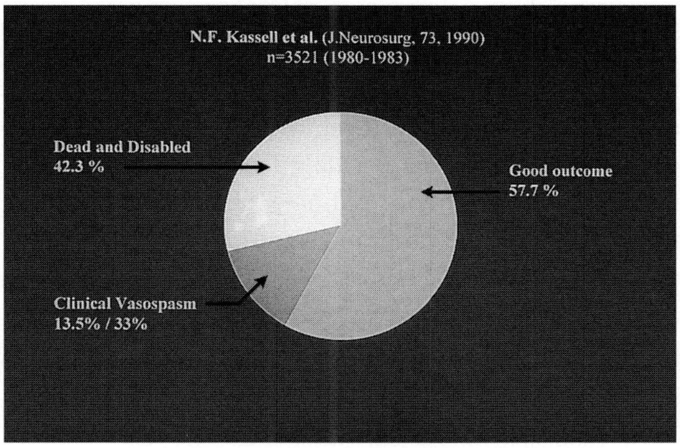

Fig. 1. Results of the International Cooperative Study, 1980–1983. Clinical vasospasm permanently affected 13.5% of all patients and accounted for 33% of deaths and disability

Table 1. *Prospective Randomized Nimodipine Studies*

Author	n	Dose	Ischemic deficits
Allen (1983)	125	30 mgq4h po	reduced (p = 0.03)
Phillipon (1986)	70	60 mgq4h po	reduced (p = 0.05)
Petruk (1987)	188	90 mgq4h po	reduced (p = 0.05)
Ohman (1988)	127	2 mg/h iv	reduced (p = 0.01)
Pickard (1989)	554	60 mgq4h po	reduced (p = 0.014)

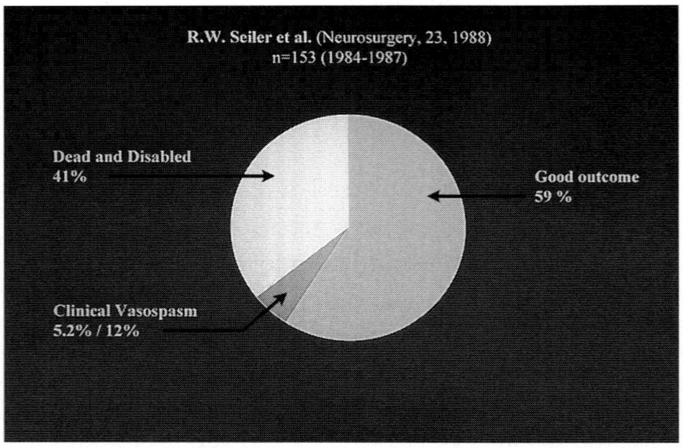

Fig. 2. Results of an outcome study in Berne between 1984 and 1987 using nimodipine and hemodynamic therapy. Clinical VSP permanently affected 5.2% of all patients and accounted for 12% of deaths and disability

treated patients and to 12% as the cause of death and disability [21] (Fig. 2). The direct effect of the initial or recurrent hemorrhage replaced VSP as the leading cause of morbidity and mortality after SAH.

In the late 1980's, aggressive prophylactic hypervolemic hemodilution therapy with a central venous pressure or a Swan-Ganz catheter combined with induced hypertension of 160–200 mmHg systolic blood pressure until the 14th day after SAH was introduced under the name of Triple-H-Therapy [2, 23]. With this treatment, delayed cerebral ischemia after SAH can be effectively reduced, but it requires expensive intensive care and has significant side effects, such as hemorrhagic brain infarction, pulmonary edema and heart failure [22]. In one randomized study, aggressive prophylactic Triple-H-Therapy was not found to confer any additional benefit over treatment with intravenous nicardipine and standard hemodynamic therapy [9]. In another randomized study, prophylactic hypervolemic therapy was not found to increase CBF or blood volume compared with normovolemic therapy [13].

It has been clearly documented that the location and amount of subarachnoid blood are directly related to the frequency and severity of cerebral VSP after subarachnoid hemorrhage. Mechanical removal of the periarterial clot has been performed in an attempt to prevent VSP and delayed ischemic deficits. However, surgical removal of subarachnoid blood in the acute stage of SAH is technically difficult and even dangerous for the patient. Therefore, nonmechanical and less traumatic methods of clearing subarachnoid blood using clot-liquefying thrombolytic agents such as tissue-type plasminogen-activator (tPA) or urokinase have been investigated in animal models and clinical studies. These methods appear to be effective in clearing subarachnoid blood and reducing VSP [6, 7, 16], especially in combination with cisternal drainage [14]. A randomized trial of intraoperative tPA in 1995 showed a 56% relative risk reduction of severe VSP only in those patients with thick subarachnoid clots. Overall hemorrhagic complications did not differ between the two groups, but there were two severe treatment-related hemorrhages from incompletely secured aneurysms [8]. It was concluded that tPA may be effective in preventing VSP, but requires reexamination in a larger randomized trial. Therefore, this treatment remains experimental.

Cerebral angioplasty was first reported by Zubkov *et al.* in 1984 [25]. In the 1990's, we witnessed the evolution of this interventional neuroradiological technique for the treatment of cerebral vasospasm. The largest series with 50 cases was published by Eskridge *et al.* in 1998. 28 patients showed sustained neurological improvement within 72 hours of angioplasty [4]. The disadvantage of angioplasty is that it requires neuroradiological expertise and is not available everywhere and at all times. Also the timing of angioplasty is critical and still controversial, and the method may have serious side effects, including arterial rupture. The benefit of interventional techniques in improving the management morbidity and mortality of patients with SAH and cerebral VSP remains to be demonstrated. In our experience between 1992–1995, the management mortality and morbidity did not change significantly (Fig. 3) which is in accordance with the experience of other centers. (Fig. 4) [20].

With modern treatment, only 5–7% of all patients with aneurysmal SAH are affected permanently by cerebral VSP. Prophylactic treatment of asymptomatic aneurysms to eliminate the devastating effect of the initial hemorrhage and early coiling or clipping of ruptured aneurysms to reduce rebleedings will have a greater impact on the outcome of patients with SAH

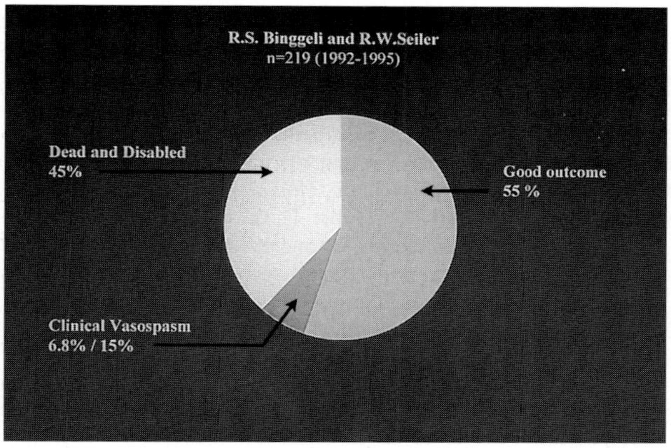

Fig. 3. Results of an outcome study in Berne between 1992 and 1995 using nimodipine, hemodynamic therapy and interventional neuroradiology. Clinical vasospasm permanently affected 6.8% of all patients and accounted for 15% of deaths and disability

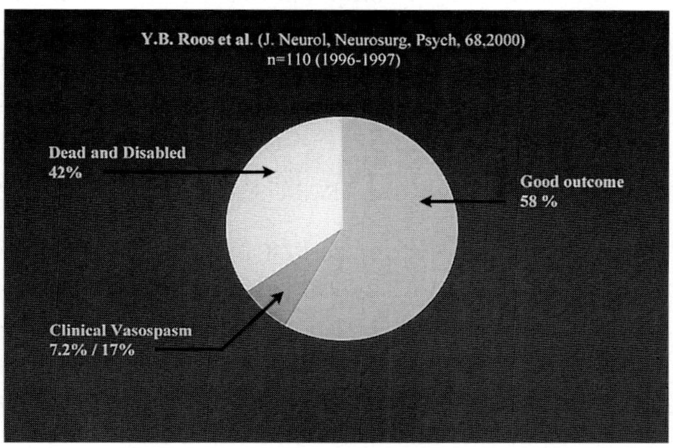

Fig. 4. Results of an outcome study in the Netherlands between 1996 and 1997 using nimodipine and hemodynamic therapy. Clinical vasospasm permanently affected 7.3% of all patients and accounted for 17% of deaths and disability

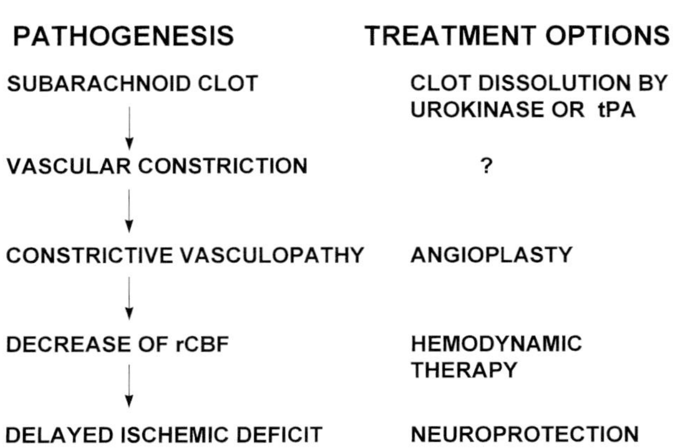

Fig. 5. The different steps in the pathogenesis of vasospasm and delayed ischemic deficits and the current treatment options. We still lack a single drug to prevent vasoconstriction

than improved treatment of delayed ischemia and VSP. But our current therapy of cerebral VSP consists of treating the consequences of the vasoconstriction, and we still lack a single drug to prevent vasospasm (Fig. 5). If we could find such a drug, we would reduce the complexity, side effects and probably also the costs of the treatment and improve the outcome of our patients. Therefore, basic research on the molecular mechanisms of vasoconstriction and vasorelaxation must be pursued further.

References

1. Allen GS, Ahn HS, Preziosi TJ, Battye R, Boone SC, Chou SN, Kelly DL, Weir BK, Crabbe RA, Lavik PJ, Rosenbloom SB, Dorsey FC, Ingram CR, Melits DE, Bertsch LA, Boisvert DPJ, Hundley M, Johnson RK, Strom JA, Transou CR (1983) Cerebral arterial spasm – a controlled trial of nimodipine in patients with subarachnoid haemorrhage. N Engl J Med 308: 619–624
2. Awad IA, Carter LPH, Spetzler RF, Medina M, William FW Jr (1987) Clinical vasospasm after subarachnoid hemorrhage: response to hypervolemic hemodilution and arterial hypertension. Stroke 18: 365–372
3. Barker FG, Ogilvy CS (1996) Efficacy of prophylactic nimodipine for delayed ischemic deficit after subarachnoid hemorrhage: meta-analysis. J Neurosurg 84: 404–414
4. Eskridge JM, McAuliffe W, Song JK, Deliganis AV, Newell DW, Lewis DH, Mayberg MR, Winn HR (1998) Balloon angioplasty for the treatment of vasospasm: results of first 50 cases. Neurosurgery 42: 510–517
5. Farhat SM, Schneider RC (1967) Observations on the effect of systemic blood pressure on intracranial circulation in patients with cerebrovascular insufficiency. J Neurosurg 27: 441–445
6. Findlay JM, Weir BKA, Steinke D, Tanabe T, Gordon P, Grace M (1988) Effect of intrathecal thrombolytic therapy on subarachnoid clot and chronic vasospasm in a primate model of SAH. J Neurosurg 69: 723–735
7. Findlay JM, Weir BKA, Kassell NF, Disney LB, Grace MGA (1991) Intracisternal recombinant tissue plasminogen activator after aneurysmal subarachnoid hemorrhage. J Neurosurg 75: 181–188
8. Findlay JM, Kassell NF, Weir BKA, Haley EC, Kongable G, Germanson T, Truskowski L, Alves WM, Holness RO, Knuckey NW, Yonas H, Steinberg GK, West M, Winn R, Ferguson G (1995) A randomized trial of intraoperative, intracisternal tissue plasminogen activator for the prevention of vasospasm. Neurosurgery 37: 168–178
9. Haley EC, Kassell NF, Torner JC, participants (1993) A randomized controlled trial of high-dose intravenous nicardipine in aneurysmal subarachnoid hemorrhage. A report of the Cooperative Aneurysm Study. J Neurosurg 78: 537–547
10. Kassell NF, Torner JC, Haley EC, Jane JA, Adams HP, Kongable GL, participants (1990) The International Cooperative Study on the Timing of Aneurysm Surgery. J Neurosurg 73: 18–36
11. Kassell NF, Peerless SJ, Durward QJ, Beck DW, Drake CG, Adams HP (1982) Treatment of ischemic deficits from vaso-

spasm with intravascular volume expansion and induced arterial hypertension. Neurosurgery 11: 337–343
12. Kosnik EJ, Hunt WE (1976) Postoperative hypertension in the management of patients with intracranial arterial aneurysms. J Neurosurg 45: 148–154
13. Lennihan L, Mayer SA, Fink ME, Beckford A, Paik MC, Zhang H, Wu YC, Klebanoff LM, Raps EC, Solomon RA (2000) Effect of hypervolemic therapy on cerebral blood flow after subarachnoid hemorrhage. A randomized controlled trial. Stroke 31: 303–391
14. Mizoi K, Yoshimoto T, Takahashi A, Fujiwara S, Koshu K, Sugawara T (1993) Prospective study on the prevention of cerebral vasospasm by intrathecal fibrinolytic therapy with tissue-type plasminogen activator. J Neurosurg 78: 430–437
15. Öhman J, Heiskanen O (1988) Effect of nimodipine on the outcome of patients after aneurysmal subarachnoid hemorrhage and surgery. J Neurosurg 69: 683–686
16. Öhman J, Servo A, Heiskanen O (1991) Effect of intrathecal fibrinolytic therapy on clot lysis and vasospasm in patients with aneurysmal subarachnoid hemorrhage. J Neurosurg 75: 197–201
17. Ljunggren B, Brandt L, Sundbärg G, Saveland H, Cronquist S, Stridbeck H (1982) Early management of aneurysmal subarachnoid hemorrhage. Neurosurgery 11: 414–418
18. Philippon J, Grob R, Dagreou F, Guggiari M, Rivierez M, Viars P (1986) Prevention of vasospasm in subarachnoid haemorrhage. A controlled study with nimodipine. Acta Neurochir (Wien) 82: 110–114
19. Pickard JD, Murray GD, Illingworth R, Shaw MDM, Teasdale GM, Foy PM, Humphrey PRD, Lang DA, Nelson R, Richards P, Sinar J, Bailey S, Skene A (1989) Effect of oral nimodipine on cerebral infarction and outcome after subarachnoid haemorrhage: British aneurysm nimodipine trial. BMJ 298: 636–642
20. Roos YBWEM, de Haan RJ, Beenen LFM, Groen RJM, Albrecht KW, Vermeulen M (2000) Complications and outcome in patients with aneurysmal subarachnoid haemorrhage: a prospective hospital based cohort study in The Netherlands. J Neurol Neurosurg Psychiatry 68: 337–341
21. Seiler RW, Reulen HJ, Huber P, Grolimund P, Ebeling U, Steiger HJ (1988) Outcome of aneurysmal subarachnoid hemorrhage in a hospital population: A prospective study including early operation, intravenous nimodipine, and transcranial Doppler ultrasound. Neurosurgery 23: 598–604
22. Shimoda M, Oda S, Tsugane R, Sato O (1993) Intracranial complications of hypervolemic therapy in patients with a delayed ischemic deficit attributed to vasospasm. J Neurosurg 78: 423–429
23. Solomon RA, Fink ME, Lennihan L (1988) Early aneurysm surgery and prophylactic hypervolemic hypertensive therapy for the treatment of aneurysmal subarachnoid hemorrhage. Neurosurgery 23: 699–704
24. Vermeulen M, Lindsay KW, Murray GD, Cheah F, Muizelaar JP, Schannong M, Teasdale GM, van Crevel H, van Gijn J (1984) Antifibrinolytic treatment in subarachnoid hemorrhage. N Engl J Med 311: 432–7
25. Zubkov YN, Nikiforov BM, Shustin VA (1984) Balloon catheter technique for dilatation of constricted cerebral arteries after aneurysmal SAH. Acta Neurochir (Wien) 70: 65–79

Correspondence: Rolf W. Seiler, Neurosurgical Department University Hospital, CH-3010 Berne, Switzerland.

Part 1: Basic Science and Experimental Vasospasm

Molecular Biology of Vasospasm

Acta Neurochir (2001) [Suppl] 77: 7–11

Pathophysiology and Molecular Genetics of Vasospasm

R. L. Macdonald

Section of Neurosurgery, University of Chicago Medical Center and Pritzker School of Medicine, Chicago, Illinois, USA

Introduction

An overview of current understanding of the vasospasm that occurs days after SAH is provided with the primary purpose being to highlight some areas where a more rigorous scientific understanding of the processes involved is required.

Keywords: SAH; cerebral vasospasm; cerebrovascular regulation; gene expression; Rho kinase; fasudil HCl.

Extracellular Processes in Vasospasm

Spasmogens

The theory that hemoglobin causes vasospasm remains viable. Inconsistencies are that hemoglobin did not produce vasospasm that was as severe as that due to whole blood, suggesting that other spasmogens are involved [10, 14]. Most hemoglobin solutions that have been used in vasospasm experiments are not pure. Contractions of arteries to hemoglobin in vitro were potentiated by a low molecular weight fraction of erythrocyte hemolysate [1]. Changes in gene expression in smooth muscle cells in response to hemolysate were different from those due to pure hemoglobin [23]. There may be multiple spasmogens independent of hemoglobin and/or generated by hemoglobin-driven reactions that are different at different times after SAH and that have different mechanisms of action. The role of interactions between the brain, cerebral arteries and clot in the generation of spasm have not been investigated. It may be difficult to replicate this situation in vitro. For example, the ability of fresh erythrocyte hemolysate to elevate $[Ca^{2+}]_i$ in smooth muscle cells was due to adenosine triphosphate (ATP) although there was not enough ATP present in the human subarachnoid space days after SAH to cause vasospasm [12].

Changes in Arterial Wall Mechanics

The mechanism by which the arteries narrow initially is active smooth muscle contraction. In the first days, experimental vasospasm can be reversed with vasodilators such as papaverine and the arteries do not show major alterations in contractility and compliance [22]. Contraction by other cells and lumen narrowing by mural thrombosis may contribute in some cases. With time, arteries exposed to subarachnoid blood become less contractile and compliant when studied under isometric tension in vitro. These changes become progressively severe with time and continue to do so even as angiographic vasospasm resolves. They contribute to vasospasm by rendering the artery less able to relax in response to a vasodilator or in response to removal of the spasmogenic stimulus. The extent to which vasospasm can be reversed by superselective intraarterial papaverine is decreased with increased time after SAH [22].

These changes are reminiscent of those occurring with vascular remodeling. Reducing blood flow by 70% through the common carotid artery of rabbits caused an endothelium-dependent 21% decrease in diameter of the artery 2 weeks later [9]. The response is lost in mice lacking endothelial NO synthase [18]. The diameter reduction was apparent within days of flow reduction and was reversible at first with papaverine but became less reversible with increasing time [9]. One difference is that in vasospasm there is a primary reduction in diameter that is associated with reduced relaxation whereas in remodeling there is a primary reduction in flow. Remodeling may be mediated by the need for endothelium to maintain constant shear stress. Vasospasm is associated with increased endothelial shear stress that should induce vasodilation.

Reports that the effect of endothelium-derived NO is reduced in vasospasm and the possibility of the endothelium mediating remodeling may be mutually exclusive events. One cannot be correct. Other key questions are whether or not remodeling occurs with prolonged constriction rather than flow reduction as the primary process. The basis for the remodeling and of the structural changes in vasospasm are uncertain. There was no fibrosis in the experiments of Langille. It was suggested that the changes in vasospasm are not due to active smooth muscle contraction and are therefore due to alteration in the extracellular matrix secondary to inflammation [22]. Other possibilities are that the muscle is set to a shorter length and/or that there is fibrosis of the extracellular matrix or the cytoskeletal domain of the smooth muscle cell. There is some evidence for increased collagen and fibronectin in the arterial wall after SAH [11]. It has not been demonstrated that pure hemoglobin can cause these structural changes. Hemoglobin can cause some of the pathological changes but the solutions used were impure [10, 14].

Hemoglobin and Endothelium

A key unanswered question is how hemoglobin causes vasospasm. Numerous mechanisms have been postulated, including direct action on smooth muscle, removal of NO, increase in endothelin, damage to perivascular nerves, effects of free radicals, production of lipid peroxides and eicosanoid-like substances, metabolism to bilirubin and other breakdown products and release of hemorphins from the globin chains. Pure hemoglobin does not readily increase $[Ca^{2+}]_i$ and is not particularly toxic to smooth muscle cells, suggesting that any vasospastic actions are indirect [13]. Prior studies showing that hemoglobin has these effects probably was because the hemoglobin solutions were impure [2].

The nitric oxide relaxation system is disrupted after SAH [5, 11]. Endothelium-dependent relaxations may be impaired by reduced endothelial NO synthase function, destruction of NO after it is released, and/or reduced responsiveness of smooth muscle to NO. Experiments supporting reduced NO release and reduced ability of the smooth muscle to relax to NO have been reported. Reports that nitrovasodilators reverse vasospasm are inconsistent with a primary defect in the smooth muscle response to NO [5]. The main effect of hemoglobin would be to remove NO. It is unclear how hemoglobin could prevent the action of NO derived from the endothelium. Hemoglobin does penetrate into the arterial wall after SAH although it would have to reach the internal elastic lamina in substantial quantities to remove all of the NO before it acted on the smooth muscle cells, a process not supported by immunohistochemical studies [6]. The process may involve free radicals formed by hemoglobin that traverse the arterial wall. Removal of NO produced by neuronal NO synthase in the arterial adventitia may be important [5].

Relaxation of vascular smooth muscle also occurs by the cyclic adenosine monophosphate (cAMP) pathway and by activation of K^+ channels. Relaxation via the cAMP pathway may be impaired after SAH [21]. Vascular smooth muscle is depolarized after SAH and this may contribute to vasospasm [5]. This could be a result of hemoglobin removing NO and reducing cGMP, an endogenous K^+ channel opener. NO also may directly activate some K^+ channels in some arteries.

The characteristics of endothelin-1 that suggest it may be involved in vasospasm are that it is a potent vasoconstrictor, it is increased in CSF after SAH in animals and man and numerous studies show that endothelin antagonists prevent or decrease vasospasm [11]. The increase in endothelin after SAH probably is secondary to brain ischemia [17]. Second, NO normally inhibits endothelin production so that removal of NO after SAH may be responsible [5]. The contribution of other mechanisms of hemoglobin-induced cerebrovascular contraction are less well defined.

Changes in Smooth Muscle Cells in Vasospasm

Studies of isolated cerebrovascular smooth muscle cells show that hemoglobin or erythrocyte hemolysate cause prolonged elevations in $[Ca^{2+}]_i$ that are associated with cell contraction, membrane bleb formation, and cell death [11]. The elevation in $[Ca^{2+}]_i$ by fresh hemolysate is due to ATP although this is not an important cause of vasospasm [12]. Pure hemoglobin may be devoid of these effects [2]; they are probably due to contaminants in the hemoglobin solutions or to interaction of other compounds in hemolysate.

There are many intracellular pathways involved in

smooth muscle contraction. Adequate assessment of their role in vasospasm is difficult at present due to lack of specific pharmacological agents, incomplete understanding of the regulatory pathways involved and lack of detailed studies of each mechanism over time in appropriate vasospasm models. There are no studies of whether pure hemoglobin causes any of the changes reported below although in some cases, hemolysate has been shown to alter the pathway in vitro.

Most smooth muscle contraction involves Ca^{2+}-calmodulin binding to the actin-myosin complex, activating myosin light chain kinase, phosphorylation of myosin light chains and contraction. Persistent contraction usually is not associated with increased myosin light chain phosphorylation. In vasospastic arteries, myosin, α-actin and caldesmon may [15, 20] or may not [11, 15] be decreased and levels of myosin light chain phosphorylation are decreased [11] or at least not markedly elevated [20]. An inhibitor of myosin light chain kinase, ML-9, prevented experimental vasospasm although the nonspecific actions of this drug and the inability of calmodulin antagonists to prevent vasospasm argues for involvement of other processes [11]. Changes in $[Ca^{2+}]_i$ are important but contraction can occur with no or only minimal increase in $[Ca^{2+}]_i$. During vasospasm in dogs, $[Ca^{2+}]_i$ in the basilar artery was unchanged or decreased [11]. The ability of smooth muscle cells to regulate $[Ca^{2+}]_i$ may be disrupted during vasospasm or the contractile apparatus may be more sensitive to a given $[Ca^{2+}]_i$, leading to Ca^{2+} sensitization [11]. The plasma membrane Ca^{2+}-ATPase that pumps Ca^{2+} out of cells and lowers $[Ca^{2+}]_i$, was significantly decreased in basilar artery smooth muscle following SAH in dogs [11].

Other processes whose involvement in smooth muscle contraction remains theoretical include latch bridges, proteins associated with thin-filaments such as calponin and caldesmon and action of phosphatases on myosin light chain. Each of these processes is modulated by complex, parallel and series cascades of kinases including tyrosine kinases, mitogen-activated protein kinases, Rho kinase and protein kinase C. Calponin may regulate contraction by inhibiting the actin-myosin interaction. Its action may be accentuated when it is phosphorylated by protein kinase C and/or Ca^{2+}-calmodulin-dependent protein kinase II. Calponin was decreased in vasospastic dog basilar arteries and there may be an increase in phosphorylation of the remaining protein, both of which could promote vasoconstriction [3, 7, 8, 15, 20].

Rho kinase may prolong contraction by inhibiting the phosphatase that dephosphorylates myosin light chain. HA1077 (fasudil) is a nonspecific inhibitor of serine/threonine kinases that is more potent against p160 Rho kinase than myosin light chain kinase. HA1077 inhibited vasospasm in dogs and humans [20]. An inhibitor of Rho kinase, Y27632, reversed established vasospasm in dogs [19]. Tyrosine and mitogen-activated kinases may be involved in hemolysate-induced contractions of rabbit [24] and cow cerebral arteries [4].

Protein kinase C, which is activated by diacyl glycerol, may be involved in tonic smooth muscle contraction and in vasospasm. There are 11 isozymes. The specific distribution and function of the various isozymes varies with species and tissue and the drugs used to inhibit protein kinase C are sufficiently nonspecific as to render a complete elucidation of the role in vasospasm poorly defined. Vasospasm was associated with a decrease in α and ε but not ζ isoforms in one study [11]. Vasospasm was associated with increased diacyl glycerol levels and increased overall protein kinase C activity and topical application of the relatively nonspecific protein kinase C inhibitors, H-7 and staurosporine, reversed vasospasm in dogs [11]. Involvement of IP_3 and protein kinase C in vasospasm also was suggested by observations that oxyhemoglobin elevates $[Ca^{2+}]_i$ and inositol trisphosphate in cultured smooth muscle cells and that these responses are blocked by neomycin, an inhibitor of phospholipase C [11].

Calpains are neutral proteases that when activated by increased $[Ca^{2+}]_i$ will break down cytoskeletal and contractile proteins and protein kinases, leading in part to activation of kinases, including protein kinase C, and possibly to smooth muscle contraction [8, 11]. The decrease in contractile proteins, the demonstrated activation of calpain proteolysis, and the efficacy of inhibitors of calpeptin against experimental vasospasm supports a role for Ca^{2+}-activated proteolysis in vasospasm [8].

Smooth muscle cells rely on high energy phosphate compounds such as ATP and guanosine triphosphate for contraction and relaxation. Deficiencies, particularly of ATP, may result in smooth muscle rigor, a state that could theoretically be involved in vasospasm [11]. Vasospasm has been associated with a progressive reduction in high-energy phosphates and there is evidence that hemoglobin and bilirubin can decrease ATP levels in cultured smooth muscle cells [11]. This also might contribute to impaired vascular relaxation in vasospasm.

Changes in Gene Expression

The average cell expresses 15,000 to 40,000 genes out of a total genome containing 60,000 to 100,000 genes. Technology such as the complimentary DNA array, is available to determine the relative levels of expression of possibly every gene expressed in a cell in response to a given stimulus. Interpreting the results is difficult unless one has a specific question in mind. Analysis of a vasospastic artery is the analysis of multiple cell types at different stages of response to perhaps hundreds of stimuli, many of no importance to arterial narrowing. Onda, *et al.*, examined changes in gene expression at different times after SAH in dogs [16]. 49 out of 588 genes examined (8%) were expressed in dog basilar artery. 18 genes were upregulated (37%) and 2 were downregulated (4%). Genes that were upregulated were vascular endothelial growth factor, BiP protein (glucose-regulated protein 78), growth-arrest and DNA-damage-inducible protein, neuromodulin, protein disulfide isomerase-related protein P5, acid sphingomyelinase-like phosphodiesterase and 5 genes related to inflammation (monocyte chemotactic protein 1, cystatin B, inter-α-trypsin inhibitor family heavy chain-related protein, serum amyloid A protein, glycoprotein 130). Frizzled-6 was downregulated. Since genes related to cell stress and inflammation were upregulated, a role for these processes was postulated in vasospasm.

References

1. Aoki T, Takenaka K, Suzuki S, Kassell NF, Sagher O, Lee KS (1994) The role of hemolysate in the facilitation of oxyhemoglobin-induced contraction in rabbit basilar arteries. J Neurosurg 81: 261–266
2. D'Agnillo F, Alayash AI (2000) Oxyhemoglobin and apoptosis (letter). J Neurosurg 92: 899–900
3. Doi M, Kasuya H, Weir B, Cook DA, Ogawa A (1997) Reduced expression of calponin in canine basilar artery after subarachnoid haemorrhage. Acta Neurochir (Wien) 139: 77–81
4. Doi M, Watanabe M, Nishikawa Y, Sasaki K, Suzuki M, Ogawa A (2000) Involvement of protein kinases in the mechanisms of contraction of cerebral arterial smooth muscle. J Stroke Cerebrovasc Dis 9 [Suppl] 1: 363–364
5. Faraci FM, Heistad DD (1998) Regulation of the cerebral circulation: role of endothelium and potassium channels. Physiol Rev 78: 53–97
6. Foley PL, Kassell NF, Hudson SB, Lee KS (1993) Hemoglobin penetration in the wall of the rabbit basilar artery after subarachnoid hemorrhage and intracisternal hemoglobin injection. Acta Neurochir (Wien) 123: 82–86
7. Fujikawa H, Tani E, Yamaura I, Miyaji K, Sato M, Takahashi K (2000) Phosphorylation of calponin of canine basilar artery in vasospasm. J Sroke Cerebrovasc Dis 9 [Suppl] 1: 225–226
8. Kim I, Leinweber BD, Morgalla M, Butler WE, Seto M, Sasaki Y, Peterson JW, Morgan KG (2000) Thin and thick filament regulation of contractility in experimental cerebral vasospasm. Neurosurgery 46: 440–447
9. Langille BL, O'Donnell F (1986) Reductions in arterial diameter produced by chronic decreases in blood flow are endothelium-dependent. Science 231: 405–407
10. Macdonald RL, Weir BK, Runzer TD, Grace MG, Saito K, Findlay JM, Cook DA, Mielke BW, Kanamaru K (1991) Etiology of cerebral vasospasm in primates. J Neurosurg 75: 415–424
11. Macdonald RL, Wang X, Zhang J, Marton LS (1996) Molecular changes with subarachnoid hemorrhage and vasospasm. The molecular basis of neurosurgical disease. In: Raffel C, Harsh GRI (eds) Williams and Wilkins, Baltimore, pp 278–293
12. Macdonald RL, Weir B, Marton LS, Zhang ZD, Sajdak M, Johns LM, Kowalczuk A (2000) Role of adenosine triphosphate in vasospasm: investigations in humans. J Neurosurg 92: 227 (Abstr)
13. Marton LS, Wang X, Kowalczuk A, Zhang ZD, Windmeyer E, Macdonald RL (2000) Effects of hemoglobin on heme oxygenase gene expression and viability of cultured smooth muscle cells. Am J Physiol (in press)
14. Mayberg MR, Okada T, Bark DH (1990) The role of hemoglobin in arterial narrowing after subarachnoid hemorrhage. J Neurosurg 72: 634–640
15. Oka Y, Ohta S, Todo H, Kohno K, Kumon Y, Sakaki S (1996) Protein synthesis and immunoreactivities of contraction-related proteins in smooth muscle cells of canine basilar artery after experimental subarachnoid hemorrhage. J Cereb Blood Flow Metab 16: 1335–1344
16. Onda H, Kasuya H, Takakura K, Hori T, Imaizumi T, Takeuchi T, Inoue I, Takeda J (1999) Identification of genes differentially expressed in canine vasospastic cerebral arteries after subarachnoid hemorrhage. J Cereb Blood Flow Metab 19: 1279–1288
17. Pluta RM, Boock RJ, Afshar JK, Clouse K, Bacic M, Ehrenreich H, Oldfield EH (1997) Source and cause of endothelin-1 release into cerebrospinal fluid after subarachnoid hemorrhage. J Neurosurg 87: 287–293
18. Rudic RD, Shesely EG, Maeda N, Smithies O, Segal SS, Sessa WC (1998) Direct evidence for the importance of endothelium-derived nitric oxide in vascular remodeling. J Clin Invest 101: 731–736
19. Sato M, Tani E, Fujikawa H, Yamaura I, Kaibuchi K (2000) Importance of Rho-kinase-mediated phosphorylation of myosin light chain in cerebral vasospasm. J Stroke Cerebrovasc Dis 9 [Suppl] 1: 223–224
20. Sun H, Kanamaru K, Ito M, Suzuki H, Kojima T, Waga S, Kureishi Y, Nakano T (1998) Myosin light chain phosphorylation and contractile proteins in a canine two-hemorrhage model of subarachnoid hemorrhage. Stroke 29: 2149–2154
21. Todo H, Ohta S, Wang J, Ichikawa H, Ohue S, Kumon Y, Sakaki S (1998) Impairment in biochemical level of arterial dilative capability of a cyclic nucleotides-dependent pathway by induced vasospasm in the canine basilar artery. J Cereb Blood Flow Metab 18: 808–817
22. Vorkapic P, Bevan RD, Bevan JA (1991) Longitudinal time course of reversible and irreversible components of chronic cerebrovasospasm of the rabbit basilar artery. J Neurosurg 74: 951–955

23. Wang X, Marton LS, Weir BK, Macdonald RL (1999) Immediate early gene expression in vascular smooth-muscle cells synergistically induced by hemolysate components. J Neurosurg 90: 1083–1090
24. Zubkov AY, Ogihara K, Tumu P, Patlolla A, Lewis AI, Parent AD, Zhang J (1999) Mitogen-activated protein kinase mediation of hemolysate-induced contraction in rabbit basilar artery. J Neurosurg 90: 1091–1097

Correspondence: R. Loch Macdonald, Section of Neurosurgery, MC 3026, University of Chicago Medical Center, 5841 South Maryland Avenue, Chicago, Illinois, USA, 60637.

Acta Neurochir (2001) [Suppl] 77: 13–16

Identification of Genes Differentially Expressed in Canine Vasospastic Cerebral Arteries after Subarachnoid Hemorrhage

H. Kasuya, H. Onda, A. Kawashima, A. Sasahara, and **T. Hori**

Department of Neurosurgery, Tokyo Women's Medical University, Tokyo, Japan

Introduction

Recently, a number of molecular biological techniques have been applied in the studies of cerebral vasospasm [2]. Most of the previous studies have focused on some known genes encoding related factors such as vasoconstriction agonists or antagonists. A single cell is estimated to express ~15,000 genes, of which several hundreds are thought to play some tissue-specific roles in the cell. However, since most of them are unknown and have not yet been characterized, it is important to identify the unknown genes which could be involved in the pathogenesis of cerebtral vasospasm. In this study, as a first step to better understand the whole molecular process of cerebral vasospasm, the two molecular biological techniques of cDNA expression array and mRNA differential display [3] were applied to identify differentially expressed genes during cerebral vasospasm.

Keywords: Cerebral vasospasm; subarachnoid hemorrhage; differential gene expression; inflammation.

Materials and Methods

Cerebral Vasospasm Models

Twenty-one dogs were divided into three groups. Group D-0 comprised control animals, sacrificed on day 0 without cisternal blood injection. Group D-2 animals were sacrificed on day 2 following the first injection on day 0. Group D-7 animals were sacrificed on day 7 following injections on days 0 and 2 (double hemorrhage model). Angiography of cerebral arteries of each animal was performed on days 0, 2 and 7, and diameters of the basilar arteries were measured on angiographic film for evaluation of vasospasm.

RNA Preparation

The animals were sacrificed by injection of 100 mg/kg pentobarbital, exsanguinated and perfused with 1,500–2,000 ml normal saline. Total RNAs were extracted from individual basilar arteries from each group using TRIzol (Gibco Brl) according to the manufacturer's instruction. Possible traces of genomic DNA contaminating RNA preparations were removed by DNase I (Promega) digestion.

cDNA Expression Array

Fifty μg of total RNA prepared from D-0 and D-7 groups was purified to poly (A) RNA. cDNA probes were synthesized from the poly (A) RNA in the presence of [α-^{32}P] dATP using random primers and M-MLV reverse transcriptase (Clontech). The two Atlas Human cDNA Expression Array membranes (Clontech) were prehybridized at 42 °C for 30 min. The two membranes were then separately hybridized at 42 °C for 16 hr in the same solution with the ^{32}P-labeled cDNA probes prepared from D-0 and D-7 samples. The membranes were washed at room temperature and then at 60 °C for 30 min, and exposed to X-ray film for 3 days with an intensifying screen. After confirming equal intensities of hybridization signals for several housekeeping genes between autoradiograms for D-0 and D-7, differentially expressed genes were evaluated by comparing intensities of specific hybridizing signals.

mRNA Differential Display

cDNA was synthesized from 1 μg total RNA using one of five oligo (dT) primers T_{12}AG, T_{12}CG, T_{12}GG, T_{12}GC, and T_{12}AC. cDNAs from at least four individual basilar arteries from each group were subjected to the same experiment to confirm reproducibility. The oligo (dT) primer was end-labeled with [γ-^{32}P] ATP. One twentieth of the cDNAs generated were amplified by PCR in the presence of labeled oligo (dT) primer and one of 21 upstream arbitrary primers. One hundred and five primer pairs were used to screen mRNAs from groups D-0, D-2 and D-7. PCR conditions used were 25 cycles of denaturation at 94 °C for 30 sec, annealing at 40 °C for 1 min and extension at 72 °C for 30 sec. The radiolabeled PCR products were separated on 5 or 6% denaturing polyacrylamide gels and the dried gels were exposed to X-ray film for 12–16 hr.

After autoradiography, the intensity of each band was compared among groups D-0, D-2 and D-7. Differentially expressed bands were excised from the gels, reamplified by PCR using the same set of primers, and subcloned into pGEM-3Z (Promega). The cDNA inserts were then sequenced using an Applied Biosystem DNA Sequencer model 377 with a Taq DyeDeoxy Termination Cycle Sequencing Kit (Perkin Elmer).

Reverse Transcription (RT) – PCR

Total RNAs (1 μg) from arteries of groups D-0, D-2 and D-7 or from several tissues were reverse-transcribed using oligo (dT) primer. One-twentieth of the cDNA synthesized was amplified by PCR in the presence of [α-^{32}P] dCTP and a pair of specific primers. PCR conditions used were 18–31 cycles of denaturation at 94 °C for 45 sec, annealing at 58 °C, 60 °C or 62 °C for 45 sec and extension at 72 °C for 45 sec. The PCR products were separated on a 6% non-denaturing polyacrylamide gel, and the dried gel was exposed to X-ray films for 3–6 hr. The relative ratio of expression patterns of mRNAs was evaluated by direct measurement of radioactivity in each band using a scintillation counter.

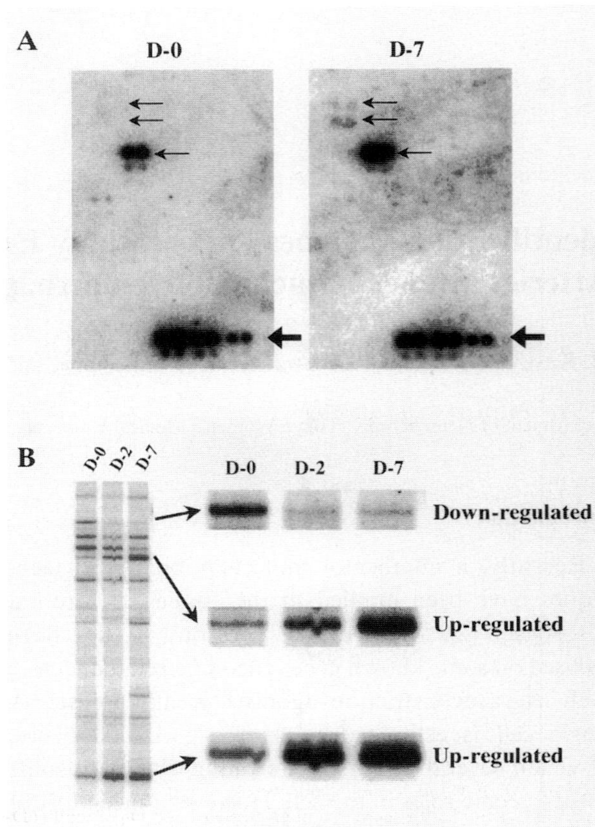

Fig. 1. Identification of differentially expressed mRNAs. (A) A representative autoradiogram of groups D-0 and D-7 in cDNA expression array. Thick arrows indicate equal intensities in duplicated hybridization signals for three housekeeping genes between D-0 and D-7 membranes. Thin arrows indicate hybridization signals for genes up-regulated in group D-7. (B) A autoradiogram of mRNA differential display. The radiolabeled PCR products derived from D-0, D-2 and D-7 groups were separated on a 5% denaturing polyacrylamide gel. The differentially expressed bands were identified by comparing the intensity of corresponding bands among three groups (reproduction from J Cereb Blood Flow Metab 19: 1279–1288, 1999 with permission)

Results

Differentially Expressed mRNAs Identified

The cDNA Atlas Array examined includes 588 human known cDNAs. High stringent hybridization indicated that 49 (8.3%) of them were found to be expressed in dog basilar arteries; a representative hybridization pattern is shown in Fig. 1A. The dots of six housekeeping genes for ubiquitin, β-actin, GAPDH, α-tubulin, 23-kDa highly basic protein, and ribosomal protein S9 generated equal intensities of hybridizing signals in both membranes for D-0 and D-7 groups, which could normalize mRNA abundance between samples. Of 49 genes, four were up-regulated in the basilar arteries with vasospasm: the genes for gadd45 (growth arrest and DNA-damage-inducible protein 45), MCP-1 (monocyte chemotactic protein-1), neuromodulin, and VEGF (vascular endothelial growth factor). RT-PCR confirmed their differential expression patterns (Fig. 2A).

Forty differentially expressed bands in groups D-2 and D-7 were identified by mRNA differential display; a representative pattern of display is shown in Fig. 1B. The bands, designated DVS 1–40, were sequenced, generating 26 non-redundant sequences. RT-PCR confirmed the differentially expressed patterns of 16 of the 26 clones obtained (Fig. 2B). Three clones (DVS 14, 26, and 27) were highly up-regulated in group D-7 compared to group D-2, and in group D-2 compared to group D-0 and six clones (DVS 3, 4, 11, 30, 31, and 37) were more mildly up-regulated. Five clones (DVS 5, 15, 16, 23, and 28) were up-regulated in groups D-2 and D-7 equally, one clone (DVS 2) was down-regulated in groups D-2 and D-7, and one clone (DVS 29) was down-regulated in only group D-2.

Database Analysis

The sequences of 16 clones obtained by mRNA differential display were compared with those in the nucleotide databases using the BLAST network service [1]. The sequences of eight clones were highly homologous to those of human known genes (Table 1). The DVS 3, 4, 5, 11, 14, 26 and 30 clones had 90%, 82%, 75%, 84%, 64%, 85% and 95% identity to human genes for glycoprortein 130 (gp130), inter-α-trypsin inhibitor family heavy chain-related protein (IHRP), cystatine B, protein disulfide isomerase-related protein P5 (PDI-

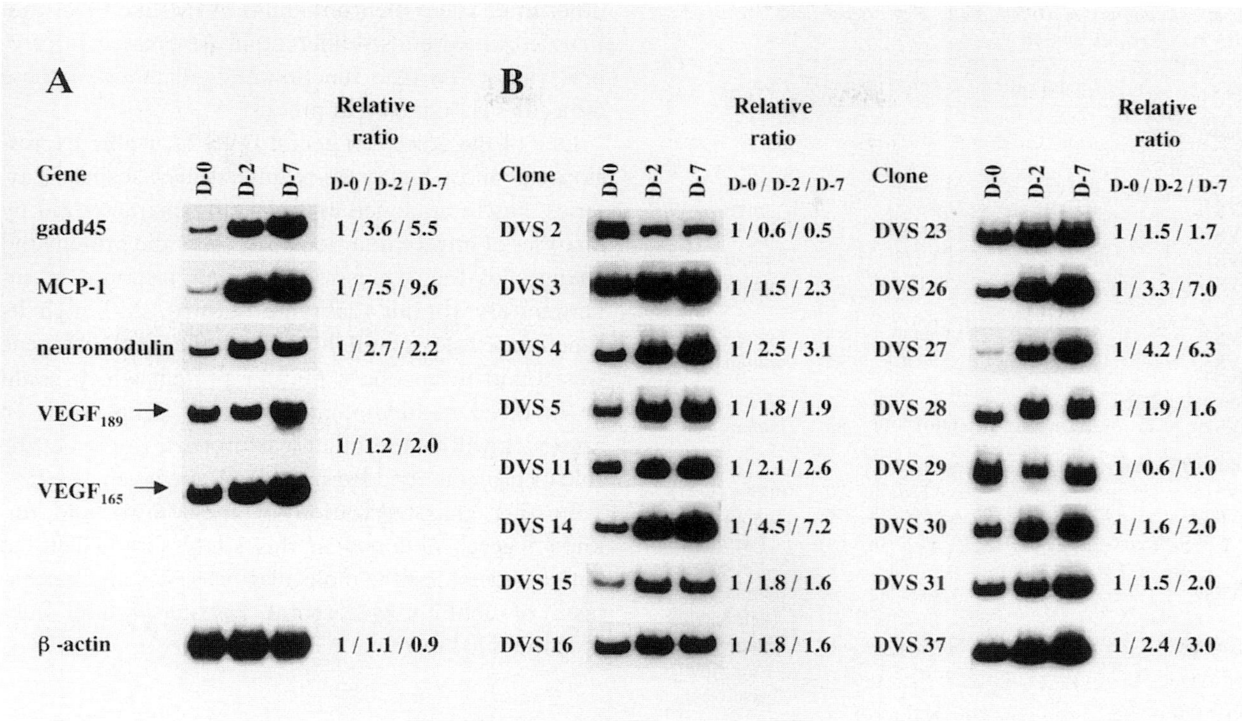

Fig. 2. (A) RT-PCR of differentially expressed mRNAs in cerebral vasospasm identified by cDNA expression array. The expression levels of gadd 45, MCP-1 and VEGF genes were strongly up-regulated in groups D-2 and D-7 (D-0 ≪ D-2 ≪ D-7). The expression level of neuromodulin was mildly up-regulated in groups D-2 and D-7 equally (D-0 < D-2 = D-7). (B) RT-PCR for sixteen differentially expressed mRNAs identified by mRNA differential display. Nine clones (DVS 3, 4, 11, 14, 26, 27, 30, 31 and 37) were up-regulated in group D-2 and D-7 (D-0 ≪ D-2 ≪ D-7). Five clones (DVS 5, 15, 16, 23, and 28) were up-regulated in groups D-2 and D-7 equally (D-0 < D-2 = D-7), one clone (DVS 2) was down-regulated in groups D-2 and D-7 (D-0 > D-2 = D-7), and one clone (DVS 29) was down-regulated in only group D-2 (D-0 > D-2 < D-7). The ratio of expression level in group D-2 and D-7 to that in group D-0 was quantified by scintillation counts (reproduction from J Cereb Blood Flow Metab 19: 1279–1288, 1999 with permission)

RP P5), acid sphingomyelinase-like phosphodiesterase (ASM-like PDE), serum amyloid A protein (SAA), and BiP protein, respectively. The DVS 29 showed 88% identity to human mRNAs for Frizzled-6. The four sequences were similar to other expression sequence tags. The other four sequences were not related to any known genes in the databases (Table 1).

Discussion

In this study, 12 genes differentially expressed during cerebral vasospasm were known. They can be classified into three groups according to their function: the genes for molecules associated with inflammation, genes whose expression can be induced by stress conditions such as hypoxia and hypoglycemia, and genes apparently not related to cerebral vasospasm. Five genes encoded MCP-1, cystatin B, IHRP, SAA, and gp130 which were closely related to inflammatory events. It has been reported that cerebral vasospasm can be inhibited by some anti-inflammatory reagents in canine cerebral vasospasm models. The expression of intercellular adhesion molecule 1 (ICAM-1), a ligand for the leukocyte adhesion receptor, increased in the endothelial and medial layer of the cerebral arteries following subarachnoid hemorrhage in rats, and monoclonal antibodies against ICAM-1 attenuated cerebral vasospasm after experimental subarachnoid hemorrhage in rabbits. Recently, Ono S. *et al.* [4] reported the successful inhibition of cerebral vasospasm in the rabbit subarachnoid hemorrhage model, using decoy synthetic DNA fragments with a high affinity to NF-κB, a transcription factor activated in inflammatory responses. The present results are consistent with these observations that inflammatory reactions are closely related to the development of cerebral vasospasm,

Table 1. *Summary of Differentially Expressed Clones Identified by mRNA Differential Display*

Gene	Identification	Account no	%ID	Species
Known genes				
Up-regulated				
DVS3	gp130	M57230	90	human
DVS4	IHRP	D38595	82	human
DVS5	cystatine B	L03558	75	human
DVS11	PDI-RP P5	U79278	84	human
DVS14	AMS-like PDE	Y08136	64	human
DVS26	SAA	M26152	85	human
DVS30	BiP protein	X87949	95	human
Down-regulated				
DVS29	frizzled-6	AB012911	88	human
Similar to other expression sequence tags				
DVS15		AA238250	70	mouse (liver)
DVS23		AA890534	76	human (parathyroid tumor)
DVS27		AA428482	73	human (embryo)
DVS28		N58809	79	human (multiple sclerosis)
No match				
DVS16				
DVS31				
DVS37				
DVS2				

%ID The identity obtained by nucleotide database search. (Reproduction from J Cereb Blood Flow Metab 19: 1279–1288, 1999 with permission).

suggesting that the functional significance of other known chemokines and their receptors should also be assessed.

The expression of three up-regulated genes for VEGF, BiP protein, and gadd45 is known to be induced under various stress conditions. Although the other three genes (neuromodulin, ASM-like PDE, and Frizzled-6) were also differentially expressed in cerebral vasospasm, the functional significance of these molecules is unknown at present.

One of the unknown genes, DVS 27, whose expression was most highly up-regulated in vasospastic arteries, has been cloned and partially characterized by analyses of intracellular localization of the protein and changes of the expression levels in response to inflammatory stimuli (data not shown). Although its functional role is still unknown, the DVS 27 gene was found to encode a nuclear protein which could be involved in inflammatory events. Thus, such an approach will be useful, at least in part, to predict the role of proteins encoded by the unknown genes.

Further characterization of the known and unknown genes obtained in this study should help to better understand the molecular processes and mechanism of continuous cerebral vasospasm after subarachnoid hemorrhage.

References

1. Altschul SF, Gish W, Miller W, Myers EW, Lipman DJ (1990) Basic local alignment search tool. J Mol Biol 215: 403–410
2. Kasuya H, Weir B, Shen Y, Hariton G, Vollrath B, Ghahary A (1993) Procollagen type I and III and transforming growth factor-beta gene expression in the arterial wall after exposure to periarterial blood. Neurosurgery 33: 716–722
3. Liang P, Pardee AB (1992) Differential display of eukaryotic messenger RNA by means of the polymerase chain reaction. Science 257: 967–971
4. Ono S, Date I, Onoda K, Shiota T, Ohmoto T, Ninomiya Y, Asari S, Morishita R (1998) Decoy administration of NFKB into the subarachnoid space for cerebral angiopathy. Hum Gene Ther 9: 1003–1011

Correspondence: Hidetoshi Kasuya, M.D., Department of Neurosurgery, Tokyo Women's Medical University, Kawada-cho 8-1, Shinjuku-ku, Tokyo 162, Japan 162-8666.

Acta Neurochir (2001) [Suppl] 77: 17–19

Complimentary Deoxyribonucleic Acid Array Analysis of Cerebral Arteries after Experimental Subarachnoid Hemorrhage

Z.-D. Zhang, L. S. Marton, S. Ono, T. Komuro, B. Weir, and **R. L. Macdonald**

Section of Neurosurgery, Department of Surgery, Pritzker School of Medicine and the University of Chicago, U.S.A.

Introduction

Cerebral vasospasm is a prolonged vasoconstriction that develops on average 3 days after subarachnoid hemorrhage (SAH), peaks 7 to 8 days after the hemorrhage and then slowly resolves over the next 5 to 7 days [6]. Vasospasm may be initiated by erythrocyte lysis with release of hemoglobin and/or breakdown products of hemoglobin. The subsequent events that cause and then lead to the onset and reversal of the vasospasm are less certain. Vasospastic arteries have an increased tendency to spontaneously contract when placed under isometric tension although they are less responsive to contractile agents [5]. This suggests that changes in the vascular wall are critical for vasospasm.

Numerous alterations of specific gene expression could be important such as changes in genes associated with relaxation or in those that influence contraction. In this study, we used a complimentary deoxyribonucleic acid (cDNA) array method to screen for changes in levels of messenger ribonucleic acid (mRNA) in vasospastic monkey cerebral arteries at different times after SAH in order to identify candidate genes that may be involved in the above-noted responses.

Keywords: SAH; vasospasm; cDNA array; gene expression.

Materials and Methods

Monkey SAH Model

The cDNA array analysis was carried out on 3 animals randomly selected from a group of 14 cynomolgus monkeys that underwent unilateral SAH by placing blood clot in the right basal cisterns along the course of the middle cerebral (MCA), anterior cerebral and internal carotid arteries [3]. The diameter of the MCA arteries was measured at angiography performed before clot placement and 3, 7 or 14 days later (n = 4 to 6 per time). After the second angiogram, animals were euthanized and the MCAs were removed and placed in liquid N_2. The Animal Care and Use Committee of the University of Chicago approved procedures on animals.

cDNA Array Analysis

cDNA arrays (GF211, Research Genetics, Huntsville, AL) contained 5184 cDNAs. Total RNA and protein were extracted from each MCA and the cDNA array was hybridized with ^{33}P labeled probe [3]. Arrays were then exposed to a phosphorimager screen for 30 hours after which the screen was scanned and the signals quantified using ImageQuant software (Molecular Dynamics, Sunnyvale, CA). The intensity of each gene was standardized by comparing to the signal obtained for spots on the array for total genomic DNA. Positive hybridization was considered present when the mRNA from clot- or control-side arteries showed a signal 5-fold higher than genomic DNA. Data were expressed as a ratio of right (clot) over control (left) side. A significant change in gene expression was considered to be present if the ratio of right/left expression was <0.8 or >1.2.

Results

The reduction in MCA diameter on days 3, 7 and 14 was 45 ± 13% ($p < 0.0005$, paired t-test), 41 ± 23% ($p < 0.05$) and 6 ± 14% ($p > 0.05$) respectively. The reduction in MCA diameter for animals used for cDNA array analysis was 33%, 44% and 11% for day 3, 7 and 14, respectively. The mean ratio (right/left) of intensities of 192 genomic DNA signals was 1.00 ± 0.10. Positive hybridization was detected for 537 genes. 164 (31%) did not change significantly after clot placement and 373 genes (69%) were differentially expressed at 3, 7 and/or 14 days after SAH. These 373 genes changed from less than 0.8-fold to greater than 1.2 to 7-fold compared to control arteries. If the threshold for change in expression was increased to greater than 2-fold, only 163 genes were altered. Only 2 genes showed a decrease to less than 0.5-fold expres-

Table 1. *Patterns of Gene Expression after SAH in Monkeys*

Number of genes change	Pattern						ANOVA
	Day 3		Day 7		Day 14		
	Value	Change	Value	Change	Value	Change	
146	normal	1.00 ± 0.10	normal	1.04 ± 0.10	↑	2.08 ± 0.85	.001 (14 > 3 = 7)
80	normal	0.97 ± 0.10	↑	1.39 ± 0.18	↑	2.78 ± 1.01	.001 (3 < 7 < 14)
33	↓	0.70 ± 0.09	↑	1.47 ± 0.18	↑	3.16 ± 1.22	.001 (3 < 7 < 14)
28	↑	1.24 ± 0.04	normal	0.98 ± 0.13	↑	1.61 ± 0.39	.001 (3 < 7 < 14)
24	↑	1.27 ± 0.07	normal	1.00 ± 0.10	normal	1.05 ± 0.09	.001 (3 > 7 = 14)
16	↓	0.73 ± 0.06	normal	1.11 ± 0.08	↑	2.32 ± 1.60	.001 (14 > 3)
14	normal	1.01 ± 0.12	↑	1.28 ± 0.05	normal	1.05 ± 0.09	.001 (7 > 3 = 14)
10	normal	1.09 ± 0.04	↓	0.72 ± 0.09	↑	1.75 ± 0.50	.001 (3 > 7 < 14)
9	↑	1.26 ± 0.08	↑	1.29 ± 0.07	↑	1.67 ± 0.42	.003 (14 > 3 = 7)

sion. Intercellular adhesion molecule-1 was decreased more than 2-fold on day 7 and PTH-R1 was reduced greater than 2-fold on day 3. The mean expression of genes was 1.00 ± 0.18 (right/left ratio) on day 3, 1.15 ± 0.24 ($P < 0.0001$, unpaired t-test versus control, $P < 0.001$, ANOVA) on day 7 and 2.14 ± 1.07 ($P < 0.0001$, unpaired t-test versus control, $P < 0.001$, ANOVA) on day 14. Of 27 possible patterns of change in gene expression, 16 patterns were observed but only 9 patterns were common (Table 1). For the 163 genes with greater than 2-fold change in expression, 93% [151] showed a pattern of progressive increase with time. The most common patterns for all genes were for progressively increasing gene expression over time. Differentially expressed genes were classified into groups according to known functions. There were alterations in genes involved in regulation of gene expression (38 genes), Ras-related (6), growth, proliferation and cell cycle (29), second messenger pathways (10), oxidative stress (12), DNA structural proteins (7), apoptosis, DNA damage and repair (9) inflammation and immune responses (22), membrane proteins and receptors (35), cell cytoskeleton (15), extracellular matrix (6), metabolic pathways (19), miscellaneous intracellular enzymes (42), kinases and phosphatases (27), miscellaneous disease-related genes (13), protein synthesis (16) and miscellaneous other functions (67). Many genes had no known or an uncertain relationship to vascular contraction or relaxation, vascular remodeling or vasospasm.

Multiple transcription factors were upregulated. There was a progressive increase in transcription factor AP-2 β, c-myc binding protein and c-jun. Ras-related and intracellular signal transduction pathway genes progressively increased including cyclic adenosine monophosphate (cAMP) responsive element binding protein, β subunit. There was an initial decrease followed by a marked increase in vascular endothelial growth factor and transforming growth factor-β. CD72 and brain-derived neurotrophic factor were increased on day 14. Stress-related proteins that were increased included superoxide dismutase-1 and genes for heat shock factor protein 2 and heat shock protein 70. Multiple regulators of inflammation were altered. There was increased expression of β-catenin, thrombomodulin, β-2 adrenergic receptor, α M integrin, glypican 1, ryanodine receptor, platelet/endothelial cell adhesion molecule (CD31), CD73, intercellular adhesion molecule 1 (CD54), paxillin, occludin, neural cell adhesion protein (NCAM21), tropomodulin, β-tubulin, α4 tubulin, myosin light chain, myosin binding protein H, dynactin, several collagens (type IV α2, type XVIII α1), matrix metalloproteinase 7 (matrilysin, uterine), cystatin B and cystatin C. There was an increase at all times in α-3 actinin and an increase at day 3 in troponin 1 (skeletal fast) and troponin T2 (cardiac). Myosin-1β was decreased at day 7 and 14. Genes for 27 protein kinases and phosphatases were altered, the most common pattern being a progressive increase with time. One of the greatest increases in gene expression was seen for parathyroid hormone receptor (PTH-R1, 7-fold increase at day 14). PTH also was increased. Whether or not changes in mRNA level were translated into changes in protein was assessed for this gene. Purified PTH-R from monkey kidney, a tissue with abundant PTH-R, was recognized as a 60 kDa protein by Western blotting. The intensity of the specific band that represented PTH-R1 was significantly increased in the right compared to the left middle cerebral artery 7 and 14 days after SAH ($P < 0.05$, ANOVA).

Discussion

Our results show that SAH is associated with change in expression of multiple genes in cerebral arteries as assessed by mRNA levels. The most common change is an increase in gene expression over time. The functions of altered genes were diverse. Since we used whole artery for RNA extractions, the sources of the altered genes may include smooth muscle, endothelial and inflammatory cells in the artery wall. Our findings are similar to those of Onda, *et al.*, who showed 49 out of 588 genes examined (8%) were expressed in dog basilar artery [2]. This is similar to our finding of 10% of genes expressed on an array containing almost 10 times as many (5184) cDNAs. We confirm that vascular endothelial growth factor and cystatin B are upregulated after SAH. Other genes detected by Onda and colleagues were not on the array we used. Our findings confirm that a common class of genes upregulated after SAH are those mediating inflammation. We extend the prior findings by noting patterns of gene expression occurring as vasospasm resolves.

A novel finding of this study was the marked induction of PTH and PTH type 1 receptor in cerebral arteries. PTH-related peptide (PTHrP) has high homology to PTH, may be produced in vascular endothelial and smooth muscle cells and has high affinity binding capacity to type 1 PTH receptor. PTHrP can lower blood pressure in experiments in vivo and directly relaxed vascular smooth muscles from peripheral and cerebral arteries by activating adenylate cyclase in studies in vitro [5, 6]. This suggests that the PTH/PTHrP pathway may modulate vascular tone. Our results suggest the possible correlation between changes in expression of PTH, PTH-R1 and the onset and resolution of vasospasm.

In this study, we did not identify a specific gene that can be used solely to explain the onset of vasospasm. There are several possible explanations. Gene(s) important in vasospasm may not be included on the array. Certain genes were expressed at a very low level so the mRNA of these genes or their changes cannot be detected. Some processes may be regulated at the level of translation or post-translationally which would not be detected by this method. Functional changes or modifications of proteins without change in their expression, such as phosphorylation, may be more important for some proteins.

The large number of mRNAs that are increased progressively over time suggest a chronic response to subarachnoid blood like that reported to occur after any other arterial injury such as balloon angioplasty. Many genes were involved in regulation of cell proliferation, smooth muscle phenotype regulation and inflammation. Further study is needed to determine what causes the changes in gene expression, whether the changes are in smooth muscle, endothelial or perivascular inflammatory cells and what role, if any, the changes have in the onset and resolution of vasospasm.

References

1. Huang M, Rorstad OP (1984) Cerebral vascular adenylate cyclase: evidence for coupling to receptors for vasoactive intestinal peptide and parathyroid hormone. J Neurochem 43: 849–856
2. Onda H, Kasuya H, Takakura K, Hori T, Imaizumi T, Takeuchi T, Inoue I, Takeda J (1999) Identification of genes differentially expressed in canine vasospastic cerebral arteries after subarachnoid hemorrhage. J Cereb Blood Flow Metab 19: 1279–1288
3. Ono S, Zhang ZD, Marton LS, Yamini B, Windmeyer E, Johns L, Kowalczuk A, Lin G, Macdonald RL (2000) Heme oxygenase-1 and ferritin are increased in cerebral arteries after subarachnoid hemorrhage in monkeys. J Cereb Blood Flow Metab 20: 1066–1076
4. Suzuki Y, Lederis K, Huang M, Leblanc FE, Rorstad OP (1983) Relaxation of bovine, porcine and human brain arteries by parathyroid hormone. Life Sci 33: 2497–2503
5. Vorkapic P, Bevan RD, Bevan JA (1991) Longitudinal time course of reversible and irreversible components of chronic cerebrovasospasm of the rabbit basilar artery. J Neurosurg 74: 951–955
6. Weir B, Grace M, Hansen J, Rothberg C (1978) Time course of vasospasm in man. J Neurosurg 48: 173–178

Correspondence: R. Loch Macdonald, M.D., Ph.D., Section of Neurosurgery, MC3026, University of Chicago Medical Center, 5841 South Maryland Avenue, Chicago, Illinois, U.S.A., 60637.

Acta Neurochir (2001) [Suppl] 77: 21–24

Which Protein Kinase C Isoforms are Involved in the Development of Vasospasm after Subarachnoid Haemorrhage?

S. Nishizawa[1], **K. Obara**[2], **K. Nakayama**[2], **M. Koide**[2], **T. Yokoyama**[1], **N. Yokota**[1], and **S. Ohta**[1]

[1] Department of Neurosurgery, Hamamatsu University School of Medicine, Japan
[2] Department of Pharmacology, School of Pharmaceutical Sciences, University of Shizuoka, Japan

Introduction

We have been investigating the role of PKC in the vascular smooth muscle cells in the development and maintenance of cerebral vasospasm after subarachnoid haemorrhage (SAH) [3, 4, 5], and our previous experimental results on the canine basilar artery showed that measurement of PKC activity was significantly enhanced in the membrane fraction of the vascular smooth muscle cells of cerebral vasospastic arteries in a canine subarachnoid haemorrhage model [4, 5], and that the time course of the development of angiographic vasospasm and increased PKC activity in the membrane fraction were closely correlated with time. PKC activity was not significantly increased in the mild vasospasm model compared to the control, but the increase was significant in the severe vasospasm model [5]. These results indicated that PKC plays a pivotal role in the development of vasospasm following SAH.

In this study, we identified the PKC isoforms expressed in canine vasospastic basilar artery by immunoblot analysis, and investigated which PKC isoforms are involved in the development of vasospasm.

Keywords: Isoform; protein kinase C; subarachnoid haemorrhage; vasospasm.

Materials and Methods

Materials

The basilar arteries of beagle dogs of either sex weighing 7–10 kg were used.

Methods

Vasospasm was conducted in a basilar artery using "two haemorrhage canine" model [7]. PKC isoforms were identified by Western blot analysis according to the modified method designed by Obara *et al.* [6]. Twelve dogs were randomly divided into three groups: a control group, a group in which the dogs were sacrificed on day 4 one hour after the second injection, and a group sacrificed on day 7. After sacrifice, the membrane fraction of the basilar artery and the cytosol fraction of the cerebellum were prepared in the same way as for assay of PKC activity, and the samples were used for Western blot analysis. In the present study, the antibodies from Sigma (St. Louis, MO, USA) were mainly used in the following experiments. The PKC isoform-specific primary antibodies from Sigma are raised in rabbits by using synthetic peptides corresponding to the C-terminal amino acid sequence of rat PKCα (659–672), PKCβ1 (658–671), PKCβ2 (660–673), PKCγ (684–697), PKCδ (662–673), PKCε (726–737), PKCη (670–683), or PKCζ (577–592). The amount of PKC was quantified by densitometric scans of immunostained nitrocellulose blots. The results were expressed as a percentage of the total amount of each PKC isoform.

Rat brain was used as a positive control. Specificity of signal was shown by the absence or presence of isoform-specific synthetic peptide (5 μg of immunizing peptide). Isoform-specific synthetic peptides of PKCζ and η were not commercially available. Therefore, the presence of isoform-specific band of PKCζ and η was evaluated according to the position of the band expressed in the rat brain extract.

Statistical Analysis

Data are expressed as mean $\pm$ standard error of the mean. Data were analyzed by paired or unpaired Student's t-test, or Dunnett's multiple comparison test after analysis of variance (ANOVA). P values less than 0.05 were considered significant.

Results

Identification of PKC Isoforms by Western Blot Analysis

We always used rat brain as a positive control in the identification of PKC isoforms, and Western blot analysis consistently showed a band associated with PKCα at 83 kDa (Figs. 1, 2 arrowheads). We exam-

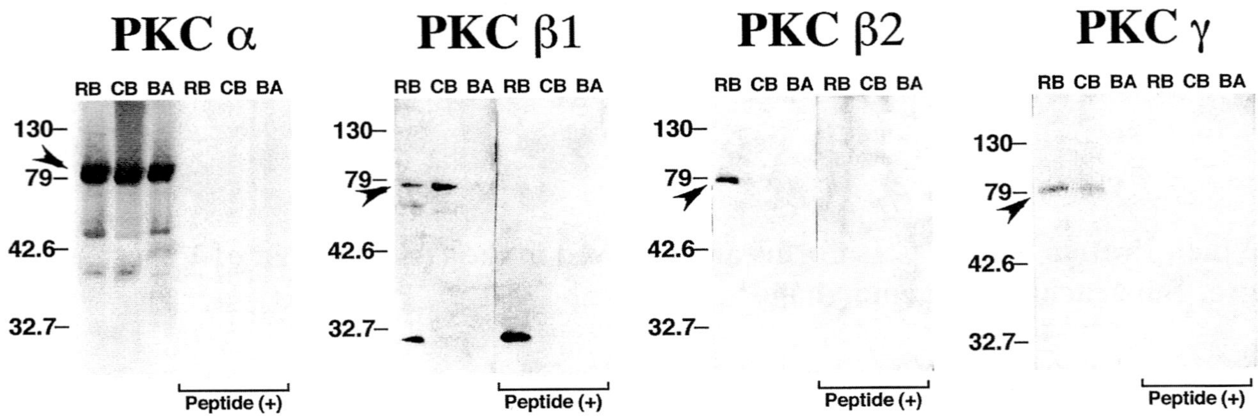

Fig. 1. PKC isoforms (PKCα, β1, β2, γ) of the rat brain, the canine cerebellum and the canine basilar artery. The cytosol fraction of rat brain was used as a positive control. Isoforms of PKC in the cytosol of the rat brain and the canine cerebellum, and those of the cytosol and the membrane fractions of the basilar artery were separated by sodium dodecyl sulfate polyacrylamide gel electrophoresis and analyzed by Western immunoblotting. The specificity was demonstrated by showing loss of the immunoreactive signal using isoform-specific synthetic peptides. peptide: isoform-specific synthetic peptide

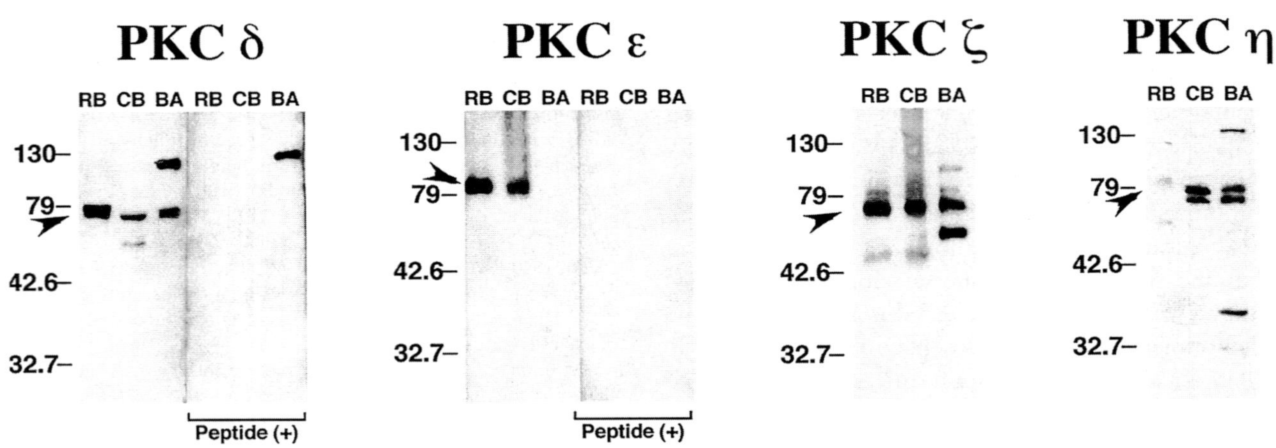

Fig. 2. PKC isoforms (PKCδ, ε, ζ and η) of the rat brain, the canine cerebellum and the canine basilar artery

ined eight PKC isoforms-specific antibodies (PKCα, β1, β2, γ, δ, ε, ζ, and η) (Figs. 1, 2). Four PKC isoforms were identified in canine basilar artery in Western blot analysis: PKCα, PKCδ, PKCζ, and PKCη, and the proteins corresponding to these PKC isoforms showed bands around 80 kDa. No other PKC isoforms were detected. Specificity, shown by loss of the immunoreactive signal, was demonstrated by inclusion of isoform-specific synthetic peptides during the primary antibody incubation stage. As for PKCα, the value on day 7 in the cytosol fraction (number of the samples; $n = 4$) was significantly lower than the control value ($n = 4$) ($p < 0.01$), and the day 4 after the injection value ($n = 4$) ($p < 0.05$). In the membrane fractions, the difference between the values in the control group ($n = 4$) and in the group on day 4 ($n = 4$) was not statistically significant, however the value on day 7 ($n = 4$) was significantly higher than the control ($p < 0.01$), and the day 4 after the injection value ($p < 0.05$). As for the PKCδ values of the cytosol fractions, the values on days 4 ($n = 4$) and 7 ($n = 4$) were significantly decreased compared to the control group ($n = 4$) ($p < 0.01$). PKCδ values of the membrane fractions on days 4 ($n = 4$) and 7 ($n = 4$) were significantly higher than the control ($p < 0.01$) (Fig. 3). In both PKCζ and η, no statistically significant differences were noted in either the cytosol or the membrane fractions ($n = 4$, respectively). Furthermore, there was no significant translocation of either PKCζ or η from the cytosol to the membrane fractions.

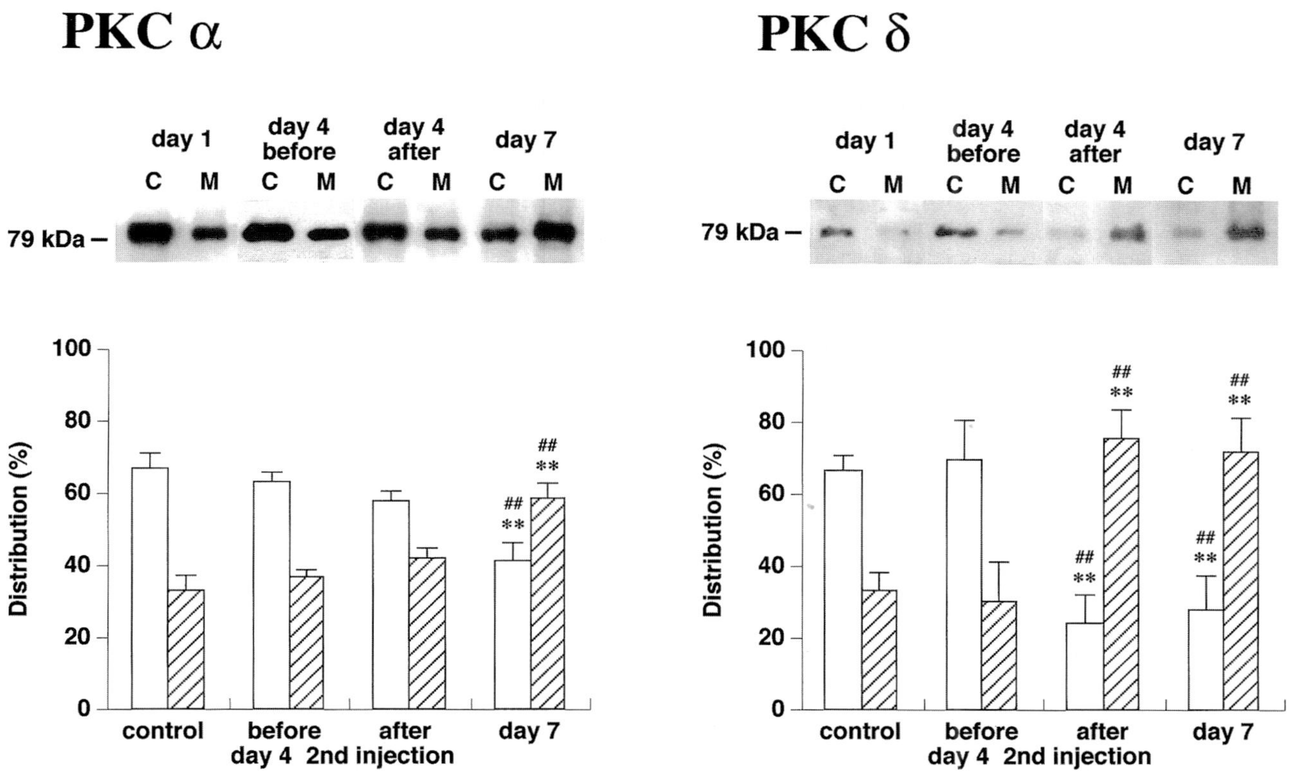

Fig. 3. Quantitative summary of chronological changes in the amounts of identified protein kinase C isoforms. The results are expressed as a percentage of the total amount of each protein kinase C isoform. Each value represents the mean ± standard error of the mean. The amounts of protein kinase Cα and protein kinase Cδ in the cytosol and the membrane fractions changed significantly as vasospasm developed ($n = 4$). open bars: cytosol fraction. shaded bars: membrane fraction. *C* Cytosol fraction, *M* membrane fraction. In protein kinase Cα, $^{**}P < 0.01$, corresponding to the control, $^{\#\#}P < 0.01$, corresponding to the day 4 before and after the second injection. In protein kinase Cδ, $^{**}P < 0.01$, corresponding to the control, $^{\#\#}P < 0.01$, corresponding to the day 4 before the second injection

Discussion

At least 12 isoforms of PKC have been identified thus far, and they have been classified into three groups: classical PKCs (PKCα, β1, β2, and γ), novel PKCs (PKCδ, ε, η, μ, θ, and ι) and atypical PKCs (ζ and λ) [1, 2]. In this study, we examined the specificity of PKC-isoform primary antibodies. We always used rat brain as a positive control. Furthermore, we confirmed the specificity of the signals using isoform-specific synthetic peptides.

We identified four PKC isoforms (PKCα, δ, ζ, and η) in the canine basilar artery and the bands corresponding to these PKCs were expressed at almost the same position as PKC in rat brain. In addition, we showed that PKCα and δ were significantly translocated from the cytosol to the membrane fractions. It is noteworthy that PKCδ was initially translocated, followed by translocation of PKCα, as angiographic vasospasm developed. We believe that this is the first report to show a clear relation between the progression of angiographic vasospasm after SAH and expression and translocation of two PKC isoforms in the canine basilar artery. Our results directly indicate that PKCδ and α play a significant role in the pathogenesis of the development and maintenance of vasospasm after SAH.

As for chronological changes, to begin with, PKCδ was translocated from the cytosol to the membrane fractions on day 4, and then PKCα followed on day 7. Accordingly, PKCδ may therefore play an important role as a Ca^{2+} sensitizer in the initiation/development of vasospasm, whereas PKCα is mainly involved in the mechanism of maintenance of severe vascular contraction.

References

1. Hug H, Sarre TF (1993) Protein kinase C isoenzymes: divergence in signal transduction? Biochem J 291: 329–343

2. Jamieson L, Carpenter L, Biden TJ, Fields AP (1999) Protein kinase Ciota activity is necessary for Bcr-Abl-mediated resistance to drug-induced apoptosis. J Biol Chem 274: 3927–3930
3. Nishizawa S, Peterson JW, Shimoyama I, Uemura K (1992) Relation between protein kinase C and calmodulin systems in cerebrovascular contraction: Investigation of the pathogenesis of vasospasm after subarachnoid hemorrhage. Neurosurgery 31: 711–716
4. Nishizawa S, Nezu N, Uemura K (1992) Direct evidence for a key role of protein kinase C in the development of vasospasm after subarachnoid hemorrhage. J Neurosurg 76: 635–639
5. Nishizawa S, Yamamoto S, Yokoyama T, Ryu H, Uemura K (1995) Chronological changes of arterial diameter, cGMP, and protein kinase C in the development of vasospasm. Stroke 26: 1916–1921
6. Obara K, Hata S, Sato K, Koide M, Ishii K, Nakayama K (1999) Contractile potentiation by endothelin-1 involves protein kinase C-δ activity in porcine artery. Jpn J Physiol 49: 175–183
7. Varsos VG, Liszczak TM, Han DH, Kistler JP, Vielma J, Black PM, Heros RC, Zervas NT (1983) Delayed cerebral vasospasm is not reversible by aminophylline, nifedipine, or papaverine in a "two-hemorrhage" canine model. J Neurosurg 58: 11–17

Correspondence: Shigeru Nishizawa, M.D., Ph.D., Department of Neurosurgery, Hamamatsu University School of Medicine, 3600 Handacho Hamamatsu Shizuoka 431-3192 Japan.

Acta Neurochir (2001) [Suppl] 77: 25–27

Role of Mitogen-Activated Protein Kinase in the Contractions of Rabbit Basilar Artery Induced by Hemolysate, Oxyhemoglobin, and Bloody CSF

A. Y. Zubkov, K. Shadon Rollins, B. McGehee, A. D. Parent, and **J. H. Zhang**

Introduction

It has been suggested that tyrosine kinases are involved in smooth muscle contraction [1] induced by hemolysate or other spasmogens and might be involved in cerebral vasospasm. Mitogen-activated protein kinase (MAPK), a tyrosine kinase substrate, was activated by oxyhemoglobin (OxyHb) [5] and hemolysate [9] and contributed to cerebral arterial contraction. MAPK inhibitor PD98059 reduced the contraction of a rabbit basilar artery by hemolysate [9] and endothelin-1 [8].

In this study, three spasmogens, hemolysate, OxyHb, and CSF, were used in the contraction and MAPK immunoprecipitation, and the inhibitory effect of a novel and potent MAPK inhibitor U0126 was tested.

Keywords: Mitogen-activated protein kinase; oxyhemoglobin; vasospasm.

Materials and Methods

Materials

U0126 was purchased from Promega (Madison, WI). Anti-MAPK (ERK1/ERK2) antibodies were purchased from Zymed Laboratories (San Francisco, CA). Other chemicals were purchased from Sigma (St. Louis, MO).

Hemolysate, Oxyhemoglobin, and Bloody CSF Preparation

Hemolysate [4], OxyHb [3] and CSF [7] were prepared as previously described.

Isometric Tension

The rabbit basilar artery rings were preincubated with U0126 (30 μM) for 30 minutes, and then dose dependent responses to hemolysate (0.1–10%), OxyHb (0.1–100 μM), or CSF (30%) were studied. In the second group, the arterial samples were contracted with hemolysate (10%), OxyHb (10 μM), or CSF (30%) and then a dose dependent relaxation was initiated with U0126 (1–100 μM). Each ring was used with only one agonist to avoid cross-reaction.

MAPK Assay

The basilar arteries were removed from the brain and were exposed to hemolysate (10%), oxyhemoglobin (10^{-4} M), or bloody CSF (30%) for 5 minutes. In another group arteries were pretreated with U0126 (30 μM) for 30 minutes and then were exposed to hemolysate (10%), oxyhemoglobin (10^{-4} M), or bloody CSF (30%) for 5 minutes. The MAPK activity was studied according to the method described in the MAPK assay (New England Biolabs, Inc., Beverly MA). The density of the bands were quantified with Quantity One software (Biorad, Hercules, CA)

Data Analysis

Data are expressed as the mean ± the standard error of the mean. Statistical differences between the control and other groups were compared using a one-way analysis of variance (ANOVA) and then the Tukey-Kramer multiple comparison procedure if significant variance was found. A probability value (P) of less than 0.05 was considered statistically significant.

Results

Effects of U0126 on the Arterial Contraction

Pre-incubation of the basilar artery rings with U0126 (30 μM) for 30 minutes significantly reduced the contractions to hemolysate and OxyHb. At a higher concentration, U0126 (100 μM) completely abolished the contraction induced by hemolysate (Fig. 1A, $P < 0.05$–0.01, ANOVA) and significantly reduced contractions to oxyhemoglobin (Fig. 1B, $P < 0.05$–0.001, ANOVA). Contractions induced by bloody CSF were significantly reduced by 1 μM of U0126 and completely abolished by 30 μM of U0126 (Fig. 1C, $P < 0.05$, ANOVA).

Effects of U0126 on the MAPK Activity

Hemolysate, oxyhemoglobin, and bloody CSF induced significant increase in MAPK activity

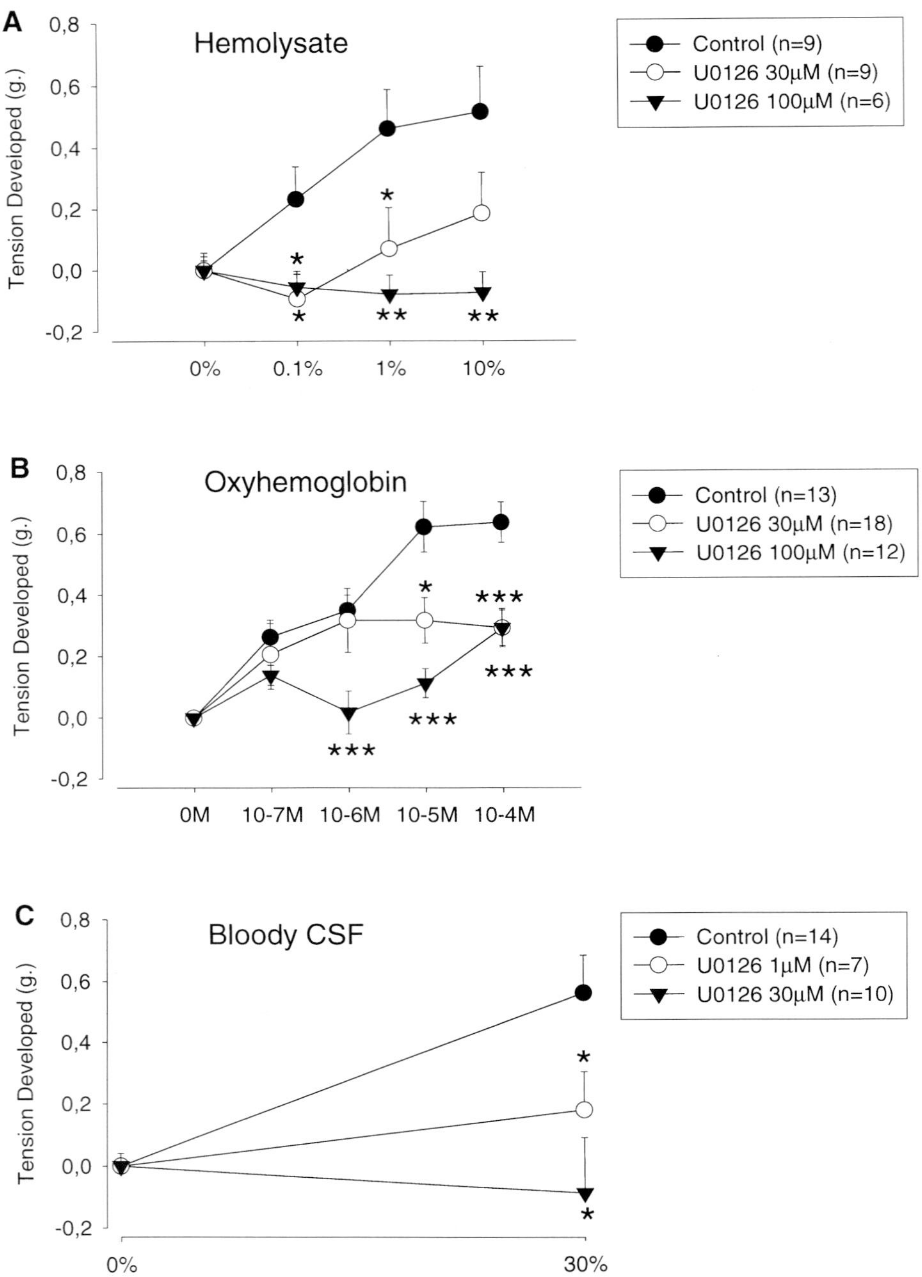

Fig. 1. U0126 inhibited contraction to hemolysate. The rings of the rabbit basilar arteries were incubated with U0126 for 30 minutes and then contracted in a dose-dependent manner with hemolysate, OxyHb, or bloody CSF. (A) U0126 significantly reduced hemolysate-induced contraction at a low dose (30 μM) and completely abolished the contraction to hemolysate at a high dose (100 μM) ($P < 0.05$–0.01, ANOVA). (B) U0126 reduced significantly OxyHb-induced contraction at 30 μM, and further reduced contraction at 100 μM ($P < 0.05$–0.001, ANOVA). (C) U0126, at 1 μM, markedly reduced contraction by bloody CSF, and, at 30 μM, completely abolished the bloody CSF-induced contraction ($P < 0.05$, ANOVA). n = number of rings tested. * and ** indicate $P < 0.05$ or 0.01 vs. control (ANOVA)

($P < 0.05$–0.001, ANOVA). Pre-treatment of the basilar arteries with U0126 (30 μM) for 30 minutes completely abolished this increase of MAPK activity caused by studied agonists. The preincubation of control vessels with U0126 non-significantly reduced the MAPK activity.

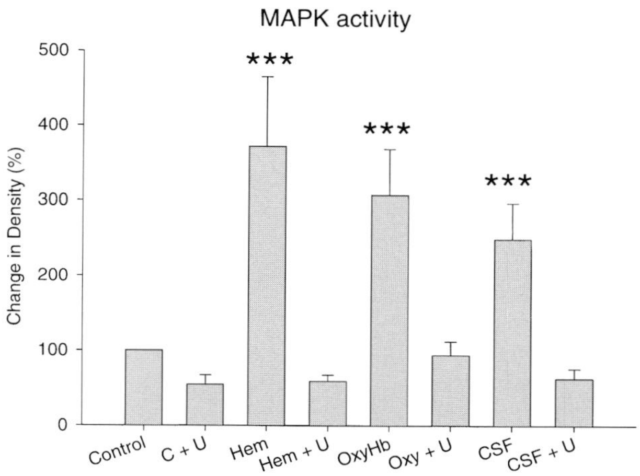

Fig. 2. MAPK activity assay. Graphical summary of six experiments, demonstrating that hemolysate, oxyhemoglobin, and bloody CSF significantly increased MAPK activity ($P < 0.001$, <0.01, <0.01, respectively, ANOVA). U0126 completely abolished the activation of MAPK. There was non-significant inhibition of MAPK activity in the control vessels after exposure to U0126. **, and *** indicate $P < 0.01$, and <0.001, respectively. *Hem* Hemolysate, *CSF* bloody CSF, *Hem + U* hemolysate + U0126, *Oxy + U* OxyHb + U0126, *CSF + U* bloody CSF + U0126, *C + U* control + U0126

Discussion

Several findings were presented in this report: (1) U0126 significantly inhibited the contractions of rabbit basilar arteries to hemolysate, OxyHb, or bloody CSF; (2) U0126 significantly relaxed all rings pre-contracted with hemolysate, OxyHb, or bloody CSF; (3) Hemolysate, oxyhemoglobin, and bloody CSF induced significant increase in MAPK activity; (4) U0126 significantly reduced MAPK activity induced by hemolysate, OxyHb, and bloody CSF.

Mechanism of MAPK Activation by Spasmogens

OxyHb is an established causative agent for vasospasm [2]. The mechanism for OxyHb-induced contraction remains unsolved despite intensive studies in the past. Oxidation of OxyHb to MetHb generates free radicals. Free radicals are involved in the activation of protein tyrosine kinase and in canine cerebral smooth muscle cells [5]. However, more evidence is needed to clarify the mechanism of OxyHb-induced MAPK activation.

The mechanism of bloody CSF-induced MAPK activation is difficult to identify. Bloody CSF induced elevation of intracellular Ca^{2+} in cerebral smooth muscle [6]. As shown in Fig. 1, 30% CSF induced a similar degree of contraction to that of hemolysate and OxyHb (Fig. 1), even though bloody CSF contains only 1.8 μM OxyHb (30% of 6 μM), and OxyHb and hemolysate solution contain 10–100 μM and 1.2 mM OxyHb, respectively. Thus, other factors in bloody CSF might produce additional contraction or enhance the effect of OxyHb.

Hemolysate is also a mixture of different substances from the lysed erythrocytes. Some small molecules of hemolysate produced an elevation of intracellular Ca^{2+} in cerebral smooth muscle cells [6]. Other unknown factors in hemolysate also might be involved in the activation of MAPK.

References

1. Kim C-J, Kim K-W, Park J-W, Lee J-C, Zhang JH (1998) Role of tyrosine kinase in erythrocyte lysate-induced contraction in rabbit cerebral arteries. J Neurosurg 89: 289–296
2. Macdonald RL, Weir BK (1991) A review of hemoglobin and the pathogenesis of cerebral vasospasm. Stroke 22: 971–982
3. Martin W, Villani GM, Jothianandan D, Furchgott RF (1985) Selective blockade of endothelium-dependent and glyceryl trinitrate-induced relaxation by hemoglobin and by methylene blue in the rabbit aorta. J Pharmacol Exp Ther 232: 708–716
4. Onoda K, Ono S, Ogihara K, Shiota T, Asari S, Ohmoto T, Ninomiya Y (1996) Inhibition of vascular contraction by intracisternal administration of preproendothelin-1 mRNA antisense oligoDNA in a rat experimental vasospasm model. J Neurosurg 85: 846–852
5. Vollrath B, Cook D, Megyesi J, Findlay J, Ohkuma H (1998) Novel mechanism by which hemoglobin induces constriction of cerebral arteries. Eur J Pharmacol 361: 311–319
6. Zhang H, Weir B, Marton LS, Macdonald RL, Bindokas V, Miller RJ, Brorson JR (1995) Mechanisms of hemolysate-induced $[Ca^{2+}]_i$ elevation in cerebral smooth muscle cells. Am J Physiol 269: H1874–H1890
7. Zubkov A, Ogihara K, Tumu P, Mandybur GD, Lewis AI, Parent AD, Zhang JH (1999) Bloody cerebrospinal fluid alters contraction of cultured arteries. Neurol Res 21: 553–558
8. Zubkov A, Rollins K, Parent A, Zhang J (2000) Mechanism of endothelin-1-induced contraction in rabbit basilar artery. Stroke 31: 526–533
9. Zubkov AY, Ogihara K, Tumu P, Patllola A, Lewis AI, Parent AD, Zhang J (1999) Mitogen-activated protein kinase mediates hemolysate-induced contraction in rabbit basilar artery. J Neurosurg 90: 1091–1097

Correspondence: John H. Zhang, M.D., Ph.D., Department of Neurosurgery, University of Mississippi Medical Center, 2500 North State Street, Jackson, MS, 39216-4505.

Acta Neurochir (2001) [Suppl] 77: 29–31

Apoptosis in Basilar Endothelial Cells in a Canine Double Hemorrhage Model

A. Y. Zubkov[1], **R. E. Tibbs**[1], **B. Clower**[2], **K. Ogihara**[1], **K. Aoki**[1], and **J. H. Zhang**[1]

[1] Department of Neurosurgery, University of Mississippi Medical Center, Jackson, Mississippi, USA
[2] Department of Anatomy, University of Mississippi Medical Center, Jackson, Mississippi, USA

Introduction

Cerebral vasospasm after subarachnoid hemorrhage (SAH) is a combination of prolonged contraction and vessel remodeling that may lead to cerebral ischemia or infarction [2]. Morphological studies of cerebral arteries affected by vasospasm often show extensive necrosis of smooth-muscle cells [1] as well as desquamation and dystrophy of endothelial cells [7, 11]. The actual mechanisms of cellular death following cerebral vasospasm are not known. Recent studies of post-SAH vasospasm in this laboratory strongly suggest that endothelial cells may be dying through apoptotic pathways [8, 10].

The dog double hemorrhage method, an established model for inducing vasospasm, was used in this study to investigate the time course of apoptotic changes in endothelial cells.

Keywords: Apoptosis; endothelium; experimental subarachnoid haemorrhage.

Materials and Methods

Dog Double Hemorrhage Model

This study utilizes a double hemorrhage dog model previously described by Varsos *et al.* [9]. The first SAH was considered as day 0. Two days later animals underwent a second SAH (day 2 SAH). The dogs were divided into three groups and were sacrificed (four per period) on days 3, 5, and 7, respectively. As stated above a second angiogram was performed on dogs just prior to their sacrifice. Three dogs were not exposed to SAH and served as controls for vessel pathology studies. Animals were sacrificed by an overdose of pentobarbital (120 mg/kg).

Morphological Studies

Brains were immediately removed, and the circle of Willis, still attached to the brain stem, was quickly perfused with 2% glutaraldehyde. After processing, the samples were examined with a LEO 906 (Leo, Thoenwood, NY) transmission electron microscope (TEM).

Data Analysis

The angiographic data is expressed as the mean ± the standard error of the mean. Statistical differences between the control and other groups were compared using a one-way analysis of variance (ANOVA), and then, if significant variance was found, the Tukey-Kramer multiple comparison procedure. A probability value (P) of less than 0.05 was considered statistically significant.

Results

Angiographic Changes of the Basilar Arteries on Days 3–7

All four dogs developed mild vasospasm on day 3 with residual diameter of 80.8 ± 13.5%, which represents a 20% reduction in luminal size. On day 5, a moderate degree of vasospasm was observed, with residual diameter of 67.3 ± 6.4%, which represents a 33% reduction in luminal size. A severe vasospasm was obtained on day 7 with residual diameter of 53.4 ± 5.5%, representing a 47% reduction in luminal size.

Morphology of Normal Basilar Arteries

The normal basilar artery consists of three layers, the intima, the media, and the adventitia. The intimal layer includes a monolayer of ovoid shaped endothelial cells attached to an underlying internal elastic lamina (IEL). Their nucleus contains peripheral heterochromatin and centrally located euchromatin. No condensation of chromatin is visible in normal nuclei. The cytoplasm contains numerous organelles. The media of the vessel consists of smooth muscle cells with

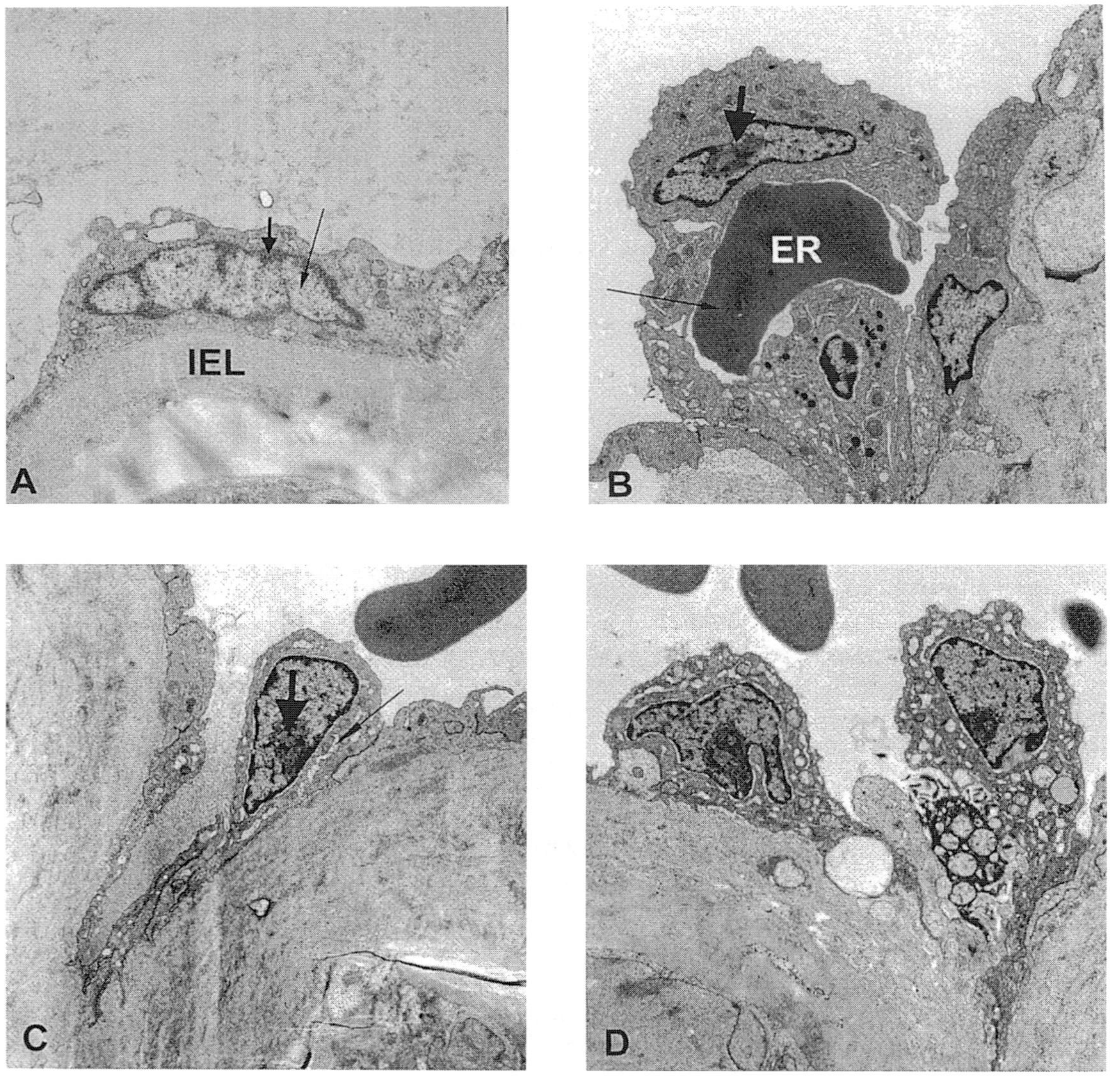

Fig. 1. The normal endothelial cells (A) were ovoid shaped, being connected with neighboring endothelial cells and the underlying internal elastic lamina (*IEL*). The nucleus, also ovoid shaped, possessed central euchromatin and peripheral heterochromatin. No condensation of chromatin, or blebbing of cell membrane were observed. Intracellular organelles appeared normal. The basilar arteries from day 3 group (B). Endothelial cells showed degenerative changes with blebbing of the cell membrane and increased condensation of peripheral nuclear chromatin (arrow). Note an erythrocyte lying between two endothelial cells, one (top) of which is detached. Note some corrugation of IEL. The basilar arteries from day-5 group (C). Note increased condensation of peripheral chromatin (wide arrow), cytoplasmic vacuolization, condensation of cytoplasm, and blebbing of the membrane in the endothelial cells. Notice dilation of endoplasmic reticulum (small arrow). The basilar arteries from day-7 group (D). Vacuolization in cytoplasm, blebbing of cell membrane, and condensation of nuclear chromatin were widespread and severe. Detachment of endothelial cells was widespread resulting in large areas of denudation (×*6000*)

small amounts of connective tissue. The adventitial layer contains mainly collagen fibers (Fig. 1A).

Changes in the Basilar Arteries on Day 3, 5 and 7 After SAH

Morphological evidence of vasospasm consists of mild corrugation of the IEL with shortening of smooth muscle cells. Some of the endothelial cells showed signs of injury consisting of detachment from the IEL, disruption of tight junctions between neighboring cells, and cytoplasmic organelle swelling. A few cells demonstrated apoptotic-like changes consisting of peripheral condensation of nuclear chromatin, and electron dense appearing cytoplasm (Fig. 1B).

On day 5, morphological presentation of vasospasm

resembled that occurring on day 3, but was more prominent. Apoptotic-like changes, particularly condensation of peripheral chromatin, clearly appeared to be more pronounced and involved more endothelial cells (Fig. 1C).

Morphological changes on day 7 in the basilar artery were similar to those on day 5, but even more severe and widespread. Both endothelial cells and smooth muscle cells showed evidence of necrotic changes. Apoptotic changes remained pronounced and appeared to involve even more endothelial cells (Fig. 1D).

Discussion

The leading cause of death and disability in patients suffering from aneurysmal subarachnoid hemorrhage (SAH) is cerebral vasospasm, a persistent, progressive constriction of cerebral arteries [4]. Despite extensive research efforts cerebral vasospasm remains largely unmanageable because of poor understanding of the pathogenesis of the disease [6].

In the present study apoptotic-like changes were observed in endothelial cells of cerebral arteries following SAH and the magnitude of their presence correlated positively with the severity of vasospasm. The results of in vitro studies indicated that oxyhemoglobin, a substance known to be involved in the production of both vasospasm [5], and endothelial injury following SAH, produce early apoptosis-like changes in bovine endothelial cells [8]. In these studies the extent of apoptotic involvement was oxyhemoglobin dosage dependent. Zubkov *et al.* demonstrated apoptotic changes in cerebral endothelial cells of a patient who died of cerebral vasospasm following SAH [10]. While the above studies only report structural evidence of apoptosis, its participating role in cell death and/or vasoconstriction following SAH is unclear. However, the mere observation of the presence of apoptotic changes in vessels exposed to subarachnoid blood is significant since there is evidence to indicate that apoptosis might be altered or manipulated. Caspases, a large group of intracellular signal transduction proteins, are known to be major players in promoting the process of apoptosis. In vitro studies have shown that when some caspases are inhibited (particularly caspases 3 and 9), there is a significant reduction in apoptotic changes in vascular endothelial cells induced by oxidized low-density lipoproteins [3].

In conclusion, the results of this study have demonstrated apoptotic like changes in endothelial cells in the basilar artery exposed to subarachnoid blood. Apoptosis coincided with the onset of basilar artery constriction and progressed along the course of vasospasm. Whether apoptosis represents a more encompassing mechanism of cell death than now considered or whether it can be manipulated to alter the final outcome of cell injury will require more studies, particularly biophysiological ones at the molecular level.

References

1. Fein JM, Flor WJ, Cohan SL, Parkhurst J (1974) Sequential changes of vascular ultrastructure in experimental cerebral vasospasm. Myonecrosis of subarachnoid arteries. J Neurosurg 41: 49–58
2. Findlay JM, Macdonald RL, Weir BK (1991) Current concepts of pathophysiology and management of cerebral vasospasm following aneurysmal subarachnoid hemorrhage. Cerebrovasc Brain Metab Rev 3: 336–361
3. He J, Xiao Y, Zhang L (2000) Cocaine induces apoptosis in human coronary artery endothelial cells. J Cardiovasc Pharmacol 35: 572–580
4. Kassell NF, Haley EC, Jr., Apperson-Hansen C, Alves WM (1996) Randomized, double-blind, vehicle-controlled trial of tirilazad mesylate in patients with aneurysmal subarachnoid hemorrhage: a cooperative study in Europe, Australia, and New Zealand. J Neurosurg 84: 221–228
5. Macdonald RL, Weir BK (1991) A review of hemoglobin and the pathogenesis of cerebral vasospasm. Stroke 22: 971–982
6. Mayberg MR (1998) Cerebral vasospasm. Neurosurg Clin N Am 9: 615–627
7. Mayberg MR, Okada T, Bark DH (1990) The significance of morphological changes in cerebral arteries after subarachnoid hemorrhage. J Neurosurg 72: 626–633
8. Ogihara K, Zubkov AY, Bernanke DH, Lewis AI, Parent AD, Zhang J (1999) Oxyhemoglobin induced apoptosis in cultured endothelial cells. J Neurosurg 91: 459–465
9. Varsos VG, Liszczak TM, Han DH, Kistler JP, Vielma J, Black PM, Heros RC, Zervas NT (1983) Delayed cerebral vasospasm is not reversible by aminophylline, nifedipine, or papaverine in a "two-hemorrhage" canine model. J Neurosurg 58: 11–17
10. Zubkov AY, Ogihara K, Bernanke DH, Parent AD, Zhang J (2000) Apoptosis of endothelial cells in vessels affected by cerebral vasospasm. Surg Neurol 53: 260–266
11. Zubkov A, Lewis AI, Scalzo D, Bernanke DH, Harkey HL (1999) Morphological changes after percutaneous transluminal angioplasty. Surg Neurol 51: 399–403

Correspondence: John H. Zhang, M.D., Ph.D., Department of Neurosurgery, University of Mississippi Medical Center, 2500 North State Street, Jackson, MS, 39216-4505.

Acta Neurochir (2001) [Suppl] 77: 33–35

Delayed Clot Removal and Experimental Vasospasm

Z.-D. Zhang, B. Yamini, T. Komuro, S. Ono, L. Johns, L. S. Marton, B. Weir, and **R. L. Macdonald**

Section of Neurosurgery, Department of Surgery, Pritzker School of Medicine, University of Chicago Medical Center, Chicago, Illinois, USA

Introduction

It is known that vasospastic arteries have reduced compliance and contractility and exhibit changes in expression of various proteins [3, 1]. It is possible that they may be altered in a manner that reduces their reactivity to blood clot and thereby contributes to the reversal of vasospasm. These experiments determined if subarachnoid blood clot induces a positive adaptive response in cerebral arteries that renders them less responsive to a subsequent challenge with subarachnoid blood.

Keywords: Preconditioning; subarachnoid hemorrhage; vasospasm.

Materials and Methods

17 cynomolgus monkeys underwent cerebral angiography and unilateral right subarachnoid blood clot placement (SAH) on day 0 using methods previously described [2]. Angiography was repeated on day 7. Animals were assigned randomly to have the subarachnoid blood clot removed and replaced with fresh clot (n = 7 arteries) or not replaced (n = 5). The removed clot was placed on the left side (n = 12). Control animals did not have clot removal on day 7 (n = 5) and/or had fresh clot placed on the left side on day 7 (n = 5). Angiography was repeated on days 8, 10, 12 and 14 after which animals were euthanized. Vasospasm was assessed by measurement of intracranial artery diameters on angiograms. The weight of all placed and removed blood clots was determined. The Animal Care and Use Committee of the University of Chicago approved procedures on animals. The possibility that there is a difference in vasospasm induced de novo by fresh clot on day 0 and that induced by fresh clot obtained from an animal on day 7 that has undergone surgical stress was studied by comparing the above groups to animals undergoing baseline angiography and bilateral SAH on day 0 followed by serial angiography on days 1, 3, 5 and 7 (n = 8 animals with bilateral SAH, n = 16 arteries). The overall results are described and analyzed separately for 3 manipulations of the right cerebral arteries (no clot removal, clot-new clot and clot removal groups) and 2 manipulations of the left cerebral arteries (placement of old clot, placement of new clot from a monkey 7 days after SAH) plus one control group with bilateral SAH (new clot, no prior manipulations). The 3 groups undergoing right-sided manipulations were analyzed together and separately from the 2 groups undergoing left-sided manipulations plus the day 0 control group undergoing bilateral manipulations. Comparisons within groups over time and between groups at each time were by analysis of variance (ANOVA). Linear regression of clot weight and per cent change in clot weight versus degree of vasospasm also was determined. Significance was taken at $p < 0.05$. All values are means ± standard deviation.

Results

There were no differences between groups in hemoglobin concentration on day 0 ($P = 0.66$, ANOVA). Since clots were derived from and placed intracranially on day 7 in some groups, the hemoglobin concentration in the blood of these groups on day 7 was compared to that on day 0 in the group undergoing bilateral SAH. Hemoglobin concentration was significantly higher in the day 0 group compared to the other groups ($P < 0.01$, ANOVA). There were no differences between groups at any other time.

Right Angiography

Groups analyzed here had undergone clot placement on day 0 followed on day 7 by: 1. no manipulation (no clot removal, n = 5), 2. removal of the old clot and placement of fresh clot (clot-new clot, n = 7) or 3. removal of the old clot (clot removal, n = 5). Analysis of angiographic middle cerebral artery (MCA) diameter over time showed that all 3 groups had significant vasospasm on day 7. If the clot was not removed, vasospasm slowly resolved and by day 14 was significantly less than on day 7 ($P < 0.001$, ANOVA). If the clot

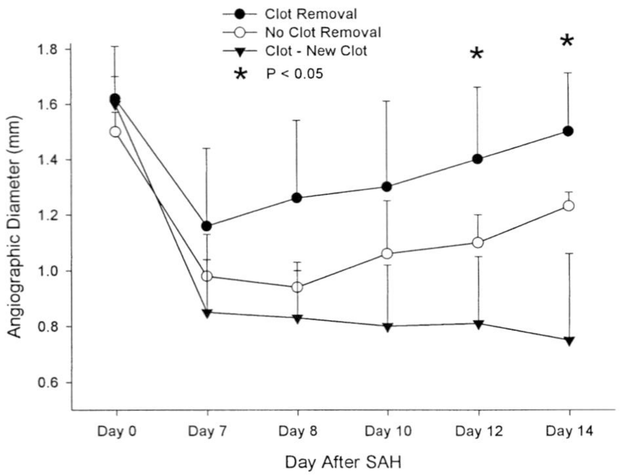

Fig. 1. Graph of angiographic MCA diameters for right sided arteries undergoing no manipulation (no clot removal, n = 5), placement of new clot (clot-new clot, n = 7) or clot removal (clot removal, n = 5). Vasospasm reverses significantly more rapidly in the clot removal group compared to the clot-new clot group by day 12 ($P < 0.05$, ANOVA) and compared to the clot-new clot and no clot removal groups by day 14 ($P < 0.05$, ANOVA)

was removed, vasospasm also resolved slowly and was significantly less than on day 7 by days 12 and 14 ($P < 0.05$, ANOVA). If fresh clot was placed, however, there was no reversal of vasospasm.

Comparisons between groups at day 0 and day 7 showed no significant differences and that each group developed significant vasospasm at day 7. Analysis between the groups over time showed no differences on days 8 and 10 but that by day 12, there was significant variance in per cent changes in MCA diameter compared to day 7 ($P < 0.05$, ANOVA, Fig. 1). The group with clot removal had significantly less vasospasm than the group with new clot placed. By day 14, all 3 groups were significantly different with clot removal resulting in less vasospasm and placement of fresh clot resulting in more vasospasm than the no clot removal group.

Left Angiography

Groups analyzed here had undergone placement of 7 day old clot removed from the right side of the head against the left arteries (4. old clot, n = 12) or placement of fresh clot (5. new clot, day 7, n = 5). The third group analyzed had bilateral clot placement followed by serial angiography (6. new clot, day 0, n = 18). Analysis of angiographic MCA diameter over time showed that all 3 groups had significant reductions in

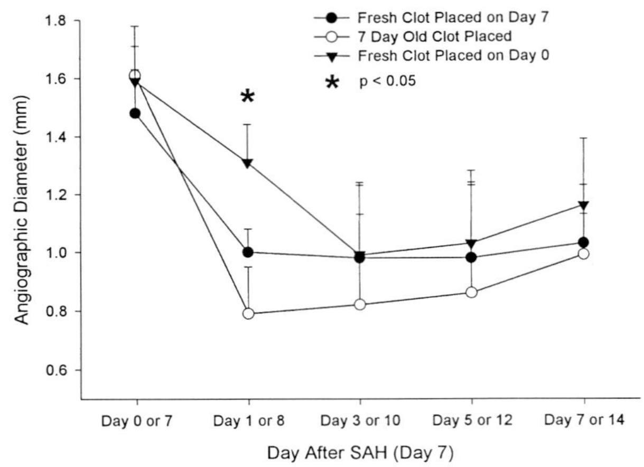

Fig. 2. Graph of angiographic MCA diameter from day 7 versus day after clot placement for left sided arteries undergoing placement of 7-day old clot removed from the right side (old clot, day 7, n = 12) or placement of new clot (new clot, day 7, n = 5) and for a control group undergoing angiography and SAH on day 0 followed by angiography on days 1, 3, 5, and 7 (new clot, day 0, n = 18). The only significant difference between the groups is one day after clot placement when there is more severe vasospasm in groups that are already 7 days after a right SAH and that have placement of old or new clot on the left side ($P < 0.001$, ANOVA). Furthermore, vasospasm is significantly more severe when old clot is placed compared to the other groups ($P < 0.001$, ANOVA)

MCA diameter starting 1 day after clot placement (day 8 or day 1, depending on the group, $P < 0.001$, ANOVA) and that vasospasm persisted without significant change until euthanasia on day 7 or 14. The trend in all 3 groups was for vasospasm to become less severe after day 3 although this was not significant.

Comparisons between groups at day 0 and day 7 prior to clot placement showed no significant differences in MCA diameters. The only significant difference between the groups was one day after clot placement when there was more severe vasospasm in groups that were already 7 days after a right SAH and that had placement of old or new clot on the left side ($P < 0.001$, ANOVA, Fig. 2). Furthermore, vasospasm was significantly more severe in animals with old clot placement compared to the other groups ($P < 0.001$, ANOVA).

Clot Weights and Relation to Vasospasm

There were no significant differences in the weights of fresh clots that were placed on day 0 or day 7. There were no differences in the weights of clots removed on day 7 although the weights of these clots were all significantly less than the weights placed on day 0

($P < 0.001$, ANOVA). Similarly, there were no differences in the weights of clots that had been present intracranially for 14 days although they were less than weights present at 7 days ($P < 0.05$, ANOVA).

In order to determine the dependence of vasospasm on the subarachnoid clot, linear regressions were conducted comparing percent reductions in angiographic arterial diameters over the 7 days after a particular clot was placed and the weight of clot placed, weight cleared over 7 days or percent of clot cleared over the same time. Separate analyses were conducted for clot placed on day 0 and for fresh and old clots placed on day 7. No significant relationships could be demonstrated in any case between any measure of clot clearance and the degree of vasospasm that developed. It was noted that small weights of day 7 clot often elicited as much spasm as fresh clots.

Discussion

This study was conducted to determine if there is a preconditioning or positive adaptive response in the subarachnoid arteries that develops during vasospasm and that leads to reversal of the spasm as well as loss of reactivity of the cerebral arteries to a second challenge with subarachnoid blood. The principle finding from the right-sided arteries is that there is no evidence for such a response. Multiple mechanisms could be involved in the maintenance and reversal of vasospasm after SAH. Vasospasm may resolve because of loss of the stimulus for the vasospasm which is the subarachnoid blood. There may be decreased release of the spasmogenic substances from the clot. There may be a positive adaptive response that allows the artery to relax even though clot still is present. Other factors that may be involved are that the spasmogen(s) could become embedded in the arterial wall such that clot removal does not have any effect on the time course of the vasospasm and that there may be a negative adaptive response that makes vasospasm more severe in response to a repeated stimulus. Adaptive responses could be local in the artery exposed to blood or general in the entire organism. One interpretation of these findings is the following. For the right arteries, the removal of clot always results in more rapid reversal of vasospasm even after 7 days, suggesting that vasospasm is always dependent to some extent on the presence of subarachnoid clot. There is no evidence for a positive adaptive response but in fact may be support for a negative adaptive response because spasm was worse when fresh blood is placed on day 7. Another possible explanation is that the systemic blood of an animal 7 days after SAH is more spasmogenic. That a spasmogen is in the arterial wall and not removed by clot removal also is possible because vasospasm reverses more slowly when clot has been there for 7 days than if it is only present for 1 or 3 days [3]. This, however, could be due to compliance changes in the arterial wall [3]. On the left side, the rapid onset of spasm with old clot would seem to contradict the results from the right but could be explained if the clot was encapsulated on the right and not releasing spasmogens at the same rate as it does when removed, broken up, and replaced on the left. The left side arteries also do not support the role of a positive adaptive response but provide some for a negative adaptive response or as mentioned above, a change in the spasmogenic activity of blood derived from an animal 7 days after SAH.

In conclusion, vasospasm resolves primarily because of loss of subarachnoid blood clot. Other factors such as decreased release of spasmogens from the persisting clot are important. There is no evidence for a positive adaptive response in the cerebral arteries that renders them less responsive to the subarachnoid clot. They are in fact more sensitive to subsequent challenges with subarachnoid blood. The importance to the pathogenesis of vasospasm of changes in arterial contractility and compliance and in expression of some genes needs to be carefully considered.

Acknowledgments

Supported by grants from the National Institutes of Health to Dr. Macdonald (K08 NS01831) and Dr. Weir (RO1 NS25946) and from the Brain Research Foundation. An American College of Surgeons Faculty Fellowship supports Dr. Macdonald.

References

1. Ono S, Zhang ZD, Marton LS, Yamini B, Windmeyer E, Johns L, Kowalczuk A, Lin G, Macdonald RL (2000) Heme oxygenase-1 and ferritin are increased in cerebral arteries after subarachnoid hemorrhage in monkeys. J Cereb Blood Flow Metab 20: 1066–1076
2. Stoodley M, Macdonald RL, Weir BK, Marton LS, Johns LM, Zhang ZD, Kowalczuk A (2000) Subarachnoid hemorrhage causes an adaptive response in cerebral arteries. J Neurosurg 93: 463–470.
3. Vorkapic P, Bevan RD, Bevan JA (1990) Pharmacologic irreversible narrowing in chronic cerebrovasospasm in rabbits is associated with functional damage. Stroke 21: 1478–1484

Correspondence: R. L. Macdonald, M.D., Ph.D., Section of Neurosurgery, MC3026, University of Chicago Medical Center, 5841 South Maryland Avenue, Chicago, Illinois, USA, 60637.

Acta Neurochir (2001) [Suppl] 77: 37–40

Influence of Brain Natriuretic Peptide on Phenotypic Change of Cerebral Vasculature

J. Hansen-Schwartz[1,2], **G. Sviri**[3], and **L. Edvinsson**[1,2]

[1] Department of Clinical Experimental Research, Glostrup Hospital, Denmark
[2] Department of Internal Medicine, Lund University Hospital, Sweden
[3] Department of Neurosurgery, Rambam Medical Center, Haifa, Israel

Introduction

Brain Natriuretic Peptide (BNP) belongs to the family of natriuretic peptides, the other members being Atrial Natriuretic Peptide (ANP) and C-type Natriuretic Peptide (CNP); each type also existing in isoforms. The average peptide length is 30 amino acid residues ranging from 20 to 54 [14]. Their systemic effects are hypotension, natriuresis and hyponatraemia, acting via specific natriuretic peptide receptors characterized on the basis of pharmacology and molecular biology [5].

The natriuretic peptides are usually considered in connection with congestive heart disease being predictive of terminal disease [4, 6]. However, increasing evidence is pointing towards a role of BNP in subarachnoid haemorrhage (SAH). Thus, increased levels have been found in plasma of patients with SAH [3, 9], indeed a correlation has been found between the degree of possible cerebral vasospasm and concentration of BNP in plasma [13]. However, the significance of this increased production of BNP in the pathophysiology of SAH and cerebral vasospasm has yet to be established.

Organ culture of entire vessel segments induces reproducible phenotypic changes in rat cerebral blood vessels. After 48 hours of organ culture the sensitivity to endothelin-1 (ET-1) in terms of the contractile response is increased 1000-fold [8]. Other changes include appearance of contractile ET_B receptors [8, 11] as well as changes in the serotonin receptors (unpublished data).

To gain further insight into the pathophysiological role of BNP we have – using vessel baths – characterized the dilatory response of the guinea pig basilar artery to the natriuretic peptides, and using organ culture, to investigate a possible change in the response to BNP as well as the possible modulatory influence of BNP on the response to endothelin.

Keywords: SAH; BNP; endothelin-1; guinea pig.

Methods

Tissue Preparation and Organ Culture Procedure

The basilar artery from guinea pigs (250–300 g) were harvested and dissected free from connective tissue, cut into circular segments of 1 mm in length and either used immediately for in vitro pharmacology (see below) or placed in sterile Dulbeccos modified Eagles's medium (DMEM) for organ culture [1].

The arterial segments were incubated for two days. Incubation was done at 37 °C in humidified atmospheric air enriched with 5% CO_2 in serum free DMEM supplemented with penicillin 100 IU/mL and streptomycin 100 μg/mL.

For experiments testing the influence of BNP during organ culture, BNP was added at a concentration of 10^{-7} M.

In vitro Pharmacology

For contractile experiments, the arteries were mounted on two wires (Myograph, J. P. Trading, Denmark) submerged in a temperature controlled buffer solution (37 °C) of the following composition (mM) NaCl 119, $NaHCO_3$ 15, KCl 4.6, MgCl 1.2, NaH_2PO_4 1.2, $CaCl_2$ 1.5 and glucose 5.5. The buffer was continuously aerated with oxygen enriched with 5% CO_2 resulting in a pH of 7.4.

Measurements were continuously recorded by a PowerLab unit (ADInstruments, Hastings, England). A tension of 2 mN was applied to the segments which were then allowed to stabilize at this tone for one hour.

Dilatation experiments were conducted using ANP, BNP and CNP (all Sigma chemicals) in fresh vessels to characterize the relaxant responses and BNP only in cultured vessels. U46619 at a concentration of 10^{-6} M was used to induce a steady level of precontraction.

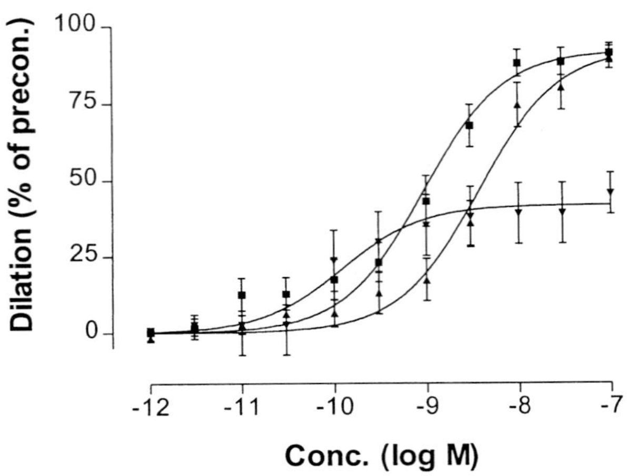

Fig. 1. Relaxant effect of ANP, BNP and CNP in fresh basilar artery segments. ■ ANP, ▲ BNP and ▼ CNP

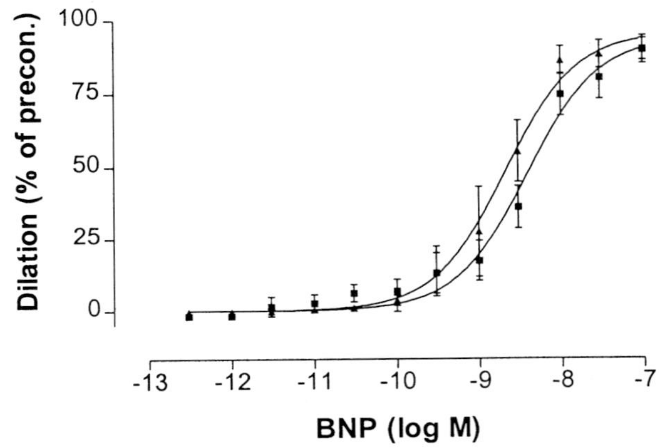

Fig. 2. Relaxant effect of BNP in fresh and cultured basilar artery segments. ■ Fresh segments and ▲ cultured segments

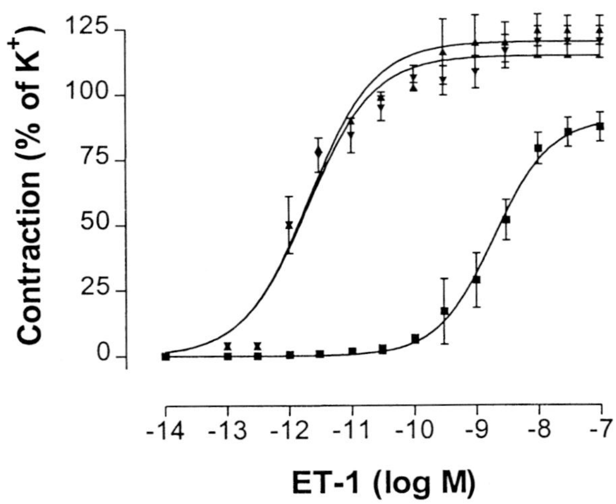

Fig. 3. ET-1 response in fresh and cultured basilar artery segments. ■ Fresh segments, ▲ cultured segments and ▼ segments cultured with BNP

Concentration-response experiments were conducted with endothelin-1 (ET-1, a general endothelin receptor agonist) (Auspep, Australia) as agonist. Concentration-response curves for the agonists were obtained by cumulative application.

Calculation and Statistics

Data are expressed as mean values ± s.e.mean. Contractile responses in each segment were expressed as a % of the contraction induced in that segment by 60 mM K^+. Dilatory responses were expressed as the % dilatation compared to the precontracted value. In a given experiment E_{max} denotes the maximum response elicited by an agonist whereas pEC_{50} denotes the negative logarithm of the concentration needed to elicit half the maximum response.

To evaluate statistical significance ($p < 0.05$) between concentration-response curves Student's t-test was used.

Results

Characterization of the Relaxant Responses Toward the Natriuretic Peptides in Fresh Basilar Arteries

All three natriuretic peptides were capable of relaxing the precontracted basilar artery in a concentration-dependant manner (Fig. 1). In terms of E_{max} and pEC_{50}, the natriuretic peptides yielded the following results: ANP 90 ± 3% and 9.4 ± 0.3, BNP 90 ± 4% ($p = 0.69$) and 8.5 ± 0.3 ($p = 0.01$), and CNP 45 ± 7% ($p < 0.01$) and 9.4 ± 1.1 ($p = 0.88$), respectively (p values are calculated with respect to ANP). The dilatation was dependant upon the presence of endothelium. Thus, removal of the endothelium almost totally abolished the NP response (data not shown).

Dilatory Effect of BNP Before and After Organ Culture

As seen in Fig. 2, organ culture did not influence the dilatory effect of BNP, thus E_{max} (90 ± 5%) and pEC_{50} (8.8 ± 0.2) after organ culture were not significantly different ($p = 0.98$ and 0.21, respectively) as compared to the values obtained in the fresh vessel segments.

Influence of BNP Added During Organ Culture on the Contractile Response to ET-1

In fresh basilar artery, ET-1 elicited a concentration-dependent contraction with an E_{max} of 95 ± 8% and a

pEC_{50} of 9.0 ± 0.3. After organ culture a highly significant 1000-fold increase in sensitivity and potency was observed with an E_{max} of $122 \pm 7\%$ ($p < 0.01$) and a pEC_{50} of 12.7 ± 0.9 ($p = 0.03$). Vessels cultured in the presence of BNP showed no difference in comparison to vessels cultured without BNP (E_{max} $119 \pm 9\%$ ($p = 0.53$) and pEC_{50} 12.5 ± 1.1 ($p = 0.61$)) (Fig. 3).

Discussion

The results of our in vitro study confirm the vasodilative effect of the natriuretic peptides on the guinea pig cerebral vessels with the sensitivity order ANP = CNP > BNP. In terms of effect both ANP and BNP are able to completely relax the precontracted vessel segments, whereas CNP only partially dilates the vessels. The response to BNP was unchanged after organ culture and BNP in itself did not have a modulatory effect on the phenotypical change of the endothelin response. This shows that the endothelial function was conserved in our experiments, also after organ culture. The capacity to change phenotypically was confirmed by the increased sensitivity and potency of ET-1 after organ culture.

So far three natriuretic peptide receptors (NPR) have been described, NPR-A, NPR-B and NPR-C. The latter is a clearance receptor and so far no pharmacological property has been ascribed to this receptor subtype. NPR-A and NPR-B belongs to the guanylyl cyclase receptors [7, 12]. NPR-A is defined by the rank order of potency ANP > BNP ≫ CNP, and the NPR-B by the rank order CNP > ANP > BNP [12]. The rank order obtained in the present experiments does not correlate perfectly with either. Since only ANP and BNP were full agonists, their difference in potency suggests the presence of the NPR-A subtype of receptors in the guinea pig basilar artery.

About one third of patients suffering from SAH experiences hyponatrieamia, a phenomenon described as the cerebral salt wasting syndrome [10]. Several studies have found a correlation between excess of BNP and observed hyponatriaemia. The source of this BNP has not been established with certainty, but it has been hypothesized that it is the hypothalamus that produces the peptide in response to hypoxic stress [3, 14]. A more recent study has also found a correlation between cerebral vasospasm and venous concentration of BNP [13]. This poses the question of whether the BNP produced alleviates the cerebral hypoxic condition. The observed concentrations of BNP in plasma are in the picomolar range. In our study the pEC_{50} value is in the nanomolar range. So far no BNP'ergic innervation of cerebral vessels has been described and thus, it would be fair to conclude that circulating BNP doesn't have any profound effect on vascular caliber.

It has earlier been shown that cerebral vessels from a rat SAH model have an increased sensitivity to ET-1 [2], and the in vitro organ culture experiments confirm this capacity of cerebral vessels [8]. This change in sensitivity may be pivotal in the events leading to CVS and cerebral ischaemia. Furthermore, in this in vitro study BNP did not alter the effect of organ culture on the response to ET-1. Thus it may be hypothesized that in the human setting, the presence of BNP in plasma doesn't have any protective influence on the vessel, while in high concentrations it may have a relaxant effect.

Conclusion

It appears that BNP produced in the course of SAH only serves to complicate the disease in terms of hyponatriaemia and hypovolaemia, a condition difficult to treat. Although further pharmacological and molecular studies are needed, it seems probable that antagonists to BNP may have a place in the treatment of associated phenomena in SAH.

Acknowledgments

The authors wish to thank the Leo Foundation and Foundation for Research in Neurology (both in Denmark) as well as the Swedish Medical Research Council (grant no. 5958) for economic support.

References

1. Adner M, Cantera L, Ehlert F, Nilsson L, Edvinsson L (1996) Plasticity of contractile endothelin-B receptors in human arteries after organ culture. Br J Pharmacol 119: 1159–1166
2. Alafaci C, Jansen I, Arbab MA, Shiokawa Y, Svendgaard NA, Edvinsson L (1990) Enhanced vasoconstrictor effect of endothelin in cerebral arteries from rats with subarachnoid haemorrhage. Acta Physiol Scand 138: 317–319
3. Berendes E, Walter M, Cullen P, Prien T, Van Aken H, Horsthemke J, Schulte M, von Wild K, Scherer R (1997) Secretion of brain natriuretic peptide in patients with aneurysmal subarachnoid haemorrhage. Lancet 349: 245–249
4. Espiner EA (1994) Physiology of natriuretic peptides. J Intern Med 235: 527–541
5. Farrell AP, Olson KR (2000) Cardiac natriuretic peptides: a physiological lineage of cardioprotective hormones? Physiol Biochem Zool 73: 1–11

6. Fyhrquist F, Tikkanen I (1988) Atrial natriuretic peptide in congestive heart failure. Am J Cardiol 62: 20A–24A
7. Garbers DL (1999) The guanylyl cyclase receptors. Methods 19: 477–484
8. Hansen-Schwartz J, Edvinsson L (2000) Increased sensitivity to ET-1 in rat cerebral arteries following organ culture. Neuroreport 11: 649–652
9. Isotani E, Suzuki R, Tomita K, Hokari M, Monma S, Marumo F, Hirakawa K (1994) Alterations in plasma concentrations of natriuretic peptides and antidiuretic hormone after subarachnoid hemorrhage. Stroke 25: 2198–2203
10. Kroll M, Juhler M, Lindholm J (1992) Hyponatraemia in acute brain disease. J Intern Med 232: 291–297
11. Leseth KH, Adner M, Berg HK, White LR, Aasly J, Edvinsson L (1999) Cytokines increase endothelin ETB receptor contractile activity in rat cerebral artery. Neuroreport 10: 2355–2359
12. Suga S, Nakao K, Hosoda K, Mukoyama M, Ogawa Y, Shirakami G, Arai H, Saito Y, Kambayashi Y, Inouye K (1992) Receptor selectivity of natriuretic peptide family, atrial natriuretic peptide, brain natriuretic peptide, and C-type natriuretic peptide. Endocrinology 130: 229–239
13. Sviri GE, Feinsod M, Soustiel JF (2000) Brain natriuretic peptide and cerebral vasospasm in subarachnoid hemorrhage: clinical and TCD correlations. Stroke 31: 118–122
14. Wijdicks EF, Schievink WI, Burnett JC, Jr. (1997) Natriuretic peptide system and endothelin in aneurysmal subarachnoid hemorrhage. J Neurosurg 87: 275–280

Correspondence: Dr. J. Hansen-Schwartz, Dept. of Clinical Experimental Research, EB 4th floor, Glostrup University Hospital, DK-2600 Glostrup, Denmark.

Acta Neurochir (2001) [Suppl] 77: 41–43

Brain Natriuretic Peptide and Cerebral Vasospasm in Subarachnoid Hemorrhage

G. E. Sviri[1], **B. Shik**[1], **B. Raz**[2], and **J. F. Soustiel**[1]

[1] Department of Neurosurgery, Rambam Medical Center, Bruce Rappaport Faculty of Medicine, The Technion Institute of Technology, Haifa, Israel
[2] Department of Endocrinology, Rambam Medical Center, Bruce Rappaport Faculty of Medicine, The Technion Institute of Technology, Haifa, Israel

Introduction

Natriuretic peptides (NPs), very potent vasodilators, are responsible for profound diuresis and natriuresis in patients with spontaneous subarachnoid hemorrhage (SSAH) [2, 6]. Okunchi *et al.* [4] reported that such a profound natriuresis precede the development of ischemic symptoms, and act therefore as a potential trigger for symptomatic cerebral arteries vasospasm (CVS) following SSAH. The present study was designed to examine the correlation between plasma levels of BNP and (CVS) following SSAH by means of transcranial Doppler (TCD) and clinical course.

Keywords: Natriuretic peptide; subarachnoid hemorrhage; cerebral vasospasm.

Material and Methods

26 patients with SSAH were recruited for the present study. There were 11 males and 15 females, ranging in age from 21 to 69 years with a mean of 49.4 years (SD: 14.6) years. Delayed neurological deterioration (DND) was defined as a worsening of the neurological condition that could not be attributed to rebleeding, systemic or post-operative complications. Intensity of SAH was determined according to the grading system proposed by Fisher. All patients underwent daily TCD recording. Mean FVs exceeding 120 cm/s and threefold that of the FVs in the internal carotid artery was selected as a criteria of vasospasm in the MCA and ACA. Patients with TCD evidence of vasospasm were further divided into two clinical subsets: 1) Nonsymptomatic vasospasm was defined by transient elevation of FVs without neurological deterioration. 2) Intense and prolonged FVs elevation associated with delayed neurological deterioration and/or ischemic deficit defined as symptomatic vasospasm.

Phlebotomy was performed for plasma sampling of BNP 4 times during the clinical course; period 1 – days 1–3 (day 1 being regarded as the day of SAH onset); period 2 – days 4–6; period 3 – days 7–9, period 4 – days 10–12. The plasma BNP levels were determined using a specific RIA (SHIONORIA BNP, Shionogi & Co, LTD).

Results

Clinical features and results are summarized in Table 1. Plasma concentrations of BNP at the first period (days 1–3) were significantly higher in the patient group (52.43 $\pm$ 48.15 pg/ml) than in the control group (5.78 $\pm$ 1.90 pg/ml, $P = 0.0023$).

Eighteen patients (69.2%) had TCD evidence for vasospasm. In ten (55%), vasospasm was only moderate and did not result in clinical worsening. In the remaining eight patients (45%), vasospasm was severe and associated with delayed neurological deterioration in all instances and hypodense ischemic lesion on CT scan was disclosed in six patients (33.3%).

As a group, SAH patients showed a progressive increase in BNP plasma concentrations between the first (days 1–3) and the third period (days 7–9). This increase in BNP plasma levels at the third period enhanced almost linearly with the intensity of the SAH. Nevertheless, the ratio of BNP levels between the third and first period was significantly higher in patients with massive SAH and those with intraparenchymal or intraventricular hemorrhage (Fisher grade 3 and 4) in comparison with patients with cryptic and slight SAH (Fisher grade 1 and 2, $P = 0.048$, Fig. 1).

Patients with symptomatic vasospasm showed a continuous elevation of BNP concentrations between the first and third period, up to six times the initial value in this group (Table 1, Fig. 2). On the other hand, in patients without CVS and with nonsymptomatic CVS, BNP plasma levels decreased progressively between the first and the third period. (Table 1, Fig. 2, $P = 0.0096$).

Table 1. *Clinical Feature and Results*

		No CVS	Non symptomatic CVS	CVS	p value
No' of patients		8	10	8	NS
Age		58.3 ± 9.1	48.3 ± 1.2	42.7 ± 15.5	$P < 0.05$
Gender M/F		3/5	5/5	3/5	NS
Hunt and Hess score	average	2.4 ± 1.26	2.7 ± 1.42	3 ± 1.47	NS
Fisher's score	average	2.3 ± 1.07	2.55 ± 1.21	3.33 ± 0.78	$P < 0.05$
BNP plasma concentration ratio	period 2/1	0.71 ± 0.46	0.85 ± 0.67	3.72 ± 5.63	NS
	period 3/1	0.66 ± 0.51	0.68 ± 0.95	6.21 ± 5.21	$P < 0.01$
	period 4/1	0.30 ± 0.27	0.34 ± 0.42	4.45 ± 4.83	$P < 0.05$
GOS	average	3.4 ± 1.91	3.5 ± 1.72	2.6 ± 1.39	NS

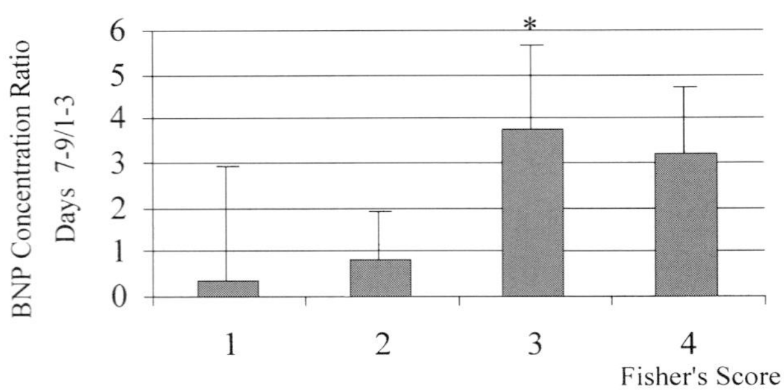

Fig. 1. BNP plasma concentrations ratio days 7–9/1–3 and hemorrhage intensity. (*$p < 0.05$)

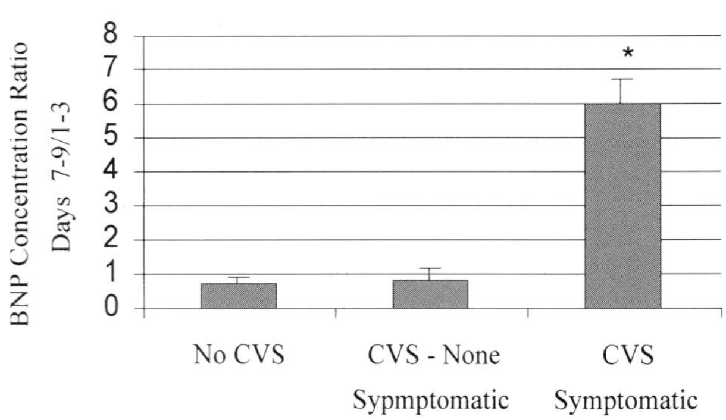

Fig. 2. BNP plasma concentration ratio days 7–9/1–3 and CVS. (*$p < 0.01$)

Discussion

Early studies have drawn attention to the frequent occurrence of hyponatremia in CVS as a cause of neurological worsening following aneurysmal SAH. BNP have been proposed as a plausible origin for the occurrence of this cerebral salt wasting syndrome [2, 6]. The results of the present study further support that BNP release is induced by SAH and may therefore, be responsible for hyponatremia and vasospasm aggravation. In the present series, however, BNP levels showed a continuous trend of elevation (630% between period 1 to 3) only in patients with symptomatic vasospasm. These findings are compatible with those reported by Morinaga *et al.* [3] in their series of 121 patients with aneurysmal SAH. These authors reported hyponatremia in 19 patients of whom 16 had symptomatic vasospasm and CT scan evidence of ischemic lesion in 8 patients. Their results as well as the results of the present study suggest that increasing release of BNP may exacerbate in some patients the hemodynamic consequences of vasospasm and lead to cerebral ischemia. These findings raise the question of the role of natriuretic peptides (NPs) and particularly the BNP in the pathogenesis of CVS. NPs have potent vasodilator effects in blood vessels, directly (using membranal receptor and cGMP as a secondary messenger) or through inhibition of vasoconstrictor signals (reduction of endothelin and its receptors expression). They also have anti-angioproliferative activities. By these local effects, NPs may play as a protective hormone counteracting the vasospastic stress in order to reduce tissue ischemia. On the other hand, by their systemic effects, (hypovolemia, veins and arterial dilatation) NPs can lead to exacerbation of cerebral blood flow reduction. Although, primarily of cardiac origin, BNP is also produced in the hypothalamus [5] in response to autocrine and paracrine stimulation [1] and from ischemic brain tissue. Nevertheless, the mechanism of BNP release in SAH and CVS remained ill defined.

Conclusion

BNP plasma concentrations are elevated shortly after SSAH, though increase markedly during the clinical course only in patients with symptomatic cerebral vasospasm. The present findings suggest that despite some protective effects on blood vessels which may be attributed to BNP, such as vasodilation, BNP through its systemic effects can exacerbate cerebral blood flow reduction secondary to CVS.

References

1. Antunes-Rodrigues J, Ramalho MJ, Reis LC, Picanco-Diniz DW, Favaretto AL, Gutkowska J, McCann SM (1993) Possible role of endothelin acting within the hypothalamus to induce the release of atrial natriuretic peptide and natriuresis. Neuroendocrinology 58: 701–708
2. Berendes E, Walter M, Cullen P, Prien T, Van Aken H, Horsthemke J, Schulte M, von Wild K, Scherer R (1997) Secretion of brain natriuretic peptide in patients with aneurysmal subarachnoid haemorrhage. Lancet 349: 245–249
3. Morinaga K, Hyashi S, Matsumoto Y, Omiya N, Mikami J, Ueda M, Sato H, Inoue Y, Okawara S (1992) [Hyponatremia and cerebral vasospasm in patients with subarachnoid hemorrhage]. No To Shinkei 44: 629–632
4. Okuchi K, Fujioka M, Fujikawa A, Nishimura A, Konobu T, Miyamoto S, Sakaki T (1996) Rapid natriuresis and preventive hypervolemia for symptomatic vasospasm after subarachnoid haemorrhage. Acta Neurochir (Wien) 138: 951–956
5. Takahashi K, Totsune K, Sone M, Ohneda M, Murakami O, Itoi K, Mouri T (1992) Human brain natriuretic peptide-like immunoreactivity in human brain. Peptides 13: 121–123
6. Wijdicks EFM, Schievink WI, Burnett JC Jr (1997) Natriuretic peptide system and endothelin in aneurysmal subarachnoid hemorrhage. J Neurosurg 87: 275–280

Correspondence: Dr. G. E. Sviri, Department of Neurosurgery, Rambam Medical Center, POB 9602, Haifa 31096, Israel.

Acta Neurochir (2001) [Suppl] 77: 45–47

Phosphatidylcholine Peroxidized by Hemoglobin Increases Intracellular Calcium in Dog Basilar Artery Smooth Muscle Cells

B. S. Jahromi, T. Komuro, R. L. Macdonald, L. S. Marton, and **B. K. Weir**

Section of Neurosurgery, Department of Surgery, Pritzker School of Medicine, University of Chicago Medical Center, Chicago, Illinois, USA

Introduction

Numerous studies in vitro and in vivo have identified hemoglobin as the primary spasmogen underlying cerebral vasospasm following subarachnoid hemorrhage (SAH) [8]. Numerous cellular mechanisms, however, remain implicated in the pathogenesis of vasospasm, and the existence of other spasmogen(s) is suggested by hemolysate fractionation studies [1, 9]. Lipid peroxides are attractive candidate spasmogens as they are key structural components of cell membranes and are abundant in the subarachnoid space after SAH, are readily formed following exposure to reactive oxygen species [3] and can have wide-ranging biological effects depending upon their putative downstream target(s) in ensuing free-radical chain reactions. We hypothesized that hemoglobin promotes the peroxidation of phosphatidylcholine (PC) to phosphatidylcholine peroxide (PCOOH), and that PCOOH contributes to cerebral vasospasm by mobilizing intracellular calcium in vascular smooth muscle cells.

Keywords: Subarachnoid hemorrhage; vasospasm; hemoglobin; oxidation.

Material and Methods

Pure human hemoglobin A_0 (Hemosol Inc., Toronto, Canada) was prepared in concentrations of 10^{-4}–10^{-7} M in 10 mM Tris-saline and incubated with pure, dried PC (Sigma) at 37 °C in the dark for 3 days. The initial hemoglobin solution was >99% ferrous oxyhemoglobin determined by spectrophotometry. Resulting peroxidized lipids were separated with thin-layer chromatography and digital densitometry (NIH Image) was used to quantify lipid fractions generated. In some experiments butylated hydroxytoluene (BHT, 1 μM), an antioxidant, was included in the reaction mixture.

Dog basilar artery smooth muscle cells were cultured by explant from basilar arteries under protocols approved by the Institutional Animal Care and Use Committee. They were cultured in Dulbecco's modified Eagle medium supplemented with 10% fetal calf serum and used on passages 2 to 4. When confluent, cultures were growth-arrested in serum free medium for 24 hours and then loaded with a calcium indicator by incubation with 5 μM fura2-AM and 0.01% pluronic acid for 45–60 minutes. Intracellular calcium concentration ($[Ca^{2+}]_i$) was measured by microfluorometry (as previously described [9]) before and after exposure to PCOOH.

Results

PC incubated in the presence of hemoglobin was peroxidized in a time- and dose-dependent manner (Fig. 1). Peroxidation of PC by hemoglobin could

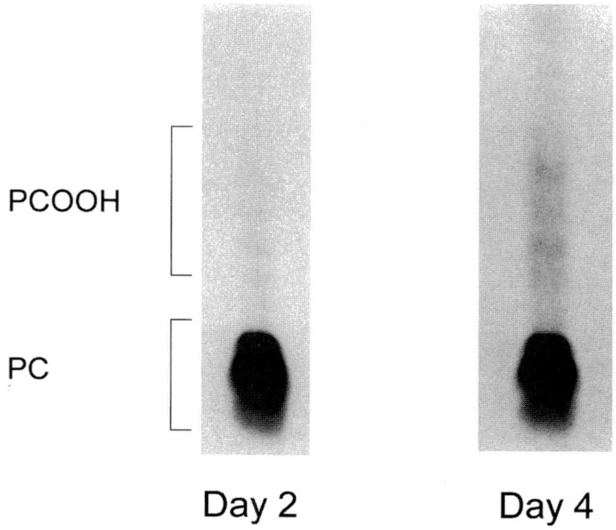

Fig. 1. Thin layer chromatographic separation of PC peroxidization products following incubation with hemoglobin for varying number of days

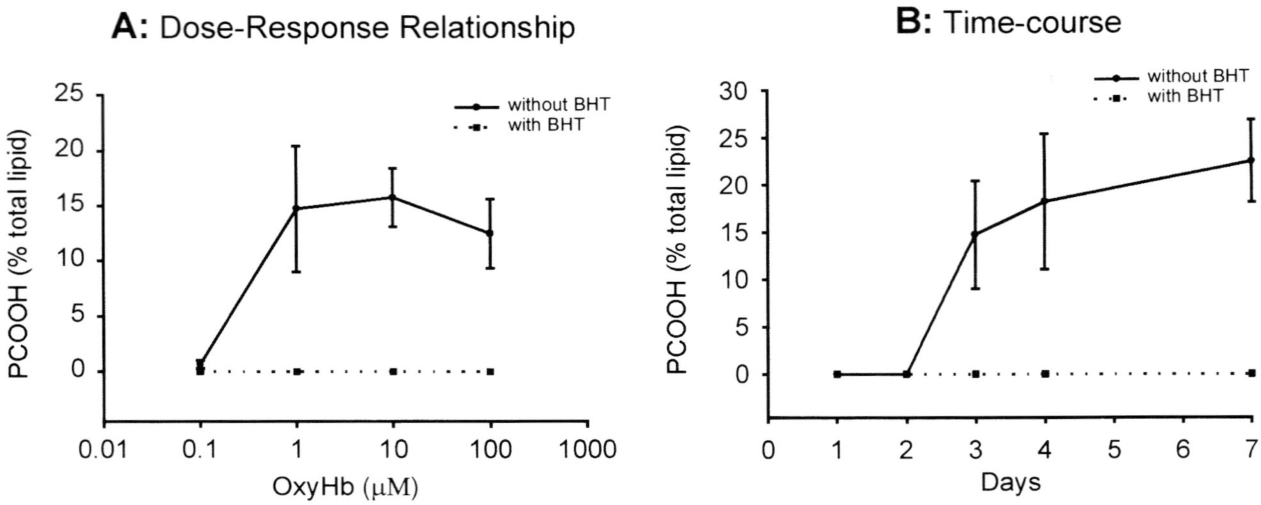

Fig. 2. Hemoglobin promotes the peroxidization of PC in a time- and dose-dependent manner. (A) PC, incubated at 37 °C in presence of increasing concentrations of hemoglobin, was peroxidized into PCOOH (solid line). This was inhibited by the presence of BHT (1 μM, dotted line). (B) The effect was near maximal by the third day of incubation. Error bars represent standard deviation, n = 4 for each data point

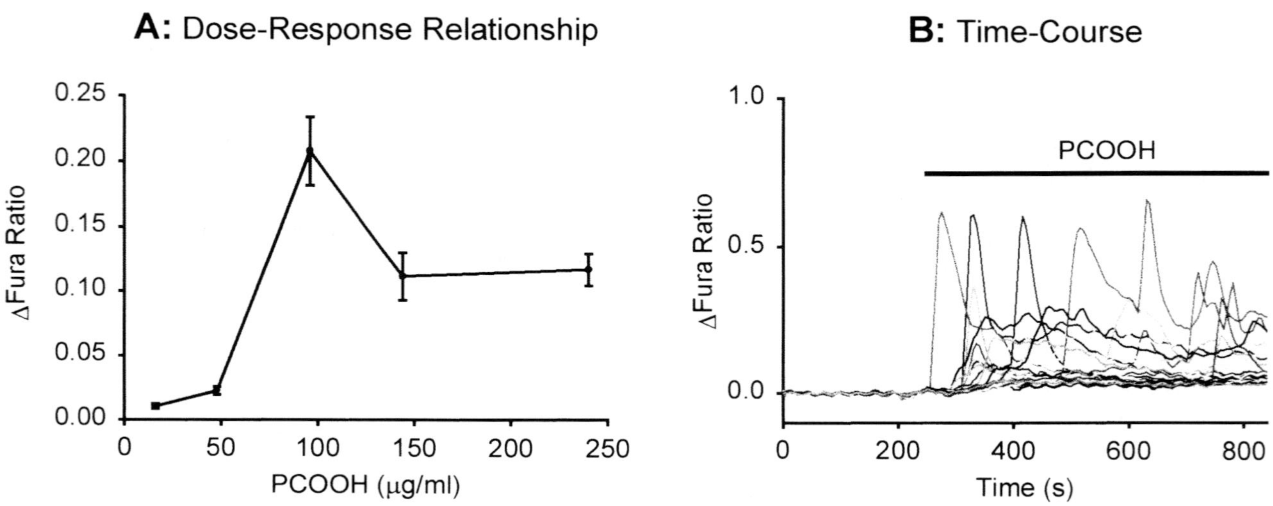

Fig. 3. PCOOH mobilizes $[Ca^{2+}]_i$ in cultured dog basilar artery smooth muscle cells. (A) Dose-response relationship. Error bars represent standard error of the mean, n = 19, 41, 48, 53 and 54 cells tested at PCOOH concentrations of 16, 48, 96, 144, & 240 μg/ml respectively. (B) A representative experiment, where basal rise and Ca^{2+} peaks and oscillations are seen in smooth muscle cells following application of PCOOH

be inhibited by inclusion of the antioxidant BHT in the reaction mixture (Fig. 2). Hemoglobin (1 μM) was sufficient to produce maximal PC peroxidation. PCOOH production was near-maximal by the third day, although peroxidized products could be detected by day 1–2 but were too small in quantity to accurately quantify.

Application of PCOOH to growth-arrested smooth muscle cells produced an increase in basal $[Ca^{2+}]_i$. Some cells also exhibited transient peaks and/or oscillations in Ca^{2+} levels (Fig. 3B). The effect was maximal at 100 ug/ml PCOOH (Fig. 3A), with concentrations beyond 1 mg/ml triggering visible cellular injury in some experiments.

Discussion

Oxyhemoglobin is known to release superoxide anion during its spontaneous conversion to methemoglobin following SAH; other reactive oxygen species are also released during the inflammatory reaction to the subarachnoid blood clot [8]. These reactive oxygen intermediates are thought to trigger further peroxidization reactions, including those involving membrane lipids. PC is the most susceptible to peroxidization amongst membrane lipids [6] and the resulting product, PCOOH, can further interact with membrane components, either directly, or by propagating a chain peroxidation reaction with resulting cleavage, cross-linking, and/or modification of other membrane proteins and lipids. Increased PC turnover has been observed in dogs following SAH [7], and the aminosteroid antioxidant tirilazad has been shown to decrease intra-arterial PCOOH levels in association with reduced vasospasm in a monkey SAH model [6].

Downstream mediators of lipid peroxides in cerebral vasospasm remain unclear. PCOOH is the preferred substrate for membrane-bound phospholipase A2 [4], leading to diacylglycerol accumulation and possibly activation of protein kinase C. The subsequent release of free arachidonic acid from cleavage of lipid peroxides by phospholipases also can stimulate the arachidonic acid cascade, generating pro-inflammatory and vasoconstricting eicosanoids [5]. Additionally, increased $[Ca^{2+}]_i$ levels are often described in vascular smooth muscle cells following free radical injury, but the exact molecular targets remain elusive and a non-specific increase in membrane permeability to external Ca^{2+} may play a role [2].

Clinically, increased levels of lipid peroxides have been detected in human cerebrospinal fluid following SAH and levels may be higher in patients with proven vasospasm. Trials of antioxidants have exhibited angiographic improvement in animal models and clinical benefits in some cases in humans [8]. The basic mechanism(s) by which such lipid peroxides might trigger vasospasm have not been definitively established. We have demonstrated that hemoglobin promotes lipid peroxidization in a time- and dose-dependent manner, which conceptually parallels the delay in cerebral vasospasm and the correlation with degree of subarachnoid blood following SAH. We have also shown that the resulting peroxide product, PCOOH, can raise $[Ca^{2+}]_i$ levels in cultured dog basilar artery smooth muscle cells. The signal transduction pathway(s) involved and the source(s) of the elevated Ca^{2+} remain as future investigative directions.

Acknowledgments

Supported by grants from the National Institutes of Health to Dr. Macdonald (K08 NS01831) and Dr. Weir (RO1 NS25946) and from the Brain Research Foundation. An American College of Surgeons Faculty Fellowship supports Dr. Macdonald. We thank Hemosol, Inc. for supplying pure hemoglobin.

References

1. YY Guan, BK Weir, LS Marton, RL Macdonald and H Zhang (1998) Effects of erythrocyte lysate of different incubation times on intracellular free calcium in rat basilar artery smooth-muscle cells. J Neurosurg 89: 1007–1014
2. RL Macdonald and BK Weir (1994) Cerebral vasospasm and free radicals. Free Radic Biol Med 16: 633–643
3. T Miyazawa, T Suzuki, K Fujimoto and T Kaneda (1990) Phospholipid hydroperoxide accumulation in liver of rats intoxicated with carbon tetrachloride and its inhibition by dietary alpha-tocopherol. J Biochem (Tokyo) 107: 689–693
4. A Sevanian, RA Stein and JF Mead (1981) Metabolism of epoxidized phosphatidylcholine by phospholipase A2 and epoxide hydrolase. Lipids 16: 781–789
5. T Shimizu, T Watanabe, T Asano, Y Seyama and K Takakura (1988) Activation of the arachidonate 5-lipoxygenase pathway in the canine basilar artery after experimental subarachnoidal hemorrhage. J Neurochem 51: 1126–1131
6. H Suzuki, K Kanamaru, M Kuroki, H Sun, S Waga and T Miyazawa (1999) Effects of tirilazad mesylate on vasospasm and phospholipid hydroperoxides in a primate model of subarachnoid hemorrhage. Stroke 30: 450–5; discussion 455–456
7. Y Takuwa, T Matsui, Y Abe, T Nagafuji, K Yamashita and T Asano (1993) Alterations in protein kinase C activity and membrane lipid metabolism in cerebral vasospasm after subarachnoid hemorrhage. J Cereb Blood Flow Metab 13: 409–415
8. B Weir, RL Macdonald and M Stoodley (1999) Etiology of cerebral vasospasm. Acta Neurochir (Wien) [Suppl] 72: 27–46
9. H Zhang, B Weir, LS Marton, RL Macdonald, V Bindokas, RJ Miller and JR Brorson (1995) Mechanisms of hemolysate-induced $[Ca^{2+}]_i$ elevation in cerebral smooth muscle cells. Am J Physiol 269: H1874–1890

Correspondence: R. L. Macdonald, M.D., Ph.D., Section of Neurosurgery, MC3026, University of Chicago Medical Center, 5841 South Maryland Avenue, Chicago, Illinois, USA, 60637.

Acta Neurochir (2001) [Suppl] 77: 49–54

Importance of Rho-Kinase-Mediated Phosphorylation of Myosin Light Chain in Vasospasm

M. Sato[1], **E. Tani**[1], **H. Fujikawa**[1], **I. Yamaura**[1], **N. Arita**[1], and **K. Kaibuchi**[2]

[1] Hyogo College of Medicine, Hyogo, Japan
[2] Nara Institute of Science and Technology, Ikoma, Nara, Japan

Introduction

Subarachnoid hemorrhage often induces a longterm narrowing of cerebral artery called vasospasm. Rho-kinase is activated by the small GTPase Rho which phosphorylates not only MLC but also myosin phosphatase at its subunit (myosin binding subunit; MBS). The present study examined 1) an activation of Rho-A and Rho-kinase in vasospasm, 2) phosphorylation of myosin binding subunit (MBS; a subunit of myosin phosphatase) in the basilar artery involved in development of vasospasm. 3) Whether these activities and phosphorylations are inhibited by kinase inhibitors (Y-27632, wortmannin, genistein)?

Keywords: vasospasm; Rho-kinase; myosin light chain.

Materials and Methods

Vasospasm was produced in the canine basilar artery by a two-hemorrhage method, which were confirmed by angiography or by use of a surgical microscope. The animals were euthanized after a perfusion with 500 mL physiological salt solution, and the basilar artery was removed together with the brain. The blood clot around the basilar artery and its branches was carefully removed without any mechanical stimulation given to the arteries. After it was washed briefly with physiological salt solution, the basilar artery was quickly frozen in liquid nitrogen until used. Rho-A and Rho-GDI (suppressor protein of Rho-A) were examined by immunoblot analysis after separated into cytosol and membrane fraction. The activation of Rho-kinase was assessed by kinase assay which was performed by SDS-PAGE with myeline basic protein (MBP) and P^{32} after immunoprecipitation with anti-Rho-kinase antibody. The phosphorylation of myosin binding subunit (MBS) was probed separately with anti-pS854 antibody which was prepared against the synthetic phosphopeptide pS854 as an antigen and with anti-GST-MBS-COOH-terminal antibody, and calculated by dividing the densitometric values of phosphorylation levels of MBS by those of immunoreactive levels of MBS. The phosphorylation of MLC was studied by urea-glycerol PAGE. Finally, after the basilar artery in vasospasm on day 7 was exposed transclivally, it was treated by a topical 30-minute application of successively increasing concentration of Y-27632; a specific Rho-kinase inhibitor, and wortmannin; a specific inhibitor of MLC kinase, and genistein; a specific tyrosine kinase inhibitor. At the end of experiment, 10 mmol/L EGTA was added, and the reduced diameter of the spastic basilar artery was expressed as a percentage of the relaxation induced by EGTA.

Results

Caliber of the Basilar Artery

No significant angiographical narrowing of the basilar artery was shown on angiographic studies before the animals in the control group were killed. The percentage of caliber reduction seen in Fig. 1, indicates the occurrence of vasospasm.

Immunoblot Analysis of RhoA and Rho-GDI

Immunoreactive RhoA and Rho-GDI were extracted from whole lysates of the basilar artery. When the immunoreactive RhoA was examined separately in the cytosolic and the membrane fractions, it was shown to be localized mainly in the cytosolic fraction in the control group, and it was increased in the membrane fraction with the passage of time after SAH whereas it was not significantly changed in level of the cytosolic fraction after SAH, as shown in Fig. 2, suggesting that RhoA is translocated from the cytosol to the plasma membrane and concomitantly produced after SAH. In contrast, Rho-GDI, which is a suppressor protein of RhoA, was decreased in the membrane fraction.

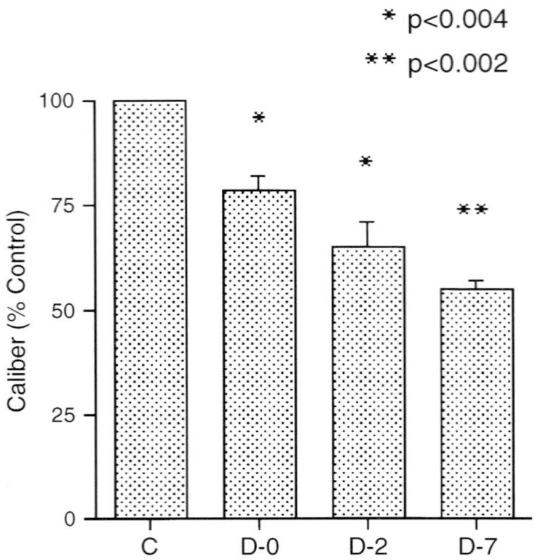

Fig. 1. Bar graph shows mean percent caliber of canine basilar artery in vasospasm on Day 0 (D-0), Day 2 (D-2), and Day 7 (D-7), as measured on angiography. Vertical lines indicate standard deviations (n = 5 per group). *C* Control

Activities of Rho-Kinase and Phosphorylations of MBS in the Spastic Basilar Artery

Rho-kinase was shown to be activated significantly with the lapse of time after SAH (Fig. 3A) whereas immunoreactive Rho-kinase, 164 kDa in size, was not changed in level after SAH (Fig. 3B), indicating that the activation of Rho-kinase was not due to an increased amount of Rho-kinase but due to the increase in activities of Rho-kinase itself. When phosphorylation of MBS of myosinphosphatase was immunologically examined using anti-pS854 antibody, phosphorylation of MBS was increased in vasospasm on day 0 and day 2, particularly on day 7 (Fig. 3C) without any changes of immunoreactive MBS levels (Fig. 3D), demonstrating significant increase in mean percent values of MBS phosphorylation and Rho-kinase activity in vasospasm, particularly on day 7 (Fig. 3E). A risen Rho-kinase activity on day 7 was decreased by topical application of the 17.2 μmol/L of genistein (tyrosine kinase inhibitor. Fig. 5).

MLC Phosphorylation in Vasospasm

We examined by urea-glycerol gel electrophoresis and subsequent immunoblot analysis whether the phosphorylation of MLC was increased or not in vasospasm. As shown in Fig. 4A and B, the monophosphorylation of MLC was increased with passage of time in vasospasm.

Dilation of Spastic Basilar Artery by Genistein, Wortmannin and Y-27632

The mean $\pm$ standard deviation diameter of the spastic basilar arteries on day 7 was reduced to $56 \pm 10\%$ of control caliber (Fig. 1). A brief washing with warm saline after a careful removal of the blood clot around the spastic basilar artery did not induce a significant change in the caliber of the spastic basilar artery. The exposed spastic basilar artery was dilated dose-dependently by a topical application of 1×10^{-6}

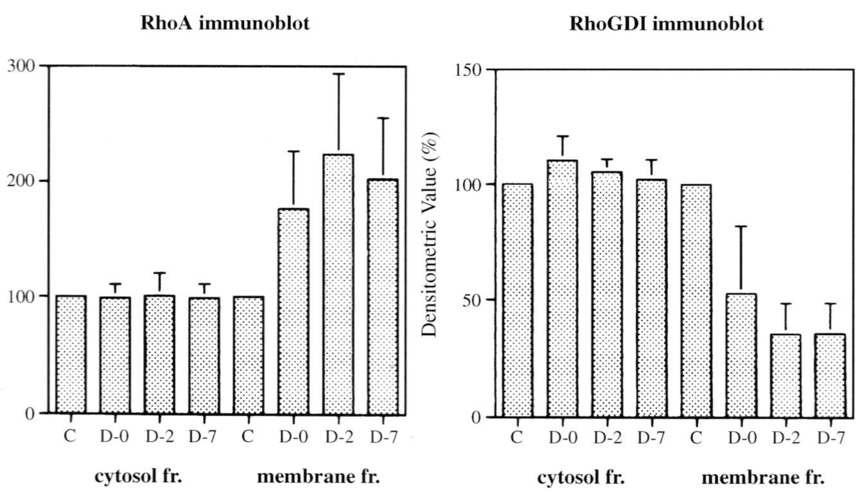

Fig. 2. Representative immunoblot analysis of Rho-A and Rho-GDI. Immunoreactive levels of Rho-A and Rho-GDI in cytosolic fraction of canine basilar artery are not so changed in vasospasm on day 0 to day 7, while those in membrane fraction of Rho-A were markedly increased with the lapse of time after SAH, but significantly decreased were Rho-GDI

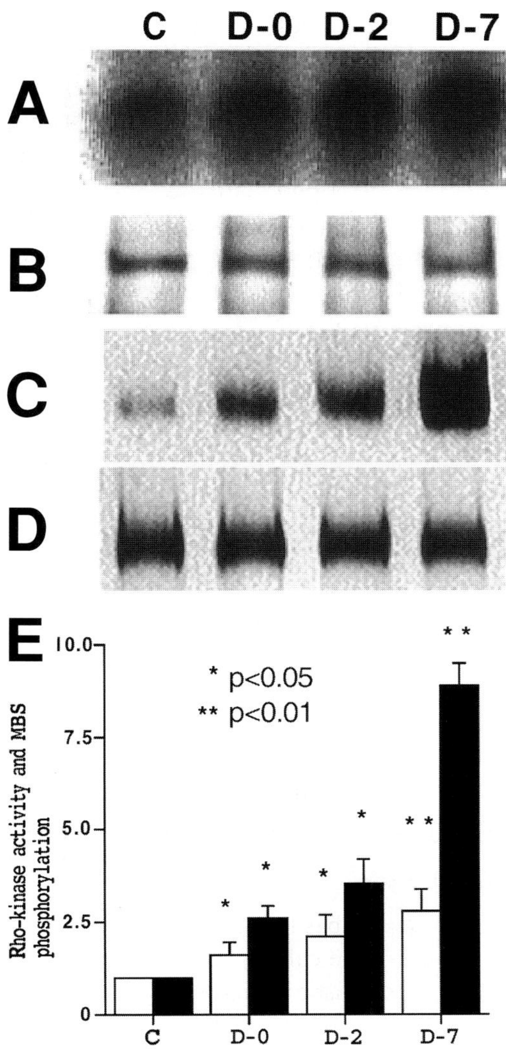

Fig. 3. A representative Rho-kinase assay (A) shows an increase in activity of Rho-kinase in canine basilar artery in vasospasm on day 0, 2, and 7 without any changes in levels of immunoreactive Rno-kinase (B), indicating an activation of Rho-kinase. Another representative immunological measurement of MBS phosphorylation (C) using anti-pS854 antibody demonstrates an enhancement of MBS phosphorylation in canine basilar artery in vasospasm on day 0, 2, and 7 without any changes in levels of immunoreactive MBS (D), indicating an increase in MBS phosphorylation. Bar graph demonstrates mean percent values of Rho-kinase activity (open bar) and MBS phosphorylation (closed bar) in vasospasm day 0, 2, and 7 (E). The mean value of Rho-kinase activity and MBS phosphorylation were calculated by dividing the densitometric values of Rho-kinase activity and MBS phosphorylation levels by those of immunoreactive Rho-kinase and MBS levels, respectively

to 3×10^{-4} mol/L genistein or wortmannin or Y-27632. Taking the relaxation induced by 10 mmol/L as 100%, the mean $\pm$ standard deviation ED_{50} value of genistein, wortmannin and Y-27632 in 5 dogs were 17.2 $\pm$ 4.5 µmol/L, 7.2 $\pm$ 0.4 µmol/L and 2.3 $\pm$ 0.3 µmol/L, respectively. The topical application of 17,2 µmol/L genistein or 10 µmol/L wortmannin or 10 µmol/L Y-27632 to the spastic basilar artery on day 7 in 5 dogs induced 50.0 $\pm$ 5.6%, 57.1 $\pm$ 5.6% and 66.2 $\pm$ 6.1% relaxation, if the relaxation induced by 10 mmol/L EGTA is taken as 100%.

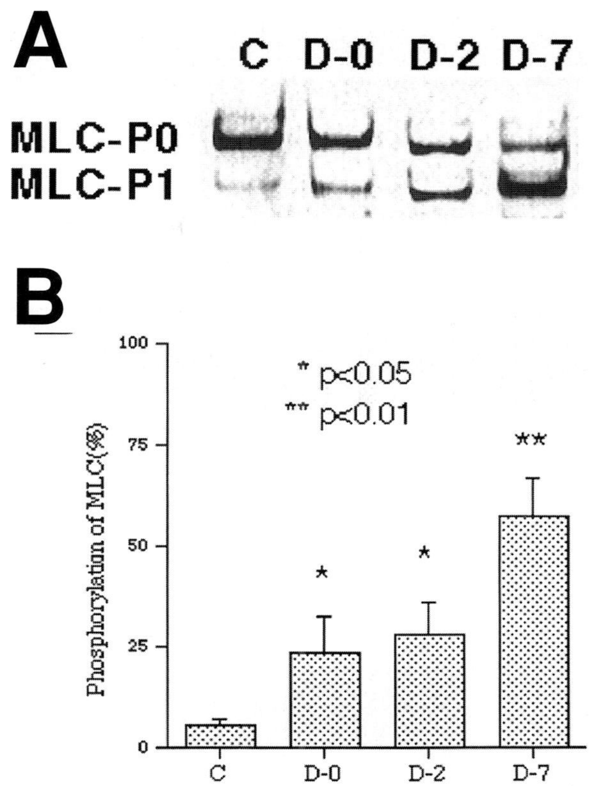

Fig. 4. Phosphorylation of MLC measured by immunoblotting following glycerol-urea polyacrylamide gel electrophoresis shows non-phosphorylated (MLC-P0) and monophosphorylated (MLC-P1) forms of 20 kDa MLC in the basilar artery, and immunoreactive MLC-P1 increases in density in vasospasm on day 0, 2, and 7 (A). (B) Densitometric quantitation of MLC phosphorylation in vasospasm was standardized as the percentage of the total ammount of immunostained MLC (MLC-P0 plus MLC-P1)

Wortmannin, Y-27632 and EGTA Produced an Affect on Rho-Kinase Activity, Phosphorylation of MBS and MLC on day 7 Spastic Basilar Artery

Rho-kinase activity and phosphorylation of MBS in vasospasm on day 7 were set as 100%, which were decreased to 34.2 $\pm$ 6.4% and 37.5 $\pm$ 7.6% by 10 µmol/L wortmannin, 13.4 $\pm$ 4.4% and 10.2 $\pm$ 4.1% by 10 µmol/L Y-27632, 90.1 $\pm$ 7.3% and 86.8 $\pm$ 9.4% by 10 mM EGTA, as shown in Fig. 6 and Fig. 7. MLC monophosphorylation in vasospasm on

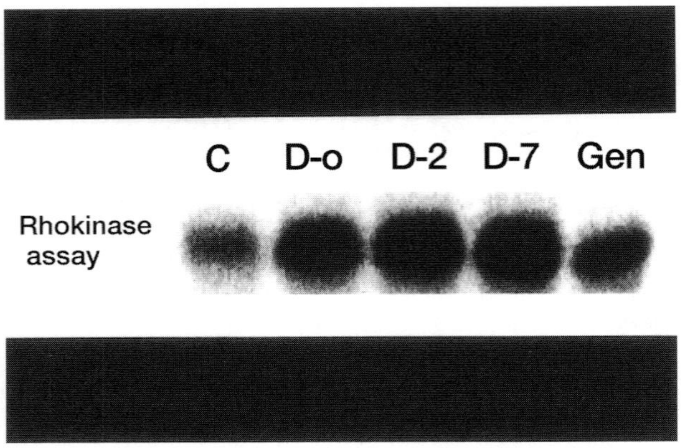

Fig. 5. Rho-kinase assay in the vasospasm group and topical application of genistein (17.2 μmol/L) on day 7 spastic basilar artery. Genistein decreased Rho-kinase activity of day 7 spastic basilar artery

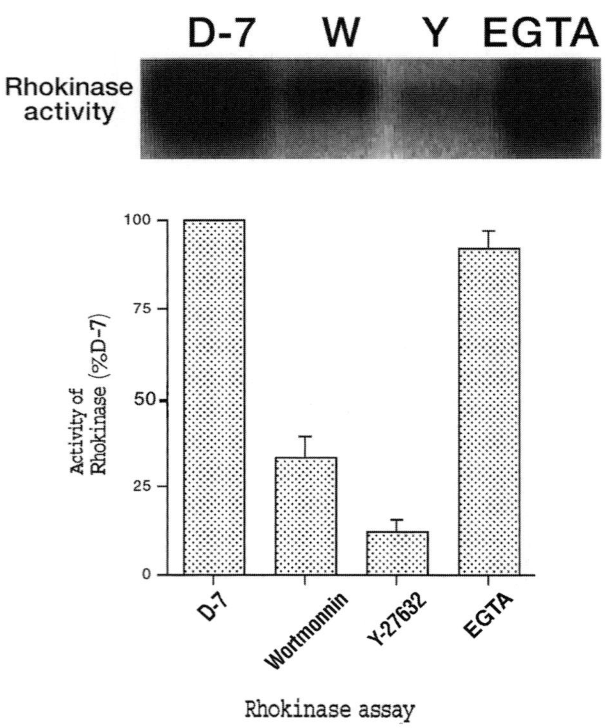

Fig. 6. Topical application of 10 μmol/L wortmannin (*WM*) and 10 μmol/L Y-27632 (*Y*) to the basilar artery in vasospasm on day 7 decrease the activity of Rho-kinase, but 10 mmol/L EGTA has little effect on the activity of Rho-kinase

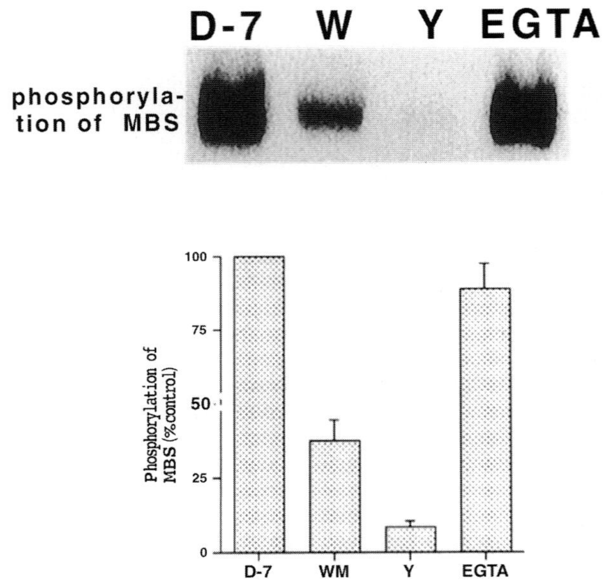

Fig. 7. Topical application of 10 μmol/L wortmannin (*WM*) and 10 μmol/L Y-27632 (*Y*) to the basilar artery in vasospasm on day 7 decrease the phosphorylation of MBS, but 10 mmol/L EGTA has little effect on phosphorylation of MBS

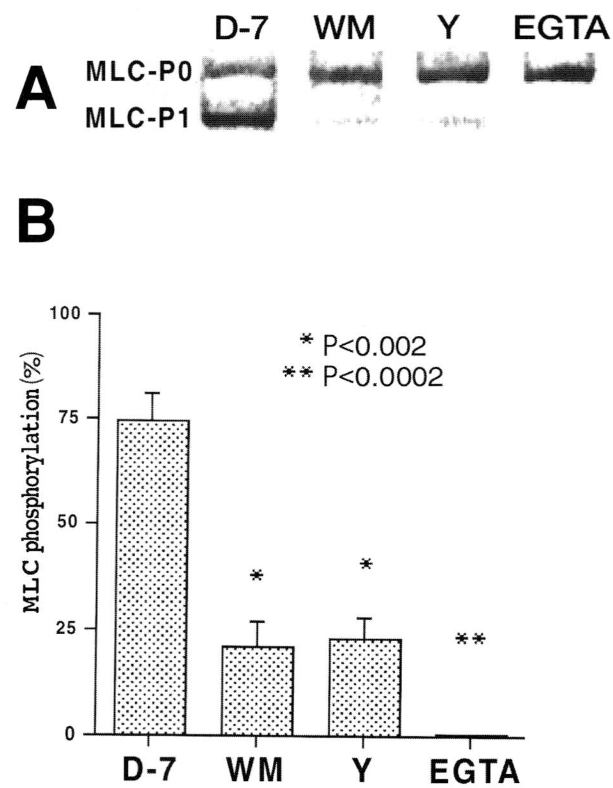

Fig. 8. Topical application of 10 μmol/L wortmannin (*WM*) and 10 μmol/L Y-27632 (*Y*) to the basilar artery in vasospasm on day 7 decrease the phosphorylation of MLC, and 10 mmol/L EGTA markedly decreases phosphorylation of MLC

day 7 was 74.4 ± 9.5% of total MLC levels, and was substantially decreased to 20.9 ± 9.2% by 10 μmol/L wortmannin, 22.8 ± 8.2% by 10 μmol/L Y-27632, and 0.5 ± 0.2% by 10 mM EGTA, as shown in Fig. 8.

Discussion

Rho family proteins act as molecular switches and are regulated by GTPase-activating proteins (GAPs), GDP-GTP exchange factors (GEFs) and GDP dissociation factor (GDI). Recently, Takahashi *et al.* have reported that Rho-GDI, complexed with inactive GDP-Rho in the cytoplasm, binds to unmasked N-terminus of ERM (Ezrin, Radixin, Moesin) for the release of inactive GDP-Rho from Rho-GDI, and the released GDP-Rho is translocated to the plasma membrane and converted to active GTP-Rho by GEFs. A serine/threonine kinase termed Rho-kinase is one of six potential targets for Rho and binds specifically to GTP-Rho in vitro. The present immunoblot analysis indicates translocation of RhoA from the cytosol to the plasma membrane after SAH, suggestive of activation of RhoA, and the Rho-kinase assay indicates activation of Rho-kinase in vasospasm which may be induced by GTP-Rho. Amano *et al.* showed the GTPγS enhanced phosphorylation of MLC in a Rho-dependent manner by inhibition of MLC phosphatase, and Matsui *et al.* demonstrated that GTPγS-RhoA stimulated the kinase activity of Rho-kinase towards the myosin-binding subunit (MBS) of myosin phosphatase about 15-fold in vitro. Using an affinity chromatography technique to isolate Rho-interacting proteins, Kimura *et al.* have shown that Rho-kinase which is activated by GTP-RhoA, phosphorylates MBS of myosin phosphatase and that the phosphorylation of MBS leads to a decrease in myosin phosphatase activity. In addition, the activated Rho-kinase stoichiometrically phosphorylates MLC at serine 19 residue, which is the site phosphorylated by MLC kinase, and results in the facilitation of the actin activation of myosin ATPase. Therefore, the activated Rho-kinase phosphorylates not only MLC, thereby activating myosin ATPase, but also myosin phosphatase, thus inactivating it in vitro. The Km value of Rho-kinase for MLC is lower than that of MLC kinase, but the molecular activity of Rho-kinase is lower than that of MLC kinase, indicating that Rho-kinase efficiently phosphorylates MLC at lower concentrations. We examined the effects of wortmannin, a potent MLC kinase inhibitor on MLC phosphorylation. Nakanishi *et al.* showed that 10 μM wortmannin used in the present study had no effect on the activities of cAMP- and cGMP-dependent protein kinase, and CaM-dependent protein kinase, little effect on PKC activity, and completely inhibited the cytosolic Ca^{2+}-provoked MLC phosphorylation of rat aorta, indicating that wortmannin demonstrates the marked selectivity of the compound for MLC kinase. In addition, wortmannin does not affect the activity of the catalytic subunit of recombinant Rho-kinase up to 100 μM in vitro. Therefore, wortmannin-sensitive MLC phosphorylation in vasospasm may be induced by activation of MLC kinase. The recombinant Rho-kinase catalytic subunit-induced smooth muscle contraction and MLC phosphorylation are insensitive to 10 μmol/L wortmannin at cytosolic Ca^{2+} at pCa 6.5, suggesting that sensitivity of Rho-kinase-induced smooth muscle contraction and MLC phosphorylation to wortmannin is dependent upon the intracellular Ca^{2+} concentrations. Contractions of the permeabilized smooth muscle induced by phosphatase inhibitor microcystin-LR at cytosolic 0 Ca^{2+} or by phosphatase inhibitor calyculin A was reduced by MLC kinase inhibitors. In contrast, Y-27632 is a specific inhibitor of Rho-kinase and selectively inhibits agonist-induced smooth muscle contraction by inhibiting Ca^{2+} sensitization (Ki: 0.14 for Rho-kinase; 26 for PKC; and >250 for MLCkinase). 10 μmol/L Y-27632 inhibits GTPγS-induced contraction of permeabilized strips of rabbit mesentery artery about 80% and phenylephrine-induced contraction of rabbit aortic strips about 90%, but it had little effect on Ca^{2+}- and calyculin A-induced contraction of permeabilized strips of rabbit mesentery artery. Therefore, Y-27632-sensitive MLC phosphorylation in vasospasm may be mediated directly by Rho-kinase and indirectly through inhibition of myosin phosphatase by Rho-kinase. The present topical application study using the spastic basilar artery on day 7 demonstrates that wortmannin and Y-27632 induce similar degree of decrease in MLC phosphorylation levels. MBS phosphorylation in the spastic basilar artery on day 7 is markedly increased, suggesting that Y-27632-sensitive MLC phosphorylation in vasospasm on day 7 is mediated largely through inhibition of myosin phosphatase. Thus, the evidence of the activation of Rho-kinase, the marked MBS phosphorylation, and the Y-27632-sensitive MLC phosphorylation in vasospasm suggests strongly the involvement of Rho-kinase, namely Ca^{2+} sensitization mechanism. The monophosphorylation of MLC in the spastic basilar artery on day 7 was more markedly reduced by 10 mmol/L EGTA than by 10 μmol/L wortmannin or 10 μmol/L Y-27632. The EGTA-sensitive component of MLC phosphorylation in vasospasm seemed to be mediated mainly by Ca^{2+}-CaM-dependent MLC kinase activity and partly by arachidonic acid-mediated inhibition of myosin phosphatase but not by Rho-kinase, because 10 mmol/L EGTA-induced nominally zero cytosolic Ca^2 inhibits not only MLC kinase but also cytosolic phospholipaseA_2 which is responsible for production of arachidonic acid in the spastic basilar artery. Rho-kinase-mediated phosphorylation of MLC, whether directly or indirectly through inhibition of myosin phosphatase, is theoretically insensitive to 10 mmol/L EGTA, but appears to be abolished by treatment with 10 mmol/L EGTA in vasospasm, suggesting that the primary effect of Rho-kinase is the inhibition of myosin phosphatase and that the direct phosphorylation of MLC by Rho-kinase play a second role, because Rho-kinase-mediated minor direct phosphorylation of MLC may be dephosphorylation by myosin phosphatase left unhibited by Rho-kinase.

References

1. Amano M, Ito M, Kimura K, Fukata Y, Chihara K, Nakano T, Matsuura Y, Kaibuchi K (1996) Phosphorylation and activation of myosin by Rho-associated kinase (Rho-kinase). J Biol Chem 271: 20246–20249
2. Kimura K, Ito M, Amano M, Chihara K, Fukata Y, Nakafune M, Yamamori B, Feng JH, Nakano T, Okawa K, Iwamatsu A, Kaibuchi K (1996) Regulation of myosin phosphatase by Rho and Rho-associated kinase (Rho-kinase). Science 273: 245–248
3. Kitazawa T, Kobayashi S, Horiuchi K, Somlyo AV, Somlyo AP (1989) Receptor-coupled, permeabilized smooth muscle: role of the phosphatidylinositol cascade, G-proteins, and modulation of the contractile response to Ca^{2+}. J Biol Chem 264: 5339–5342
4. Kureishi Y, Kobayashi S, Amano M, Kimura K, Kanaide H, Nakano T, Kaibuchi K, Ito M (1997) Rho-associated kinase directly induces smooth muscle contraction through myosin light chain phosphorylation. J Biol Chem 272: 12257–12260
5. Marchesky LM, Hall A (1996) Rho: a connection between membrane receptor signaling and cytoskelton. Trends Cell Biol 6: 304–310
6. Matsui T, Amano M, Yamamoto T, Chihara K, Nakafune M, Ito M, Nakano T, Okawa K, Iwamatsu A, Kaibuchi K (1996) Rho-associated kinase, a novel serine/threonine kinase, as a putative target for the small GTP binding protein Rho. EMBO J 15: 2208–2216
7. Nakanishi S, Kakita S, Takahashi I, Kawahara K, tsukuda E, Sano T, Yamada K, Yoshida M, Kase H, Matsuda Y, Hashimoto Y, Nonomura Y (1992) Wortmannin, a microbial product inhibitor of myosin light chain kinase. J Biol Chem 267: 2157–2163
8. Noda M, Yasuda-Fukuzawa C, Moriishi K, Kato T, Okuda T, Kurokawa K, Takuwa Y (1995) Involvement of rho in GTPγS-induced enhancement of phosphorylation of 20 kDa myosin light chain in vascular smooth muscle cells: inhibition of phosphatase activity. FEBS Lett 367: 246–250

Correspondence: Dr. M. Sato, Hyogo College of Medicine, Hyogo, Japan.

Acta Neurochir (2001) [Suppl] 77: 55–57

Role of MAPK in Chronic Cerebral Vasospasm

K. Aoki, A. Y. Zubkov, R. E. Tibbs, T. Meguro, and **J. H. Zhang**

Department of Neurosurgery, University of Mississippi Medical Center, MS, USA

Introduction

Many extracellular stimuli (including growth factors, hormones, stress, elevated temperature and G-protein coupled receptor agonists) initialize the phosphorylation cascades leading to the activation of mitogen-activated protein kinase (p44/42 MAPK) [2]. p44/42 MAPK activation may lead to an expression of the early genes, such as *c-jun* or *c-fos*, thus leading to the cellular proliferation [3]. p44/42 MAPK can cause the phosphorylation of caldesmon, thus promoting prolonged contraction [1]. It has been reported in several in vitro studies that p44/42 MAPK is involved in the prolonged contraction of the cerebral arteries, caused by hemolysate [8] and endothelin-1 [9], the most important causative agents for vasospasm. The levels of *c-fos*, and *c-jun* were increased in the presence of hemolysate, reaching maximum expression between 30 and 60 minutes in rat aorta smooth muscle cells [7].

In this study, we used an established canine double hemorrhage model of SAH to evaluate the role of p44/42 MAPK in the pathogenesis of vasospasm.

Keywords: Mitogen-activated protein kinase; cerebral vasospasm.

Materials and Methods

Subarachnoid Hemorrhage Model

Fourteen adult mongrel dogs of either sex, weighing 18–24 kg, were used in this canine double-hemorrhage model. The dogs were anesthetized with thiopental (10 mg/kg) and mechanically ventilated during the procedures. Experimental SAH was induced according to the method described by Varsos *et al.* [6]. Cerebral angiography was performed on the Exposcop 7000 (Ziehm International Medical Systems, Riverside, CA). The cisterna magna was punctured transcutaneously, and 0.4 ml/kg of CSF was withdrawn. The equivalent amount of arterial blood was withdrawn from the femoral artery and immediately injected into the cisterna magna. This first injection was considered to be the Day 0 SAH. On Day 2, this blood injection procedure was repeated without angiography.

Dogs were sacrificed on Day 3 (n = 4), Day 5 (n = 3), and Day 7 (n = 4) after blood injection (for the investigation of the time course of vasospasm and p44/42 MAPK immunoprecipitation). A control group of dogs (n = 3) was sacrificed without blood injection. The brains were removed within 10 minutes after euthanasia. The basilar arteries were carefully removed from the brain stem and were cleansed of branches, the excess tissue and blood, and then immediately frozen in the liquid nitrogen. The samples were kept in −80 °C until Western blot analysis was conducted.

Western Blot Analysis

The frozen arteries were homogenized with ultrasonic waves (10 seconds, 3 times) in an extraction buffer containing (in mmol/L) 50 Tris-HCl (pH 7.5); 100 NaCl; 5 ethylenediamine tetraacetic acid; 1 phenylmethylsulfonyl fluoride; and 100 ml of IGEPAL CA-630 for 20 minutes at 4 °C. The insoluble material was removed by centrifugation at 4 °C and 13,000 G for 10 minutes. The samples (30 µg protein) were separated by sodium dodecyl sulfate-polyacrylanide gel electrophoresis (SDS-PAGE) using 12.5% poliacrylamide gel. Detailed method was described previously [8].

Data Analysis

Data are expressed as the mean ± standard error of the mean. Statistical differences between the control and other groups were compared using the one-way analysis of variance (ANOVA) and then the Tukey-Kramer multiple comparison procedure (95% lower and upper confidence interval) if significant variance was found. A probability value (P) of less than 0.05 was considered statistically significant.

Results

Time Course of Cerebral Vasospasm

The caliber of the basilar artery was calculated as the ratio of the mean basilar artery diameter on day 3–7, as a percentage of that on day 0. Figure 1 shows the time course of the development of vasospasm. The residual diameter of the basilar arteries was 80.8 ± 13.4% ($P > 0.05$), 67.3 ± 6.4% ($P < 0.05$,

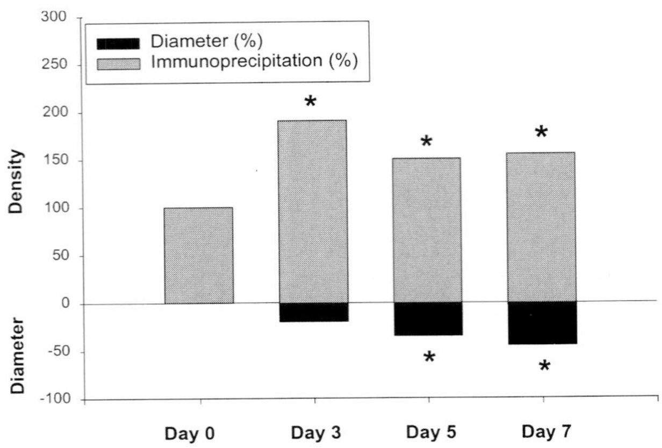

Fig. 1. The time course of cerebral vasospasm and MAPK immunoprecipitation. The onset of cerebral vasospasm was on day 3 with subsequent progression to significant narrowing of the basilar arteries on days 5 ($P < 0.05$, ANOVA) and 7 ($P < 0.005$, ANOVA). The graphical representation of the Western blot analysis, demonstrating the significant SAH-induced enhancement of p44/42 MAPK peaking on day 3 ($P < 0.001$, ANOVA). The SAH-induced enhancement of p44/42 MAPK lasted up to day 7 ($P < 0.05$, ANOVA). *** – $P < 0.001$, * – $P < 0.05$

ANOVA) and 53.4 ± 5.5% ($P < 0.005$, ANOVA) on day 3, 5, and 7, respectively.

p44/42 MAPK Immunoprecipitation

The time course of the p44/42 MAPK immunoprecipitation was calculated as the ratio of the MAPK immunoprecipitation from normal dogs. p44/42 MAPK immunoprecipitation was enhanced in the basilar arteries of the SAH dogs, peaking on day 3 ($P < 0.001$ vs. control, ANOVA) and remaining enhanced on days 5 and 7 ($P < 0.05$, ANOVA). There was no statistical difference between day 5 and day 7 ($P > 0.5$, ANOVA).

Discussion

MAPK (p44/42) is a proline-directed serine/threonine kinase, which is activated by a dual phosphorylation of threonine and tyrosine residues in response to a variety of extracellular stimuli. The MAPK (p44/42) pathway is one of the MAPK groups (the others are P56 and P38), and it is phosphorylated by mitogen-activated protein kinase kinase. It is well documented that the p44/42 MAPK pathway plays an important role in cell proliferation, differentiation, and smooth muscle contraction [2, 3]. Several studies have demonstrated the significant role of p44/42 MAPK in the contraction of peripheral smooth muscle cells, as well as cerebral arteries [4, 8, 9]. Activation of the G-protein-coupled receptors or receptor tyrosine kinases will activate the intracellular signaling cascade resulting in activation of $p21^{ras}$ protein. The phosphorylation of $p21^{ras}$ will lead to activation of Raf-1 with subsequent activation of p44/42 MAPK kinase. p44/42 MAPK phosphorylates the actin-binding protein caldesmon which was suggested to play an important role in the prolonged smooth-muscle contraction [1].

Macdonald *et al.* [5] believe that multiple factors cause cerebral vasospasm. OxyHb (hemolysate) released from blood clot and endothelin-1 (ET-1) released from the vessel wall are among the main spasmogens for vasospasm. In a previous study, we demonstrated that hemolysate enhanced MAPK immunoprecipitation in rabbit basilar arteries [8]. Another proposed spasmogen for cerebral vasospasm (endothelin-1) was tested and found to enhance MAPK immunoprecipitation and produce contraction of rabbit basilar artery [9]. In this study, p44/42 MAPK immunoprecipitation was significantly enhanced in the spastic arteries. The peak immunoprecipitation occurred on day 3, and the enhanced p44/42 MAPK immunoprecipitation sustained for up to 7 days after the SAH. Fujikawa *et al.* [4] demonstrated in a similar dog model that p44/42 MAPK immunoprecipitation peaked on day 2 (before the second injection), and this enhancement of p44/42 MAPK immunoprecipitation sustained above the baseline up to day 7. These two studies indicate that the activation of p44/42 MAPK appears to peak early in the course of vasospasm and remain elevated up to day 7 after SAH.

In conclusion, p44/42 MAPK immunoprecipitation enhanced during experimental SAH, and the peak immunoprecipitation occurred at an early stage of vasospasm. MAPK kinase inhibitor PD98059, but not U0126, attenuated the p44/42 MAPK immunoprecipitation and vasoconstriction. Signal transduction mechanism via the p44/42 MAPK pathway probably not only regulates the onset but also the prolonged phase of vasospasm. PD98059 might be useful in the management of cerebral vasospasm.

Acknowledgment

This work was partially supported by a grant-in-aid to J.H.Z. from the American Heart Association, and a grant from American Heart Association Bugher Foundation for Stroke Award.

References

1. Adam LP, Hathaway DR (1993) Identification of mitogen-activated protein kinase phosphorylation sequences in mammalian h-Caldesmon. FEBS Lett 322: 56–60
2. Di Salvo J, Kaplan N, Semenchuk LA (1996) Protein tyrosine phosphorylation and regulation of intracellular calcium in smooth muscle cells. In: Barany M (ed) Biochemistry of smooth muscle contraction. Academic Press, San Diego, pp 283–293
3. Force T, Bonventre JV (1998) Growth factors and mitogen-activated protein kinases. Hypertension 31: 152–161
4. Fujikawa H, Tani E, Yamaura I, Ozaki I, Miyaji K, Sato M, Takahashi K, Imajoh-Ohmi S (1999) Activation of protein kinases in canine basilar artery in vasospasm. J Cereb Blood Flow Metab 19: 44–52
5. Macdonald RL, Weir BK, Runzer TD, Grace MG, Findlay JM, Saito K, Cook DA, Mielke BW, Kanamaru K (1991) Etiology of cerebral vasospasm in primates. J Neurosurg 75: 415–424
6. Varsos VG, Liszczak TM, Han DH, Kistler JP, Vielma J, Black PM, Heros RC, Zervas NT (1983) Delayed cerebral vasospasm is not reversible by aminophylline, nifedipine, or papaverine in a "two-hemorrhage" canine model. J Neurosurg 58: 11–17
7. Wang X, Marton LS, Weir BK, Macdonald RL (1999) Immediate early gene expression in vascular smooth-muscle cells synergistically induced by hemolysate components. J Neurosurg 90: 1083–1090
8. Zubkov AY, Ogihara K, Tumu P, Patllola A, Lewis AI, Parent AD, Zhang J (1999) Mitogen-activated protein kinase mediates hemolysate-induced contraction in rabbit basilar artery. J Neurosurg 90: 1091–1097
9. Zubkov A, Rollins K, Parent A, Zhang J (2000) Mechanism of endothelin-1-induced contraction in rabbit basilar artery. Stroke 31: 526–533

Correspondence: John H. Zhang, M.D., Ph.D., Department of Neurosurgery, University Mississippi Medical Center, 2500 North State Street, Jackson, MS, 39216-4505, USA.

Endothelin and Nitric Oxide

Acta Neurochir (2001) [Suppl] 77: 61–65

Endothelin: The "Prime Suspect" in Cerebral Vasospasm

M. Zuccarello

Department of Neurosurgery, The Neuroscience Institute, Mayfield Clinic and Spine Institute, University of Cincinnati College of Medicine, Cincinnati, OH

Introduction

Endothelin (ET)-1 has demonstrated a wide variety of effects throughout the body. Studies have shown effects on bronchial constriction, on the kidneys, even as a potential neurotransmitter [20, 27, 40, 44]. Its effects on the vasculature have been widely studied [8, 32, 45]. Specifically, ET-1 has been studied with respect to its role in the development of subarachnoid hemorrhage (SAH)-induced vasospasm. Following is a summary of ET-1 and its role in SAH-induced vasospasm.

Keywords: Subarachnoid hemorrhage; endothelin-1; vasospasm.

Materials and Methods

We used the following procedures in our laboratory to test the role of ET-1 in the development of SAH-induced cerebral vasospasm.

General

Procedures are approved by the Institutional Animal Care and Use Committee. Conditioned New Zealand white male rabbits (3 to 4 kg) are anesthetized with ketamine HCl (30 mg/kg IM) and xylazine (6 mg/kg IM) and is maintained with sodium pentobarbital (25 mg/kg) through a catheter inserted into the ear vein (*in vivo* studies) and femoral vein (*in situ* studies).

Angiography

Vertebrobasilar angiograms are obtained on day 0 (pre-SAH) and on day 6 as follows. The left or right subclavian artery is catheterized, and the tip of a 5F catheter is directed toward the ipsilateral vertebral artery to obtain a selected injection of the vertebrobasilar system. Basilar artery diameter is measured by placing angiograms on a light box, above which is fixed a video camera connected to an image analysis computer. The angiographic image is captured by the camera, digitized, and reproduced on the video monitor. Three observers blind to the experiment measure basilar artery diameter just below the basilar-posterior cerebral artery junction, just above the basilar-vertebral artery junction, and the midpoint between these two locations. Three measurements are obtained at each position, and the mean of all nine measurements is used as the diameter of the basilar artery.

Mini-Osmotic Pump

Immediately after the day 0 angiogram, a mini-osmotic pump (10 μL/h), containing either the compound to be tested or the vehicle, is implanted in the neck, with the catheter placed in the cisterna magna.

Subarachnoid Hemorrhage

On days 1 and 3 after angiography, arterial blood is withdrawn from the central ear artery and injected (0.75 mL/kg) into the cisterna magna over 3 minutes through an additional catheter. For the *in situ* studies (no angiography or mini-osmotic pump implantation), on days 0 and 2, blood is injected through a 21-gauge butterfly needle into the cisterna magna. Similar magnitudes of spasm are induced by blood injected through a catheter or needle inserted into the cisterna magna.

In Situ Studies

Rabbits are anesthetized and mechanically ventilated with room air supplemented by O_2. The respiratory rate and volume are adjusted to maintain expiratory pCO_2 between 35 and 37 mm Hg. Heart rate and systemic pressure are measured with the use of a femoral artery catheter. Arterial pO_2 and pCO_2 are monitored and maintained within normal levels by adjusting the respiratory rate and/or tidal volume. Core body temperature is monitored rectally and maintained at 37 °C with a heating pad.

Basilar Artery Cranial Window

Rabbits are placed in a headholder in the supine position, the clivus is exposed by blunt dissection between the carotid sheath and the trachea, and the trachea and esophagus are retracted laterally. Compression of the carotid arteries and the descending vagus nerves is avoided. The muscle covering the basioccipital bone is removed by electrocautery. A rectangular osteotomy is then made at the base of the skull between the tympanic bullae with the use of a microdrill and microrongeur under an operating microscope. A perfect hemostasis is achieved, the dura is opened and excised with microscissors, and the basilar artery is exposed. The blood clot is gently removed with microforceps.

Contractility Studies

The surgical field is illuminated with a 100-W halogen lamp, which is fitted with a heat filter to avoid warming the cranial window, and is visualized through a trinocular microscope (Zeiss OPMI-1). Basilar artery diameter is measured with a personal computer image analysis system (ImagePro).

The cranial window is suffused (1 mL/min) with artificial spinal fluid (mM: NaCl 121.8, KCl 3.2, $CaCl_2$ 2.5, $MgCl_2$ 1.26, $NaHCO_3$ 25.0, D-glucose 3.7, urea 6.0), maintained at 37 °C, and gassed with 7% O_2/6% CO_2/87% N_2. Vessel diameter, blood pressure, heart rate, and arterial pO_2 and pCO_2 stabilized within 45 minutes after CSF suffusion, and agents are then suffused over the craniotomy. Vessel diameter is recorded at the time of the plateau response of each agent. Each value of vessel diameter is the mean of 13 consecutive measurements taken approximately at 10-second intervals.

Discussion

Endothelin

ET-1 is a 21 amino acid peptide [47]. It is synthesized from mRNA, which produces a precursor called prepro-ET-1, which is cleaved into a molecule called big ET-1 by a specific endopeptidase. Big ET-1 is further cleaved into ET-1 by an endopeptidase called ET-converting enzyme [24, 26, 39]. ET-1 is expressed in a variety of tissues in the brain, including the endothelium, neurons, glial cells, choroid plexus, and hypothalamic cells [9, 10, 14, 21, 22, 48]. ET-1, when injected systemically in rats, causes an initial decrease in blood pressure, which is believed to be mediated via stimulation of prostacyclin and release of endothelium-derived relaxing factor. This decrease in blood pressure is quickly followed by a prolonged increase in the blood pressure [8]. This constrictive effect was also demonstrated in the cerebral vasculature [2, 19].

Role of ET-1 in SAH-Induced Vasospasm: Review of the Literature

Clinical Studies. The presence of ET-1 in the plasma and CSF of healthy subjects and patients with SAH both with and without vasospasm has been studied. Masaoka *et al.* found the plasma concentration of ET-1 in patients with SAH was significantly higher than that in healthy subjects [25]. In addition, in patients with SAH-induced vasospasm, the plasma concentrations of ET-1 were higher than in patients with SAH but without vasospasm [25]. Fujimori *et al.* also discovered that in all patients with SAH, those with vasospasm had significantly higher concentrations of ET-1 in the plasma 8–14 days after SAH compared with patients without vasospasm. Fujimori *et al.*, however, failed to find a significant difference in the CSF concentrations of ET-1 [12].

Ehrenreich *et al.* demonstrated a peak in the CSF concentrations of ET-1 in patients with SAH-induced vasospasm, and that this peak coincided with the onset of vasospasm. This peak was absent in those patients with SAH who did not develop vasospasm [11]. Suzuki *et al.* had similar findings of ET-1 concentrations in CSF of patients with SAH [37, 38]. Seifert *et al.* reported that the postoperative relative concentration of CSF ET-1 and big ET-1 were correlated to post-SAH vasospasm [34]. Finally, Juvela *et al.* studied ET-1 immunoreactivity in plasma of 70 patients with aneurysmal SAH and 25 healthy volunteers. They found that ET concentrations correlate with delayed cerebral ischemia and vasospasm after SAH [16]. These clinical findings support the theory that ET-1 plays a role in SAH-induced vasospasm.

Mechanisms of ET-1 Stimulation. The stimulus for production of ET-1 in SAH was investigated in experimental models. Oxyhemoglobin and methemoglobin were both found to be associated with the production of ET-1 [7, 17, 30]. Studies reveal a possible protein kinase C and a cyclic adenosine monophosphate-dependent pathway for oxyhemoglobin's effect of increased ET-1 production. This pathway most likely leads to an increase in ET-1 mRNA production and, hence, ET-1 production [17]. After SAH, ET-1 release from endothelial cells can be stimulated by thrombin, epinephrine, TGF_β, angiotensin II, vasopressin, cytokines, and platelets [3, 23, 43, 47, 49].

Animal Studies. ET-1 intracisternal infusion leads to a significant vasoconstriction in experimental animals [2], contrasting with studies revealing that intravertebral artery injection of ET-1 fails to induce vasoconstriction [28]. Elevated CSF ET-1 concentrations could also be reproduced via SAH models, as could vasospasm [46]. In SAH models, a hyperreactivity to ET-1 was also noted [1]. Calcium-free mediums and calcium entry blockers significantly reduced the amount of vasoconstriction induced by ET-1, indicating the importance of the role of calcium in ET-1 induced constriction [1]. Extracellular calcium is essential for ET activity, which cannot be inhibited by the dihydropyridine class of calcium channel antagonists [52]. ET-1 binds to specific membrane receptors (ET_A and ET_{B2} in smooth muscle cells and ET_{B1} in endothelial cells), leading to intracellular biochemical signals that release calcium from intracellular calcium stores [52]. ET vasoconstriction has also been shown to be mediated through a calcium sensitization process [15].

A variety of compounds have been developed elucidating the role of ET-1 in the SAH-induced vasospasm. These compounds have been administered topically, intracisternally, intravenously, and orally.

A) Inhibitors of ET-1 production: Phosphoramidon and CGS 26303, compounds that inhibit the ET-converting enzyme [4, 36].
B) ET-1 receptor antagonists: a) ET_A receptor antagonists such as BQ123, BQ610, PD155080, SB209670, TA-0201, TBC 11251, and S-0139; b) $ET_{A/B}$ receptor antagonist, Bosentan (RO 47-0203); c) ET_{B1} and ET_{B2} receptor antagonists such as BQ788, an ET_B receptor antagonist, and RES-701-1, an ET_{B1} receptor antagonist [5, 6, 18, 33, 42, 53–57].
C) Inhibitor of mRNA synthesis: actinomycin D [35].
D) Antisense preproendothelin-oligoDNA therapy [29, 31].

Most experimental studies have shown that vasospasm was prevented and/or reduced.

Role of ET-1 in SAH-Induced Vasospasm: Our Laboratory Work

In the past 7 years, our laboratory has investigated the role of ET-1 in SAH-induced cerebral vasospasm using a two-hemorrhage rabbit model.

First, we suggested that the ET-1-dependent vasospasm was mediated by ET_A receptor activation as well as ET_B receptor activation [50]. This suggestion was supported by the *in situ* demonstration that vasospasm of the rabbit basilar artery was only partially reversed by a selective ET_A receptor antagonist, BQ123, and subsequent addition of an $ET_{A/B}$ receptor antagonist, PD 145065, was required to induce complete relaxation [50]. Similar findings were also found in an *in vivo* rabbit model of SAH in which the use of Bosentan, an $ET_{A/B}$ receptor antagonist, effectively prevented the onset of vasospasm [53]. Although evidence supports the involvement of smooth muscle ET_{B2} receptors in the mechanism of ET-induced constriction and in the development of vasospasm [54], the role of endothelial ET_{B1} receptor is still unclear.

Using our rabbit basilar artery *in situ* model, we recently demonstrated the presence of endothelin ET_{B1} receptors [55]. We also recently suggested that endothelial ET_B receptor activation maintains the spasm by the further release of ET-1 [51]. This important finding was based on the demonstration that intracisternal infusion of ET-1, as well as the cessation of the infusion, still induced ET-1-dependent spasm of the rabbit basilar artery. Lending support to the possibility that endothelial ET_B receptor activation causes further ET-1 release of newly synthesized ET-1 is our recent demonstration that ET_B receptor antagonists (BQ788 and RES-701-1) prevent and reverse SAH-induced cerebral vasospasm in rabbits [57]. The role of ET_B receptors in the development and maintenance of post-SAH vasospasm has also been confirmed by using an ET_B receptor-deficient rat strain [13].

Animals with naturally occurring or targeted mutation of ET_B exhibit coat color spotting and distal intestinal aganglionosis. Spotting lethal (sl) rats carry a 301-bp deletion in ET_B that leads to death shortly after birth. To investigate the role of ET_B receptors in adult physiology, a transgenic "rescue" of the intestinal phenotype in the (sl) rat was undertaken. The resulting rats have a normal enteric development, but they lack expression of ET_B elsewhere. Using an *in vivo* rat model of SAH, we found no vasospasm in sl/sl and sl/+ rats compared with $14.2\% \pm 2\%$ reduction in basilar artery diameter in Wistar rats [Unpublished data].

Conclusions

Our proposed working model of the role of ET-1 in SAH-induced cerebral vasospasm follows: In response to SAH, numerous factors (e.g., serotonin, hemoglobin, ATP, hypoxia) act on the endothelium to cause the initial release of ET. ET-1 then induces (1) spasm through the activation of smooth muscle ET_A and ET_{B2} receptors; (2) further ET-1 release through the activation of endothelial ET_{B1} receptors; and (3) nitric oxide release through activation of endothelial ET_{B1} receptors. Under normal physiological conditions, nitric oxide release inhibits both the magnitude of ET-1 constriction and ET-1-induced ET-1 release; however, after SAH these negative modulator effects are inhibited by the presence of hemoglobin. Desensitization of endothelial ET_{B1} receptors following continual exposure of ET after SAH has been also reported [41]. Thus, once ET-1-induced ET-1 release is established, the spasm no longer depends on the presence of hemoglobin and is not inhibited by nitric oxide with consequent chronic ET-1-dependent vasospasm.

References

1. Alabadi JA, Salom JB, Torregrosa G, Miranda FJ, Jover T, Alborch E (1993) Changes in the cerebrovascular effects of endothelin-1 and nicardipine after experimental subarachnoid hemorrhage. Neurosurgery 33: 707–715
2. Asano T, Ikegaki I, Susuki Y, Satoh S, Shibuya M (1989) Endothelin and the production of vasospasm in dogs. Biochem Biophys Res Commun 159: 1345–1351
3. Battistini B, D'Orleans-Juste P, Siriois P (1993) Endothelins: Circulating plasma levels and presence in other biologic fluids. Lab Invest 68: 600–628
4. Caner HH, Kwan AL, Arthur A, Jeng AY, Lappe RW, Kassell NF, Lee KS (1996) Systemic administration of an inhibitor of endothelin-converting enzyme for attenuation of cerebral vasospasm following experimental subarachnoid hemorrhage. J Neurosurg 85: 917–922
5. Clozel M, Watanabe H (1993) BQ-123, a peptidic endothelin receptor antagonist, prevents the early cerebral vasospasm following subarachnoid hemorrhage after intracisternal but not intravenous injection. Life Sci 52: 825–834
6. Clozel M, Breu V, Gray GA, Kalina B, Loffler BM, Burri K, Cassal JM, Hirth G, Muller M, Neidhart W, Ramuz H (1994) Pharmacological characterization of bosetan, a new potent orally active nonpeptidic endothelin receptor antagonist. J Pharmacol Exp Ther 270: 228–235
7. Cocks T, Malta E, King S, Woods R, Angus J (1991) Oxyhemoglobin increases the production of endothelin-1 by endothelial cells in culture. Eur J Pharmacol 196: 177–182
8. De Nucci G, Thomas R, D'Orleans-Juste P, Antunes E, Walder C, Warner TD, Vane JR (1988) Pressor effects of circulating endothelin are limited by its removal in the pulmonary circulation and by the release of prostacyclin and endothelium-derived relaxing factor. Proc Natl Acad Sci USA 85: 9797–9800
9. Ehrenreich H, Anderson RW, Fox CH, Rieckmann P, Hoffman GS, Travis WD, Coligan JE, Kehrl JH, Fauci AS (1990) Endothelins, peptides with potent vasoactive properties, are produced by human macrophages. J Exp Med 172: 1741–1748
10. Ehrenreich H, Kehrl JH, Anderson W, Rieckmann P, Vitkovic L, Colian JE, Fauci AS (1991) A vasoactive peptide, endothelin-3, is produced by and specifically binds to primary astrocytes. Brain Res 538: 54–58
11. Ehrenreich H, Lange M, Near KA, Anneser F, Schoeller LAC, Schmid R, Winkler PA, Kehrl JH, Schmiedek P, Goebel FD (1992) Long-term monitoring of immunoreactive endothelin-1 and endothelin-3 in ventricular cerebrospinal fluid, plasma and 24-h urine of patients with subarachnoid hemorrhage. Res Exp Med (Berl) 192: 257–268
12. Fujimori A, Yanagisawa M, Saito A, Goto K, Masaki T, Mima T, Takakura K, Shigeno T (1989) Endothelin in plasma and cerebrospinal fluid of patients with subarachnoid hemorrhage. Lancet 336: 633 (letter)
13. Gariepy CE, Cass DT, Yanagisawa M (1996) Null mutation of endothelin receptor type B gene in spotting lethal rats causes aganglionic megacolon and white coat color. Proc Natl Acad Sci USA 93: 867–872
14. Giaid A, Gibson SJ, Ibrahim NBN, Legon S, Bloom SR, Yanagisawa M, Masaki T, Varndell IM, Polak JM (1989) Endothelin-1, an endothelium-derived peptide, is expressed in neurons of the human spinal cord and the dorsal root ganglia. Proc Natl Acad Sci USA 86: 7634–7638
15. Hori M, Sato K, Sakata K, Ozaki H, Takano-Ohmuro H, Tsuchiya T, Sugi H, Kato I, Karaki H (1992) Receptor agonists induce myosin phosphorylation-dependent and phosphorylation-independent contractions in vascular smooth muscle. J Pharmacol Exp Ther 261(2): 506–512
16. Juvela S (2000) Plasma endothelin concentrations after aneurysmal subarachnoid hemorrhage. J Neurosurg 92: 390–400
17. Kasuya H, Weir BKA, White DM, Stefanson K (1993) Mechanism of oxyhemoglobin-induced release of endothelin-1 from cultured vascular endothelial cells and smooth muscle cells. J Neurosurg 79: 892–898
18. Kikkawa K, Saito A, Iwasaki H, Ban Y, Yasoshima A, Yamauchi-Kohno R, Hoshino T, Murata S (1999) Prevention of cerebral vasospasm by a novel receptor antagonist, TA-0201. J Cardiovasc Pharmacol 34(5): 666–673
19. Kobayashi H, Hayashi M, Kobayashi S, Kabuto M, Handa Y, Kawano H (1990) Effect of endothelin on the canine basilar artery. Neurosurgery 27: 357–361
20. Lagente V, Chabrier PE, Mencia-Huerta JA, Braquet P (1989) Aerosol administration of endothelin induces bronchoconstriction in the guinea pig. Biochem Biophys Res Commun 158: 625–632
21. Lee ME, de la Monte SM, Ng SC, Bloch DB, Quertermous T (1990) Expression of the potent vasoconstrictor endothelin in the human central nervous system. J Clin Invest 86: 141–147
22. MacCumber MW, Ross CA, Snyder SH (1990) Endothelin in brain: Receptors, mitogenesis, and biosynthesis in glial cells. Proc Natl Acad Sci USA 87: 2359–2363
23. Macdonald RL (1995) Cerebral vasospasm. Neurosurg Q 5: 73–97
24. MacMahon EG, Fok KF, Moore WM, Smith CE, Siegel NR, Trapani AJ (1989) In vitro and in vivo activity of chymotrypsin activated big-endothelin (porcine 1–40). Biochem Biophys Res Commun 161: 406–413
25. Masaoka H, Susuki R, Hirata Y, Emori T, Marumo F, Hirakawa K (1989) Raised plasma endothelin in aneurysmal subarachnoid hemorrhage. Lancet 336: 1402 (letter)
26. Matsumura Y, Ikegawa R, Tsukahara Y, Takaoka M, Morimoto S (1990) Conversion of big endothelin-1 to endothelin-1 by two types of metalloproteinases derived from porcine aortic endothelial cells. FEBS Lett 272: 166–172
27. Miller WL, Redfield MM, Burnett JC (1989) Integrated cardiac, renal, and endocrine actions of endothelin. J Clin Invest 83: 317–320
28. Mima T, Yanagisawa M, Shigeno T, Saito A, Goto K, Takakura K, Masaki T (1989) Endothelin acts in feline and canine cerebral arteries from the adventitial side. Stroke 20: 1553–1556
29. Ohkuma H, Parney I, Megyesi J, Ghahary A, Findlay JM (1999) Antisense preproendothelin-oligoDNA therapy for vasospasm in a canine model of subarachnoid hemorrhage. J Neurosurg 90: 1105–1114
30. Ohlstein EH, Storer BL (1992) Oxyhemoglobin stimulation of endothelin production in cultured endothelial cells. J Neurosurg 77: 274–278
31. Onoda K, Ono S, Ogihara K, Shiota T, Asari S, Ohmoto T, Ninomiya Y (1996) Inhibition of vascular contraction by intracisternal administration of preproendothelin-1 mRNA antisense oligoDNA in a rat experimental vasospasm model. J Neurosurg 85: 846–852
32. Papadopoulos S, Gilbert L, Webb C, Amato C (1990) Characterization of contractile responses to endothelin in human cerebral arteries: Implications for cerebral vasospasm. Neurosurgery 26: 810–815
33. Sato S, Yonetani Y, Fujimoto M, Kita T, Kubo K, Nakashima T (1998) Effects of an endothelin ET(A)-receptor antagonist, S-0139, on cerebral vasospasm and behavioral changes in dogs intracisternally administered endothelin-1. Life Sci 62: 191–197

34. Seifert V, Löffler BM, Zimmermann M, Roux S, Stolke D (1995) Endothelin concentrations in patients with aneurysmal subarachnoid hemorrhage. Correlation with cerebral vasospasm, delayed ischemic neurological deficits, and volume of hematoma. J Neurosurg 82: 55–62
35. Shigeno T, Mima T, Yanagisawa M, Saito A, Goto K, Yamashita K, Takenouchi T, Matsuura N, Yamasaki Y, Yamada K (1991) Prevention of cerebral vasospasm by actinomycin D. J Neurosurg 74: 940–943
36. Shinyama H, Uchida T, Kido H, Hayashi K, Watanabe M, Matsumura Y, Ikegawa R, Takaoka M, Morimoto S (1991) Phosphoramidon inhibits the conversion of intracisternally administrated big endothelin to endothelin-1. Biochem Biophys Res Commun 178: 24–30
37. Suzuki R, Masaoka E, Hirata H, Marumo F, Isotani E, Hirakawa K (1992) The role of endothelin-1 in the origin of cerebral vasospasm in patients with aneurysmal subarachnoid hemorrhage. J Neurosurg 77: 96–100
38. Suzuki K, Meguro K, Sakurai T, Saitoh Y, Takeuchi S, Nose T (2000) Endothelin-1 concentration increases in the cerebrospinal fluid in cerebral vasospasm caused by subarachnoid hemorrhage. Surg Neurol 53: 131–135
39. Takaoka M, Takenobu Y, Miyata Y, Ikegawa R, Matsumura Y, Morimoto S (1990) Pepsin, an aspartic protease, converts porcine big endothelin to 21-residue endothelin. Biochem Biophys Res Commun 166: 436–442
40. Touvay C, Vilain B, Pons F, Chabrier PE, Mencia-Huerta JM, Braquet P (1990) Bronchopulmonary and vascular effect of endothelin in the guinea pig. Eur J Pharmacol 176: 23–33
41. Touzani O, Galbraith S, Siegl P, McCulloch J (1997) Endothelin-B receptors in cerebral resistance arterioles and their functional significance after focal cerebral ischemia in cats. J Cereb Blood Flow Metab 17: 1157–1165
42. Wanebo JE, Arthur AS, Louis HG, West K, Kassell NF, Lee KS, Helm GA (1998) Systemic administration of the endothelin-A receptor antagonist TBC 11251 attenuates cerebral vasospasm after experimental subarachnoid hemorrhage: dose study and review of endothelin-based therapies in the literature on cerebral vasospasm Neurosurgery 43: 1409–1417
43. Weir B (1995) The pathophysiology of cerebral vasospasm. Br J Neurosurg 9: 375–390
44. Wiklund NP, Ohln A, Cederqvist B (1989) Adrenergic neuromodulation by endothelin in guinea pig artery. Neurosci Lett 101: 269–273
45. Yamamati T, Johshita H, Takaku F, Ohno H, Susuki N, Matsumoto H, Fugino M (1990) Endothelin family in human plasma and cerebrospinal fluid. J Clin Endocrinol Metab 71: 1611–1615
46. Yamaura I, Tani E, Maeda Y, Minami N, Shindo H (1992) Endothelin-1 of canine basilar artery. J Neurosurg 76: 99–105
47. Yanagisawa M, Kurihara H, Kimura S, Tomobe Y, Kabayashi M, Mitsui Y, Yazaki Y, Goto K, Masaki T (1988) A novel potent vasoconstrictor peptide produced by the vascular endothelial cells. Nature 332: 411–415
48. Yoshizawa T, Shimni O, Giaid A, Yanagisawa M, Gibson SJ, Kimura S, Uchiyama Y, Polak JM, Masaki T, Kanazawa I (1990) Endothelin: A novel peptide in the posterior pituitary system. Science 247: 462–464
49. Zimmermann M, Seifert V (1998) Endothelin and subarachnoid hemorrhage: an overview. Neurosurgery 43: 863–876
50. Zuccarello M, Lewis AI, Rapoport RM (1994) Endothelin ETA and ETB receptors in subarachnoid hemorrhage-induced cerebral vasospasm. Eur J Pharmacol 259: R1–R2
51. Zuccarello M, Romano A, Passalacqua M, Rapoport RM (1995) Endothelin-1-induced endothelin-1 release causes cerebral vasospasm in vivo. J Pharm Pharmacol 47: 702
52. Zuccarello M, Boccaletti R, Tosun M, Rapoport RM (1996) Role of extracellular Ca^{2+} in subarachnoid hemorrhage-induced spasm of the rabbit basilar artery. Stroke 27(10): 1896–1902
53. Zuccarello M, Soattin GB, Lewis AI, Breu V, Hallak H, Rapoport RM (1996) Prevention of subarachnoid hemorrhage-induced cerebral vasospasm by oral administration of endothelin receptor antagonists. J Neurosurg 84: 503–507
54. Zuccarello M, Boccaletti R, Rapoport RM (1998) Endothelin ETB receptor-mediated constriction in the rabbit basilar artery. Eur J Pharmacol 350: R7–R9
55. Zuccarello M, Boccaletti R, Rapoport RM (1998) Endothelin ETB1 receptor-mediated relaxation of rabbit basilar artery. Eur J Pharmacol 357: 67–71
56. Zuccarello M, Boccaletti R, Rapoport RM (1998) Endothelium-derived nitric oxide regulates endothelin A versus endothelin B receptor-mediated constriction in rabbit basilar artery in situ. Stroke 29: 323A
57. Zuccarello M, Boccaletti R, Romano A, Rapoport RM (1998) Endothelin B receptor antagonists attenuate subarachnoid hemorrhage-induced cerebral vasospasm. Stroke 29: 1924–1929

Correspondence: Mario Zuccarello, M.D., Department of Neurosurgery, University of Cincinnati College of Medicine, 231 Albert Sabin Way, Box 670515, Cincinnati, OH 45267-0515.

Acta Neurochir (2001) [Suppl] 77: 67–72

Nitric Oxide and Vasospasm

R. M. Pluta, B. G. Thompson, J. K. Afshar, R. J. Boock, B. Iuliano, and **E. H. Oldfield**

Surgical Neurology Branch, National Institute of Neurological Disorders and Stroke, Bethesda, Maryland, U.S.A.

Introduction

Delayed release of hemoglobin from the subarachnoid clot in the vicinity of conductive arteries leads to cerebral vasospasm after SAH. The mechanism of vasospasm however remains unclear. The one thousand times higher affinity of ferrous heme for nitric oxide, a potent vasodilator of cerebral vessels, than to oxygen, has led to the concept that hemoglobin scavenges nitric oxide and produces delayed cerebral vasospasm after SAH. For several years we have investigated the pathological mechanism(s) behind this event using in vivo experiments. We summarize experimental data and discuss the clinical value of the observations for the development of a new treatment for vasospasm after SAH.

Keywords: Nitric oxide; SAH; non-human primate; vasospasm.

Materials and Methods

A well-established primate model of vasospasm after SAH was used in all experiments [3, 15]. Arteriographic vasospasm was quantified relative to each animal's baseline arteriogram.

Endothelial NOS, Inducible NOS and Neuronal NOS Staining [14]

The cerebral arteries of the circle of Willis were exposed overnight at 4 °C to polyclonal antibody against purified rat cerebellar nitric oxide synthase (NOS; 1 : 25) [10] or monoclonal antibody against endothelial or inducible NOS. The reaction was developed by placement in 0.004% 3.3′-diaminobenzidine tetrahydrochloride (Sigma) and 0.003% hydrogen peroxide in TBS.

Internal Carotid Artery Cannulization for ICA NO-Donor/L-Arginine Infusion

Polyethylene radiopaque tubing (Pert −3.0; Cook Group Co, Bloomington, IN) was advanced via the external carotid artery to place the catheter tip at the bifurcation of the common carotid artery. The monkeys were fitted in a jacket containing an infusion pump (D-infusor; 2 × 20 ml/24 h; Disetronic Medical Systems, Minneapolis, MN) and the proximal end of the catheter was connected to the pump. Continuous infusion of normal saline with 250 i.u. heparin was started after priming the pump for 30 min. The set delivery volume was 40 ml/day.

Femoral Vein Cannulization for Continuous Intravenous L-Arginine Infusion

No. 6.6 French Broviac catheter was placed in the left femoral vein and advanced to the inferior vena cava. The monkey was fitted in a jacket containing an infusion pump (D-infusor or D-10 infusor; Disetronic Medical Systems, Minneapolis, MN) and the proximal end of the catheter was connected to the pump. The set delivery volume was 10 ml/day.

Cerebral Blood Flow Measurement During L-Arginine/NO Donor Infusion [16]

A CBF probe (Saber thermomonitoring, Flowtronics, Phoenix, AZ) was slipped between the dura and the brain over a region perfused by the R MCA. To compare rCBF among groups of monkeys CBF ratios were used, which were obtained for each monkey by normalizing the CBF measured during the saline and L-arginine infusions to the mean CBF of that monkey (at pCO_2 of 40 mm Hg) directly before starting the infusion.

Preparation of Nitric Oxide Donor Solutions [13]

Acute Infusion Study. Sterile normal saline was buffered with PBS to a pH of 6.8 to 7.2. The NONOate used was diethylamine-NO (half life, 2.3 min). Directly before infusion, the diethylamine-NO solution was diluted to 10 μM with sterile buffered saline. Control solution consisted of buffered sterile saline and diethylamine solution (10 μM) in saline.

Long-Term Infusion Study. The NONOate used was proli-NO (half life, 1.8 seconds at final concentration of 1 μM). After sterile filtering, the solution was placed in the D-infusor pump, primed for 20 min, and then connected to the proximal end of the intracarotid catheter.

L-Arginine Preparation and Delivery [12]

The L-arginine solution was prepared to achieve an intracarotid concentration of 10^{-6} M during a 3 min ICA administration. In the chronic infusion group, L-arginine (10^{-3} M) was delivered using a D-infusor pump via an indwelling catheter in the femoral vein. Saline was infused using the same method in the control group.

L-Arginine Levels [12]

L-arginine levels in plasma samples, collected in the chronic experiment at surgery and during postoperative arteriograms, were measured using HPLC.

In Vitro Study of NONOate Influence on H_2O_2 Toxicity

Astrocyte Cell Culture. Confluent human fetal astrocytes ($3.4 \pm 0.83 \times 10^6$ cells/well) between passages 4 and 9 were used.

Preparation of Hydrogen Peroxide. In the H_2O_2 experiments a 10^{-4} M stock solution of H_2O_2 was diluted in PBS and added to the media to produce a 10^{-6} M concentration. Media was taken for HPLC analysis after 2 h exposure. The NONOate used was diethylamine-NO (half life, 2.3 min). Directly before infusion, the diethylamine-NO solution was diluted to 10 μM with the sterile buffered saline. Control solution consisted of buffered sterile saline and diethylamine solution (10 μM) in saline.

Statistics

For statistical analysis of data we used ANOVA, the paired *t*-test, and a Wilcoxon signed-rank test (Statview + Graphics, Abacus Concepts, Inc., Berkeley, CA). The results of the staining were analyzed with non-parametric Kruskall-Wallis analysis of variance, and vasospasm was assessed with analysis of variance (StatView SE + Graphics, Abacus Concept Inc.). Significance was accepted at $P < 0.05$.

Results

Experiment 1

NOS presence in cerebral arteries after SAH [14].

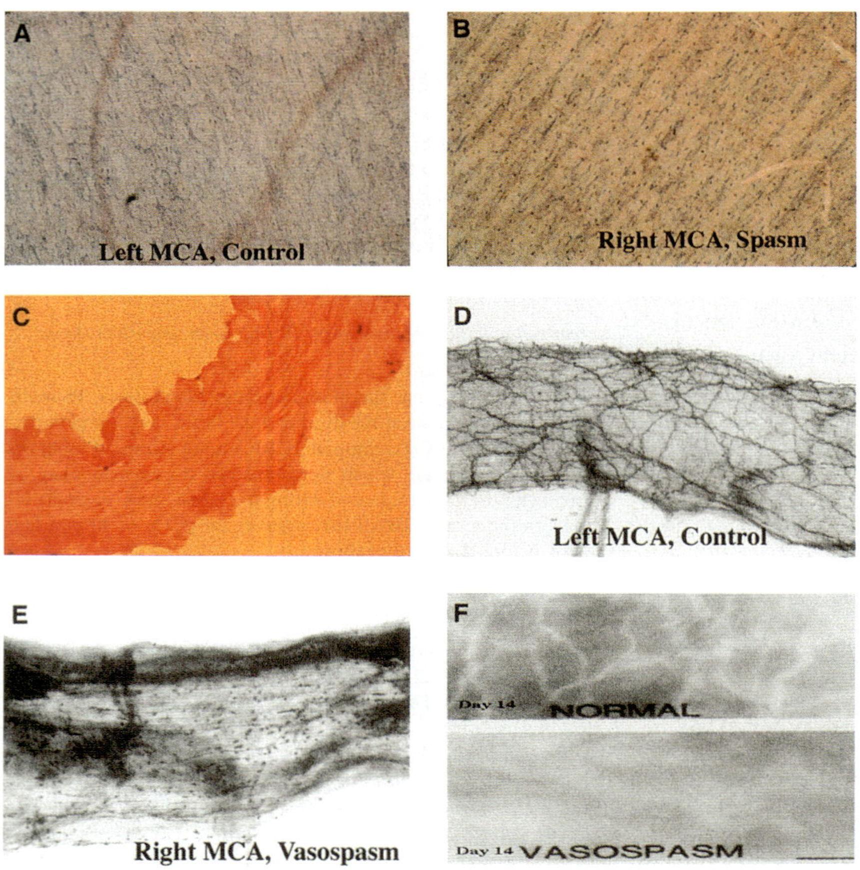

Fig. 1. Photomicrographs of the cerebral arteries of monkeys on day 7 or 14 after SAH. (A, B) Immunoreactivity of endothelial nitric oxide synthase (monoclonal antibody) in the right middle cerebral artery in spasm (B) after subarachnoid hemorrhage in a primate model on day 7 after SAH, which was unchanged, in comparison to the left middle cerebral artery (A, control). (C) Sparse immunoreactivity of inducible nitric oxide synthase (monoclonal antibody) in the right middle cerebral artery in spasm after subarachnoid hemorrhage in a primate model on day 7 after SAH. The same degree of staining was observed in the left (control) middle cerebral artery (not shown). (D) Immunoreactivity of neuronal nitric oxide synthase (polyclonal antibody) in the neural plexus of the adventitia of the left (control) middle cerebral artery on day 7 after subarachnoid hemorrhage. (E) In contrast, immunoreactivity of neuronal nitric oxide synthase was completely absent in the adventitia of the right middle cerebral artery in vasospasm after subarachnoid hemorrhage on day 7 after SAH. (F) Immunoreactivity of neuronal nitric oxide synthase in the right middle cerebral artery was less than in the left middle cerebral artery (control) despite resolution of vasospasm

Immunostaining against endothelial nitric oxide synthase and neuronal nitric oxide synthase revealed that the enzymes were present in the wall of conductive arteries of the primate brain. The endothelial NOS immunoreactivity remained present in the intima of the MCA in spasm (Fig. 1A, B), and sparse inducible NOS was present in all layers of the arterial wall (Fig. 1C). Neuronal NOS-immunoreactivity significantly decreased in the right MCA (Fig. 1E), which was in spasm, in comparison to the left MCA of the same monkey (Fig. 1D; $P < 0.04$). Furthermore, nNOS immunoreactivity did not return to normal levels when vasospasm resolved (Fig. 1F) on Day 14 after SAH.

Experiment 2

Intracarotid (acute) and intravenous (long-lasting) infusion of L-arginine as a treatment of vasospasm [12].

On arteriograms performed immediately after intracarotid infusion of saline ($n = 5$) the mean reduction of the R MCA area in the AP view was $44 \pm 7\%$ compared with the before SAH area. The vessel AP area did not change in response to intracarotid L-arginine infusion ($n = 5$; mean reduction of the R MCA area of $45\% \pm 9\%$; $P = 0.2$ between saline and L-arginine infusion groups). Intracarotid L-arginine infusion, however, increased cortical rCBF by $21 \pm 9.6\%$ compared with saline infusion ($P < 0.015$) and decreased cerebrovascular resistance from 1.64 ± 0.1 mmHg/ml/100 g/min to 1.43 ± 0.4 mmHg/ml/100 g/min ($P < 0.001$). There was no change in systemic mean arterial blood pressure during intracarotid L-arginine infusion compared with saline infusion.

In the chronic continuous intravenous infusion group, the mean reduction of the R MCA AP area was $45 \pm 4\%$ in the control group ($n = 5$) and $36 \pm 14\%$ in the L-arginine group ($n = 6$; $P = 0.16$). Vasospasm resolved, as is the normal course in this model, on day 14 (the mean reduction of the R MCA area on the AP view was $3 \pm 13\%$ in saline group and $2 \pm 12\%$ in L-arginine group; $P = 0.2$). Also, the difference in the degree of vasospasm on day 14 between the control and L-arginine groups was not significant ($P = 0.4$). The plasma L-arginine level (12.7 ± 4.0 μg/ml on day 0, before the intracarotid infusion of L-arginine) increased to 21.9 ± 13.1 μg/ml on day 7 of the infusion ($P < 0.05$) and 18.5 ± 3.1 μg/ml on day 14 ($P < 0.03$). Plasma L-citrulline, a by-product of NO production from L-arginine was unchanged on days 7, and 14.

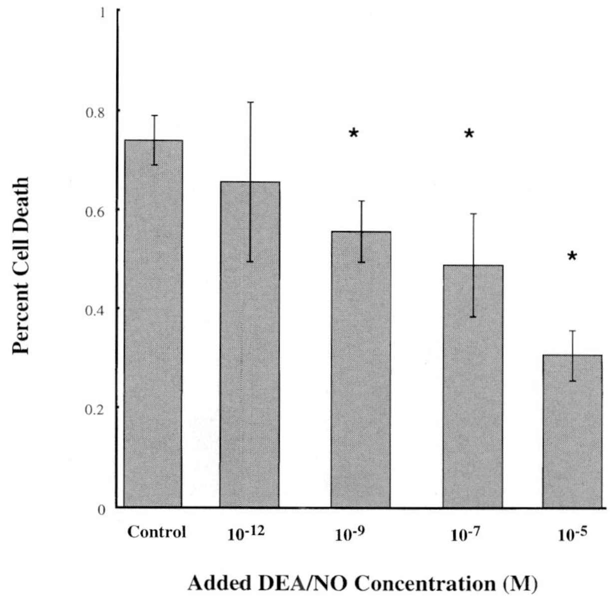

Fig. 2. This graph depicts an increased viability of astrocytes exposed to H_2O_2 (10^{-6} M) in the presence of increasing concentrations of NO donor (DEA/NO; 10^{-12} M to 10^{-5} M)

Experiment 3

In vitro study of the influence of NONOate on H_2O_2 toxicity.

To examine the cytotoxic role of increased NO levels human fetal astrocytes were exposed for 2 h to the reactive oxygen species precursor H_2O_2 in the presence of increasing concentrations of DEA/NO. When cell viability was determined, increasing concentrations of the NO donor provided increased protection in a deose-response relationship (Fig. 2; $P < 0.05$).

Experiment 4

Intracarotid delivery of Nitric oxide donor as a treatment of vasospasm [13].

In the acute infusion experiment, four monkeys with the right MCA in spasm received intracarotid infusion of a NO donor with a short serum half-life (diethylamine-NO). Cerebral arteriograms in the AP projection were obtained to assess the degree of vasospasm before and after infusion of the NO donor. Immediately after the infusion, the narrowing of the vessels decreased from $35\% \pm 12\%$ to $8.4\% \pm 4.3\%$ (Fig. 3A; $P < 0.04$).

In the long-term infusion experiment four control

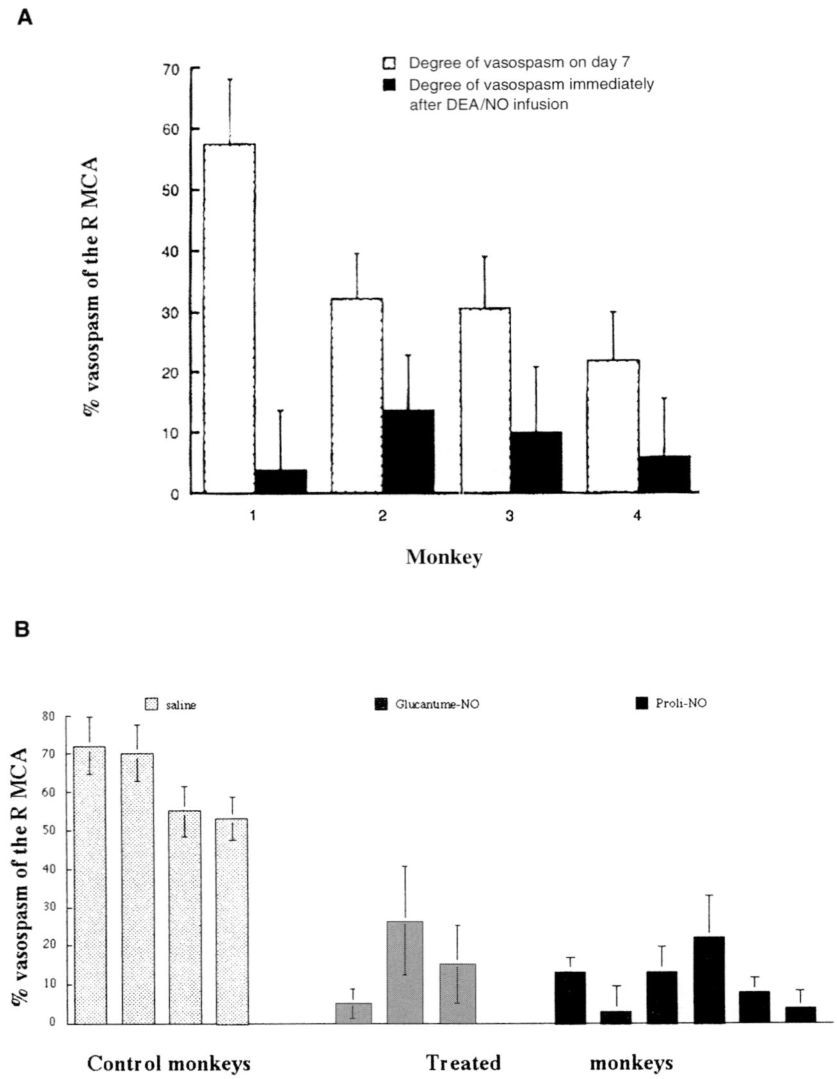

Fig. 3. (A) Bar graph depicts the immediate reversal of cerebral vasospasm during intracarotid infusion of the NO donor (DEA/NO). (B) Bar graph depicts the degree of vasospasm of the right middle cerebral artery on Day 7 after SAH in monkeys that received continuous 7-day intracarotid infusions of saline, glucantime-NO, or proliNO. Both NO donors prevented the development of vasospasm

monkeys had intracarotid infusion of alkalynized saline and six monkeys received an intracarotid infusion of NO donor (proliNO). The infusion started 24 h after clot placement and was continued for seven days when arteriography was repeated. Fig. 3B depicts the degree of arteriographic vasospasm of the right MCA on Day 7 (mean value of the right MCA area reduction compared with the preoperative area on the AP arteriogram). In control monkeys the area of the right MCA was reduced by 65% ± 5%, and in the proliNO group the area of the right MCA decreased by only 11% ± 2.9% ($P < 0.05$).

Discussion

Nitric oxide (NO) is involved in the functional regulation of cerebral blood flow [9, 16]. Furthermore, ferrous hemoglobin is contiguous with the wall of the cerebral arteries after SAH [8, 11]. The thousand times higher affinity of the ferrous heme moiety to nitric oxide than to oxygen suggests that delayed cerebral vasospasm develops in response to a release of ferrous hemoglobin from the subarachnoid clot in the vicinity of the cerebral arteries. This hemoglobin scavenges NO [18] produced in the vessel wall by NOS [10, 14], and decrease cGMP levels in the smooth muscle cells of the arterial media [7], leading to constriction of the artery. However, it seems unlikely that endothelial NOS is directly involved in the process because, despite a decrease of cGMP in the vessel wall, immunoreactivity of endothelial NOS remains the same [7] or increases (Fig. 1A, B). Disappearance of nNOS from the arterial wall at the time of vasospasm (Fig. 1E) [14] supports the idea of an NO decrease and an imbalance between vasoconstricting and vasodilating agents as the cause of vasospasm [1, 14, 19]. This hypothesis is supported by the recent observation by Toda *et al.* showing direct vasodilation of conductive vessels by stimulation of nitroxidergic neurons in the sphenopalatine ganglion [17]. To overcome the decreased availability of NO in the arterial wall, we administered ICA, an ultrafast NO donor to reverse (Fig. 3A) and prevent (Fig. 3B) vasospasm. However, to our disappointment, an easier route of NO donor administration, intravenous, did not provide the same effect despite the high doses used, which led to a decrease of systemic blood pressure. Furthermore, L-arginine, which is known to correct endothelial NOS dysfunction [2], delivered ICA in high doses (short-term infusion) or intravenously (long-term infusion) did not reverse or prevent vasospasm, despite increasing CBF and decreasing arterial blood pressure.

The sum of these observations, as well as the fact that L-arginine delivered intrathecally reverses vasospasm [4, 6], suggest that eNOS dysfunction is not a direct cause of vasospasm. They also support the possibility that decreased levels of NO in the vessel wall, most likely due to damage to nNOS in the adventitia of the artery, is responsible for spasm of cerebral vessels, which is correctable by NO donor infusion. The direct mechanism of smooth muscle contraction is not clear. Decreased levels of NO, leading to a lower concentration of cGMP, may actually enhance the constrictive action of endothelin-1 (ET-1) [14, 19] or weaken the effect of endothelium derived hyperpolarizing factor (EDHF) [1, 5]. Correction of NO supply in the vessel in spasm was achieved by the ICA delivery of an ultrafast NO donor and consistently produced complete or nearly complete reversal of vasospasm. However, other methods, such as quenching of ET-1, blockade of the $ET\text{-}1_A$ receptor, stimulation of the $ET\text{-}1_B$ receptor [19], up-regulation of EDHF, or inhibition of phosphodiesterase V, may produce the same effect, i.e. reversal and prevention of delayed cerebral vasospasm.

Despite the incompletely understood role of NO in the development of vasospasm, intracarotid delivery of an ultrafast NO donor provides a new treatment approach for vasospasm.

References

1. Brayden JE, Wellman GC (1991) Endothelium-dependent dilatation of feline cerebral arteries: role of membrane potential and cyclic-nucleotides. J Cereb Blood Flow Metabol 9: 256–263
2. Drexler H, Zeiher A, Meinzer K, Just H (1991) Correction of endothelial dysfunction in coronary microcirculation of hypercholesterolemic patients by L-arginine. Lancet 338: 1546–1550
3. Espinosa F, Weir B, Overton T, Castor W, Grace M, Boisvert O (1984) A randomized placebo-controlled double-blind trial of nimodipine after SAH in monkeys. Part I: clinical and radiological findings. J Neurosurg 60: 1167–1175
4. Findlay J, Weir B, Steinke D, Tanabe T, Gordon P, Grace M (1988) Effect of intrathecal thrombolytic therapy on subarachnoid clot and chronic vasospasm in primate model of SAH. J Neurosurg 69: 723–735
5. Huang AH, Busse R, Bassenge E (1988) Endothelium-dependent hyperpolarization of smooth muscle cells in rabbit femoral arteries is not mediated by EDRF (nitric oxide). Naunyn Schmiedebergs Arch Pharmacol 338: 438–442
6. Kajita Y, Suzuki Y, Oyama H, Tanazawa T, Takayasu M, Shibuya M, Sugita K (1994) Combined effect of L-arginine and superoxide dismutase on the spastic basilar artery after subarachnoid hemorrhage in dogs. J Neurosurg 80: 476–483
7. Kasuya H, Weir B, Nakane M, Pollock J, Johns L, Marton L, Stefansson K (1995) Nitric oxide synthase and guanylate cyclase levels in canine basilar artery after subarachnoid hemorrhage. J Neurosurg 82: 250–255
8. Macdonald R, Weir B (1991) A review of hemoglobin and the pathogenesis of cerebral vasospasm. Stroke 22: 971–982
9. McPherson R, Kirsch J, Ghaly R, Traystman R (1995) Effect of nitric oxide synthase inhibition on the cerebral vascular response to hypercapnia in primates. Stroke 26: 682–687
10. Nozaki K, Moskowitz MA, Maynard KI, Koketsu N, Dawson TM, Bredt DS, Snyder SH (1993) Possible origins and distribution of immunoreactive nitric oxide synthase-containing nerve fibers in cerebral arteries. J Cereb Blood Flow Metab 13: 70–79
11. Pluta R, Afshar J, Boock R, Oldfield E (1997) Temporal changes in perivascular concentrations of oxyhemoglobin, deoxyhemoglobin and, methemoglobin in subarachnoid hemorrhage. J Neurosurg 88: 557–561
12. Pluta R, Afshar J, Thompson B, Boock R, Harvey-White J, Oldfield E (2000) L-arginine increases cerebral blood flow but does not reverse or prevent vasospasm after subarachnoid hemorrhage. J Neurosurg 92: 121–126
13. Pluta R, Oldfield E, Boock R (1997) Reversal and prevention of cerebral vasospasm by intracarotid infusions of nitric oxide donors in a primate model of subarachnoid hemorrhage. J Neurosurg 87: 746–751
14. Pluta R, Thompson B, Dawson T, Snyder S, Oldfield E (1996) Loss of Nitric Oxide synthase immunoreactivity in cerebral vasospasm. J Neurosurg 84: 648–654
15. Pluta R, Zauner A, Morgan J, Muraszko K, Oldfield E (1992) Is vasospasm related to proliferative arteriopathy? J Neurosurg 77: 740–748
16. Thompson BG, Pluta RM, Girton M, Oldfield EH (1995) Nitric Oxide mediation of chemoregulation but not autoregulation of cerebral blood flow in primates. J Neurosurg 84: 71–78

17. Toda N, Tanaka T, Ayajiki K, Okamura T (2000) Cerebral vasodilatation induced by stimulation of the sphenopalatine ganglion and greater petrosal nerve in anesthetized monkeys. Neuroscience 96: 393–398
18. Vane JR, Anggard EE, Botting RM (1990) Regulatory Functions of the Vascular Endothelium. N Engl J Med 323: 27–36
19. Zuccarello M, Boccaletti R, Romano A, Rapoport R (1998) Endothelin B receptor antagonists attenuate subarachnoid hemorrhage-induced cerebral vasospasm. Stroke 29: 1924–1929

Correspondence: Ryszard M. Pluta, M.B. Ph.D., Surgical Neurology Branch, National Institute of Neurological Disorders and Stroke, 10 Center Drive, Bld 10, Room 5037 Bethesda, MD 20892, USA.

Acta Neurochir (2001) [Suppl] 77: 73–75

Effect of Endothelin-Converting Enzyme Inhibitors on big Endothelin-1 Induced Contraction of Rabbit Basilar Artery

M. Zimmermann[1], **C. Jung**[1], **A. Raabe**[1], **O. Spanehl**[2], and **V. Seifert**[1]

[1] Neurosurgical Clinic, Johann Wolfgang Goethe-University, Frankfurt am Main, Germany
[2] Neurological Clinic, University of Leipzig, University of Leibzig, Germany

Introduction

In 1988, a novel family of endothelium derived extremely potent vasoconstrictor peptides, named endothelins, were isolated from cultured porcine endothelial cells. ET-1, a 21-amino acid peptide, is synthesized by vascular endothelial or smooth muscle cells by specific proteolytic cleavage at Trp-21-Val-22 of a precursor 38 amino-acid peptide, big ET-1 [6]. When applied to the adventitial side of blood vessels, endothelins cause a dose dependent, long lasting vasoconstriction, similar to cerebral vasospasm following aneurysmal SAH. Increased levels of big ET-1, ET-1 and ET-3 were detected in the cerebrospinal fluid and plasma of patients after aneurysmal SAH [5]. In cerebral vessels, endothelins bind to two different receptor subtypes. The ET_A receptor is present in vascular smooth muscle cells and mediates vasoconstriction. The ET_B receptor is present in brain, endothelium, and smooth muscle cells and mediates endothelium dependent vasodilatation, but can also cause vasoconstriction. The protease that catalyzes the conversion is the so called endothelin-converting-enzyme (ECE), a membrane bound, neutral zinc metallo-endopeptidase like angiotensin-converting enzyme (ACE) and E-24.11 [4, 7]. Blocking the ECE activity may be one way to suppress or even stop the transformation of big ET-1 to vasoactive ET-1. Therefore the effects of two different putative ECE inhibitors were investigated in this experimental study.

Keywords: Angiotensin-converting-enzyme; big endothelin-1; endothelin-converting-enzyme; cerebral vasospasm.

Material and Methods

Thirty rabbits (Chinchilla-Bastard) with a body weight ranging from 2500 to 3500 g were used in this laboratory experiment. Eight animals each were assigned to the control group ($2*10^{-6}$ M big ET-1 and phyiologic saline solution), to the captopril treatment group ($2*10^{-4}$ M captopril and $2*10^{-6}$ M big ET-1), and to the [D-Val^{22}] big ET-1 [16–38] treatment group ($2*10^{-5}$ M [D-Val^{22}] big ET-1 [16–38] and $2*10^{-6}$ M big ET-1). Three animals each were used as therapeutic controls for captopril ($2*10^{-4}$ M captopril) and [D-Val^{22}] big ET-1 [16–38] ($2*10^{-5}$ M), in order to exclude any constrictive effects of these drugs to the basilar artery. Anesthesia was induced by intramuscular injection of 0.186 mg/kg dormitor and 26.25 mg/kg ketamine. After an intramuscular injection of 0.1 mg/kg atropine trachotomy was performed. The animals were ventilated with a 40% O_2 concentration using an ADS 1000 veterinary anaesthesia delivery system (Engler Engineering Corporation, Germany). Anesthesia was maintained with an intravenous infusion of 0.15 mg/kg/hr dormitor and 21,0 mg/ml/hr ketamine. After achieving normal vital parameters, the left femoral artery was dissected and a 16 G vygon catheter (Vygon, Aachen, Germany) was inserted. The catheter was placed in the vertebral artery under fluoroscopic control. An angiogram of the basilar artery was performed by manual injection of 3.0 ml of L-lysinamidotrizoat (Peritrast 300®, Dr. Franz Köhler Chemie, Alsbach-Hähnlein, Germany).

In the control group 0.5 ml of physiologic saline solution were slowly injected into the cerebello-medullary cistern. Thereafter the animals were kept in headdown position of 30 degrees for 30 minutes. Afterwards 0.5 ml $2*10^{-6}$ M big ET-1, dissolved in physiologic saline solution, were slowly injected into the cerebello-medullary cistern. After that the animals were again kept in headdown position of 30 degrees for 30 minutes. In the [D-Val^{22}] big ET-1 [16–38] and the captopril treatment groups 0.5 ml of $2*10^{-5}$ M [D-Val^{22}] big ET-1 [16–38] or 0.5 ml of $2*10^{-4}$ M captopril were slowly injected into the cerebello-medullary cistern. Afterwards the animals were kept in headdown position of 30 degrees for 30 minutes. Thereafter 0.5 ml $2*10^{-6}$ M big ET-1, dissolved in physiologic saline solution, were slowly injected into the cerebello-medullary cistern. After that the animals were again kept in headdown position of 30 degrees for 30 minutes. In the captopril and [D-Val^{22}] big ET-1 [16–38] control groups 0.5 ml of $2*10^{-4}$ M captopril or $2*10^{-5}$ M

[D-Val[22]] big ET-1 [16–38] were slowly injected into the cerebellomedullary cistern. Thereafter the animals were kept in headdown position of 30 degrees for 60 minutes. These groups served as internal controls to exclude any intrinsic activities of the test medication. After finishing the special procedures, the animals were replaced in prone position and a second angiography was performed as described above.

The data are presented as means and their standard deviations. One-way-analysis of variance were performed to calculate the difference of vessel diameter between the first and second angiography in both treatment groups (captopril/[D-Val[22]] big ET-1 [16–38]) and the control group as dependent variable, whereas the time factor served as independent variable in all calculations.

Results

In the [D-Val[22]] big ET-1 [16–38] treatment group ($n = 8$) the angiographically measured diameter of the basilar artery slightly increased from 0.63 ± 0.12 mm to 0.66 ± 0.12 mm ($p = 0.635$). These results corresponded to an increase of vessel diameter of $5.24 \pm 9.89\%$ (Fig. 1). In the [D-Val[22]] big ET-1 [16–38] control group ($n = 3$) no significant changes in the diameter of the basilar arteries occurred (0.65 ± 0.14 mm to 0.67 ± 0.11 mm; $p = 0.820$). In the captopril treatment group the angiographically measured diameter of the basilar artery slightly increased from 0.64 ± 0.11 mm to 0.71 ± 0.10 mm ($p = 0.172$). These results corresponded to an increase of vessel diameter of $13.53 \pm 19.08\%$ (Fig. 1). In the captopril control group ($n = 3$) no significant changes in the diameter of the basilar arteries occurred (0.78 ± 0.16 mm to 0.95 ± 0.11 mm; $p = 0.198$). In the control group the angiographically measured diameter of the basilar artery significantly decreased from 0.71 ± 0.13 mm to 0.57 ± 0.15 mm ($p = 0.031$) These results corresponded to a decrease of vessel diameter of $19.54 \pm 15.81\%$ (Fig. 1). Comparing the angiographic vessel diameter of the second angiographies of the [D-Val[22]] big ET-1 [16–38] treatment group and the control group, the differences (percent) between the two groups were statistically significant ($80.46 \pm 15.81\%$ in the control group and $113.53 \pm 19.08\%$ in the [D-Val[22]] big ET-1 [16–38] treatment group ($p = 0.002$). Comparing the angiographic vessel diameter of the second angiographies of the captopril treatment group and the control group, the differences (percent) between the two groups were statistically significant ($80.46 \pm 15.81\%$ in the control group and $105.24 \pm 9.89\%$ in the captopril treatment group ($p = 0.002$).

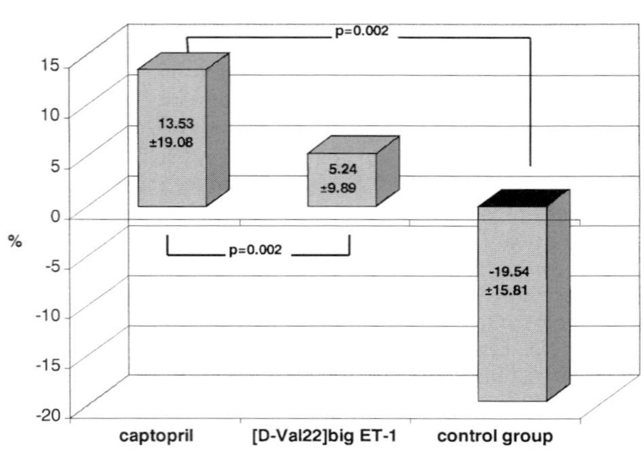

Fig. 1. Changes in the diameter of rabbit basilar artery (percent)

Discussion

The current concept of the complex etiology of cerebral vasospasm after aneurysmal subarachnoid hemorrhage is based on the presumption of a multifactorial origin, including the liberation of spasmogenic metabolites during posthemorrhage clot lysis in the basal cisterns and impairment of cerebral vasodilatation related to endothelial dysfunction and posthemorrhagic structural changes in the arterial wall. The balance between the release of endothelium-derived-constricting-factors and endothelium-derived-relaxing-factors plays an important role in the preservation of the tonus of the cerebral vascular system under normal and pathological conditions. During the past decade a number of clinical and experimental studies demonstrated the important role of endothelin as a keyfactor in the development of cerebral vasospasm and delayed ischemic neurological deficits after aneurysmal SAH. A new approach in the prophylaxis and therapy of cerebral vasospasm may therefore be the inhibition of the contractile action or activation of ET-1. This might be achieved by blocking the ET_A receptor, which had been effective in a number of experimental studies. Another level of interaction might be the inhibition of ET-1 synthesis and release. According to the literature, the results of the present study can demonstrate that [D-Val[22]] big ET-1 [16–38] significantly reduced ECE activity, resulting in a prevention of basilar artery constriction after intracisternal application of big ET-1 [1, 2]. Comparable results were obtained for captopril, an inhibitor of the angiotensin-converting-enzyme (ACE) [3]. These results, in combination with those of other investigators, demonstrate the important role of endothelins in the development of cerebral vasospasm. The efficacy of captopril and

[D-Val[22]] big ET-1 [16–38] in the prevention of ET-1 formation was clearly demonstrated by our data. It can be suggested that the application of selective ECE-inhibitors will lead to useful preventive and therapeutic concepts of cerebral vasospasm.

References

1. Caner HH, Kwan AL, Arthur A, Jeng AY, Lappe RW, Kassell NF, Lee KS (1996) Systemic administration of an inhibitor of endothelin-converting enzyme for attenuation of cerebral vasospasm following experimental subarachnoid hemorrhage. J Neurosurg 85: 917–922
2. Claing A, Neugebauer W, Yano M, Rae GA, D'Orleans-Juste P (1995) [Phe22]-big endothelin-1 [19–37]: a new and potent inhibitor of the endothelin-converting enzyme. J Cardiovasc Pharmacol 26 [Suppl] 3: 72–74
3. Iplikcioglu AC, Bayar MA, Sav A, Erbengi T (1994) Angiotensin-converting enzyme inhibitor cilazapril prevents chronic morphologic vasospasm in rat. Surg Neurol 41: 294–298
4. Matsumura Y, Ikegawa R, Tsukahara Y, Takaoka M, Morimoto S (1991) Conversion of big endothelin-1 to endothelin-1 by two-types of metalloproteinases of cultured porcine vascular smooth muscle cells. Biochem Biophys Res Commun 178: 899–905
5. Seifert V, Loffler BM, Zimmermann M, Roux S, Stolke D (1995) Endothelin concentrations in patients with aneurysmal subarachnoid hemorrhage. Correlation with cerebral vasospasm, delayed ischemic neurological deficits, and volume of hematoma. J Neurosurg 82: 55–62
6. Yanagisawa M, Kurihara H, Kimura S, Goto K, Masaki T (1988) A novel peptide vasoconstrictor, endothelin, is produced by vascular endothelium and modulates smooth muscle Ca2+ channels. J Hypertens [Suppl] 6: 188–191
7. Zimmermann M, Seifert V (1998) Endothelin and subarachnoid hemorrhage: an overview. Neurosurgery 43: 863–875

Correspondence: Michael Zimmermann, M.D., Ph.D., Neurosurgical Clinic, Johann Wolfgang Goethe-University, Schleusenweg 2-16, 60528 Frankfurt, Germany.

Acta Neurochir (2001) [Suppl] 77: 77–79

The Role of Endothelin-1 as Predictor of the Symptomatic Vasospasm in Acute Stage of Subarachnoid Haemorrhage

J. M. Kim[1], **K. H. Bak**[1], **C. H. Kim**[1], **I. K. Park**[2], **S. J. Oh**[3], and **H. K. Choi**[4]

[1] Department of Neurosurgery, Hanyang University Kuri Hospital, Kuri, Korea
[2] Department of Clinical Pathology, Hanyang University Kuri Hospital, Kuri, Korea
[3] Department of Neurosurgery, Hanyang University Medical Center, Seoul, Korea
[4] Department of Neurosurgery, College of Medicine, Pochon CHA University, Pochon, Korea

Introduction

Up to now, the pathogenesis of delayed cerebral vasospasm after subarachnoid haemorrhage (SAH) is unclear and seems to be a multifactorial event [8, 10]. Recently, endothelin-1 (ET-1) has been well known as one of key substances in the development of delayed vasospasm [6, 7, 10]. Many authors have already reported about its main function [3, 4, 9, 10] and its increased level in a subacute or late stage of SAH in delayed vasospasm patients [2, 6, 7]. On the contrary, there were only a few reports concerning its role in the prediction of subsequent vasospasm in hyperacute or acute stage of SAH.

We measured the ET-1 concentrations in both plasma and cerebrospinal fluid (CSF) in 21 consecutive aneurysmal SAH patients during the first three days after initial haemorrhagic stroke, and evaluated the predictive values for the subsequent vasospasm after early aneurysmal surgery.

Keywords: Endothelin-1 (ET-1); vasospasm; subarachnoid haemorrhage (SAH); predictor.

Patients and Methods

Study Groups

Non-SAH Patients. The ET-1 levels in the plasma and CSF without SAH were determined in seven consecutive patients who underwent lumbar myelography for detecting spinal disease. There were four women and three men, with a mean age of 40 years (range 20 to 58 years).

SAH Patients. Twenty-one patients admitted within 24 hours after initial SAH were studied. There were twelve women and nine men, with a mean age of 56 years (range 25 to 76 years). Neurological conditions on admission and at discharge were evaluated using the Glasgow coma scale (GCS), Hunt and Hess grading scale, and Glasgow outcome scale (GOS). According to Fisher grading scale, the degree of SAH on CT scan was categorized. Flow velocities in the cerebral basal arteries were documented daily by using transcranial Doppler sonography (TCD). Neurological examinations were performed daily after the admission. The occurrence of vasospsm and resulting ischaemic neurological deficits were diagnosed by the TCD characteristics and from the postoperative clinical signs worsening after exclusion of other possible causes with CT scan. The SAH patients were divided into two groups according to the presence of either clinical symptomatic and/or angiographic vasospasm. Group I (n = 14) was vasospasm group; whereas group II (n = 7) was non-vasospasm group.

All patients underwent surgical clippings for the ruptured aneurysm within two days after bleeding. A cisternal drainage was routinely placed in the sylvian cistern during craniotomy. Fourteen (66.7%) patients were in good condition (GCS score 15–13) and the rest (33.3%) were in poor condition (GCS score 11–4). Routine postoperative angiography was performed from 10 to 28 days (mean 14 days) after aneurysmal surgery in 18 patients. Three patients were missed due to two deaths and one severe disability, resulting from initial poor clinical condition (GCS score 4–6). Among seven patients who had multiple aneurysms, all the aneurysms were clipped in one-stage operation in five patients and the remaining two patients underwent second-stage operation for clipping of contralateral unruptured aneurysms. Therefore, the postoperative angiography was taken later in two patients due to the second operation time.

Laboratory Procedures

A total of 168 plasma and CSF samples were collected daily from twenty-one SAH patients from zero to three days after operation via cisternal drainage. Seven of each plasma and CSF samples were also collected from the control persons. A double-antibody sandwich-enzyme immunoassay was performed using a commercially available kit (Endothelin ELISA, The next generation®; Biomedica, Wien, Germany) for studying ET-1 immunoreactivity. Freshly collected plasma samples within potassium-ethylenediamine tetraacetic acid (EDTA) bottles were centrifuged within one hour and stored at −20 °C until the assay. The CSF samples were also stored at −20 °C until the assay after the centrifuge. According to the manufacturer, intra- and interassay coefficients of variation are less than 10%. Crossreactivity was 100% for ET-1, 100% for ET-2, less than 5% for ET-3 and less than 1% for big ET-1.

Statistical Methods

Statistical analysis was performed using multivariate analysis of variance (MANOVA) (Statistical Analysis System, SAS Institute, Cary, NC) to determine the degree to which each variable was independently correlated with vasospasm. In all cases, P values of <0.05 were considered significant. The Mann-Whitney *U* test and chi-square test were used to compare continuous variables and categorical variables, respectively. Pearson rank correlation was investigated to determine the degree to which each variable was correlated with clinical symptomatic vasospasm.

Results

Mean plasma and CSF ET-1 concentrations in patients with SAH (mean $\pm$ standard deviation, 1.02 ± 0.42 fmol/ml, 1.00 ± 0.30 fmol/ml, respectively) were higher than the control group (0.44 ± 0.17 fmol/ml, 0.35 ± 0.11 fmol/ml, respectively) and showed statistical significance ($p < 0.005$). The plasma and the CSF levels of ET-1 didn't change over time and didn't show any difference between two groups of aneurysmal SAH patients during acute stage (Figs. 1, 2). On operation day, the ET-1 levels in plasma and CSF of Group I and Group II were 1.06 ± 0.47 fmol/ml, 1.04 ± 0.35 fmol/ml and 0.94 ± 0.33 fmol/ml, 0.94 ± 0.17 fmol/ml, respectively. Three days after surgery, the ET-1 levels in plasma and CSF in two groups were 0.79 ± 0.22 fmol/ml, 0.74 ± 0.26 fmol/ml and 1.03 ± 0.21 fmol/ml, 0.96 ± 0.26 fmol/ml, respectively. There were no statistical significances in ET-1 levels in plasma and CSF between two groups in acute stage of SAH ($p > 0.05$) (Figs. 1, 2). Among the several variables which related to the clinical grade, only Glasgow outcome score (GOS) was correlated with the delayed vasospasm, statistically ($p = 0.029$). Using multivariate analysis, the correlation between vasospasm and various neurological grading scales were also studied, and there was a good correlation between GOS and vasospasm ($r = 0.447$, $p = 0.042$) (Table 1).

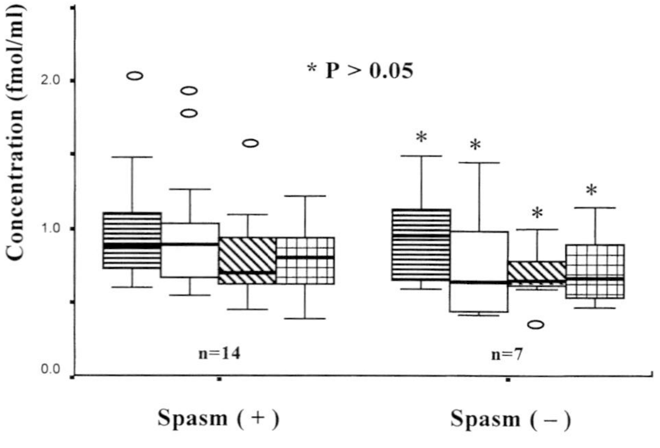

Fig. 1. Boxplot showing ET-1 concentrations in plasma between SAH and non-SAH patients. The dark line in the center of each box represents the median value; the ends of the boxes represent the quartile values; and the bars represent outliers whose values are between 1.5 and 3 times from the upper or lower edge of the box. Circles outside the bars represent extremes whose values are more than 3 times from the upper or lower edge of the box. *P value by analysis of multivariate analysis of variance for means. #POD = postoperative days; n = number of patients. #POD 0, #POD 1, #POD 2, #POD 3

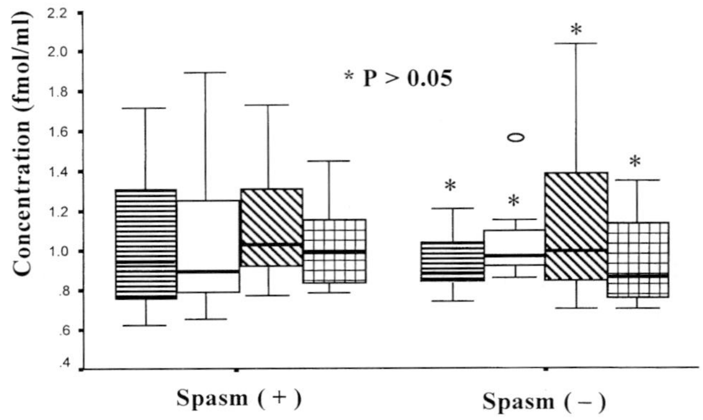

Fig. 2. Boxplot showing ET-1 concentrations in CSF between SAH and non-SAH patients. The dark line in the center of each box represents the median value; the ends of the boxes represent the quartile values; and the bars represent outliers whose values are between 1.5 and 3 times from the upper or lower edge of the box. Circles outside the bars represent extremes whose values are more than 3 times from the upper or lower edge of the box. *P value by analysis of multivariate analysis of variance for means. #POD = postoperative days; n = number of patients. #POD 0, #POD 1, #POD 2, #POD 3

Table 1. *Vasospasm Correlations with Neurological and Neuroimaging Grading System*[a]

Scale	Pearson correlation (r)	p value
GCS	0.388	0.082
Hunt-Hess grade	0.306	0.177
Fisher grade	0.239	0.297
GOS	0.447	0.042[b]

[a] GCS Glasgow coma scale; GOS Glasgow outcome scale.
[b] $P < 0.05$ by univariate analysis of variance.

Discussion

Among three iso-forms of ETs, the ET-1, which is modulated by intracellular calcium has been regarded as the most potent and long-lasting vasoconstrictor [4, 9, 10]. The ET-1 is released locally [4], and its levels in plasma and CSF are low. However, the measurements of ET-1 are a useful method to evaluate the severity [4] and the possibility of vasospasm.

According to the levels of ET-1 in plasma and CSF, the positive correlation between ET-1 level and vasospasm has been demonstrated in some studies [2, 7]; but, other reports had shown that there are no correlation between them [5, 6]. The plasma ET-1 concentrations were highest shortly after SAH and gradually decreased with time [2, 7]. These elevations of ET-1 levels are strongly associated with symptomatic and/or angiographic vasospasm [2, 6, 7]. The increase in CSF ET-1 levels is usually observed in SAH patients with cerebral vasospasm and delayed ischaemia [1, 6, 7]. CSF levels of ET-1 in those patients mainly increased during the second week after bleeding [6, 7], and this delayed rise of CSF ET-1 levels was correlated with the astrocytes releasing ET-1 into CSF following cerebral ischaemia [5]. In the present study, regardless of the presence of cerebral vasospasm, the plasma and the CSF ET-1 concentrations in SAH patients were higher than in the non-SAH control group and remained high without only gradual decline with time during the acute phase of SAH.

Suzuki *et al.* [7] reported that the CSF ET-1 levels in SAH patients with vasospasm were not increased on the first three days after SAH onset. If early CSF ET-1 levels could predict the occurrence of cerebral vasospasm following SAH, the delayed catastrophic ischaemia can be protected by a simple measurement of CSF ET-1 concentrations. In our study, there was no significant difference in CSF and plasma ET-1 levels in the acute phase of SAH between the vasospasm and the non-vasospasm groups. We only measured the concentrations of plasma and CSF ET-1 in the acute stage of SAH because it was unable to keep the cisternal drainage for a long time due to the possibility of infection. And this may contribute to the reason why the CSF ET-1 levels were not correlated with the possibility of cerebral vasospasm. Therefore, further serial long-term study will be needed to evaluate the potential role of ET-1 in SAH-associated vasospasm and the delayed ischaemic deficits in the future.

Conclusions

The levels of ET-1 in plasma and CSF of the SAH patients were higher than in the control group and there was statistical significance. However, the measurement of the levels of ET-1 in plasma and CSF in acute stage of SAH patients does not play a role as predictor of subsequent vasospasm either in the early or in late phase of post-SAH.

References

1. Ehrenreich H, Lange M, Near KA, Anneser F, Schoeller LAC, Schmid R, Winkler PA, Kehrl JH, Schmiedek P, Goebel FD (1992) Long-term monitoring of immunoreactive endothelin-1 and endothelin-3 in ventricular cerebrospinal fluid, plasma, and 24-h urine of patients with subarachnoid hemorrhage. Res Exp Med 192: 257–268
2. Juvela S (2000) Plasma endothelin concentrations after aneurysmal subarachnoid hemorrhage. J Neurosurg 92: 390–400
3. Kobayashi H, Hayashi M, Kobayashi S, Kabuto M, Handa Y, Kawano H, Ide H (1991) Cerebral vasospasm and vasoconstriction caused by endothelin. Neurosurgery 28: 673–679
4. Levin ER (1995) Endothelins. N Engl J Med 333: 356–363
5. Pluta RM, Boock RJ, Afshar JK, Clouse K, Bacic M, Ehrenreich H, Oldfield EH (1997) Source and cause of endothelin-1 release into cerebrospinal fluid after subarachnoid hemorrhage. J Neurosurg 87: 287–293
6. Seifert V, Löffler BM, Zimmermann M, Roux S, Stolke D (1995) Endothelin concentrations in patients with aneurysmal subarachnoid hemorrhage. Correlation with cerebral vasospasm, delayed ischemic neurological deficits, and volume of hematoma. J Neurosurg 82: 55–62
7. Suzuki R, Masaoka H, Hirata Y, Marumo F, Isotani E, Hirakawa K (1992) The role of endothelin-1 in the origin of cerebral vasospasm in patients with aneurysmal subarachnoid hemorrhage. J Neurosurg 77: 96–100
8. Weir B (1995) The pathophysiology of cerebral vasospasm. Br J Neurosurg 9: 375–390
9. Yanagisawa M, Kurihara H, Kimura S, Tomobe Y, Kobayashi M, Mitsui T, Yazaki Y, Goto K, Masaki T (1988) A novel potent vasoconstrictor peptide produced by vascular endothelial cells. Nature 332: 411–415
10. Zimmermann M, Seifert V (1998) Endothelin and subarachnoid hemorrhage; an overview. Neurosurgery 43: 863–876

Correspondence: Jae Min Kim, M.D., Ph.D., Department of Neurosurgery, Hanyang University Kuri Hospital, 249-1 Kyomun-dong, Kuri, Kyunggi-do, 471-701, Korea.

Gene Therapy

Acta Neurochir (2001) [Suppl] 77: 83–87

Gene Therapy for Vasospasm

J. M. Findlay

Department of Surgery, Division of Neurosurgery, University of Alberta, Edmonton

Introduction

The introduction of genetic material, nucleic acid, into cells in order to modify protein production and thereby prevent or treat disease, is known as gene therapy. A common form of this new treatment has been the introduction of a gene carried by a virus capable of penetrating eukaryotic cells, hoping that new gene will become incorporated into the genomic composition of the cell and become expressed, augmenting or adding a protein to the cell. This is referred to as a somatic gene therapy. Another is the inhibition of gene expression through the application of short sequences of DNA which can bind either to the gene directly or to the normal RNA message and prevent its transcription, amplification or translation. This blocking of gene expression is known as antisense gene therapy. Both of these types of gene therapy have been tested for the prevention of vasospasm in animal models, and antisense treatment directed at reducing endothelin synthesis has in particular shown some promise.

Keywords: Vasospasm; cerebral aneurysm; subarachnoid hemorrhage; gene therapy; endothelin; nitric oxide.

Gene Therapy

Gene therapy is the introduction of genetic material into cells intended to direct those cells to prevent or treat disease. The genetic material is nucleic acid, either deoxynucleic acid (DNA) or ribonucleic acid (RNA), and the molecular goal of gene therapy is to modify cellular protein production. In general, gene therapy attempts to either activate or inhibit the production of specific proteins.

The seeds of gene therapy were sewn a mere half-century ago when James Watson and Frederick Crick published their seminal report on the molecular structure of DNA [26], and the ability now to genetically manipulate cells and tissues is a direct product of the explosive field of molecular biology. Molecular biology is a science resulting from the merging of genetics, physical chemistry, microbiology and biochemistry. The potential advantages of gene therapy over conventional drug treatments include the possibility of replacing a defective gene in a germ line for disease prevention, the elimination of the need for repeated drug administration to control a disease, and the potential to manipulate the synthesis of a single protein, providing an extremely targeted therapeutic intervention.

There are a number of different types of gene therapy that exist at this time, and more under development. "Germ line" gene therapy is the transfer of a gene into zygotes to replace a single defective gene, so that the whole tissue or organism derived from that germ cell line would have a permanent and functioning copy of the gene. The disease caused by the protein's absence would therefore be prevented, and it would not be transmitted to future generations during reproduction.

The addition of a gene to mature cells is called "somatic" gene therapy, and the goal here may be to manufacture a "correct" protein (the native gene being somehow defective), increase the production of a beneficial protein, or to produce a new protein that is useful to the organism. Since naked nucleic acid is very inefficient at entering (or "transfecting") most eukaryotic cells, with the exception of skeletal and cardiac muscle, a "vector" or carrier is usually needed to deliver a gene into a cell and then alter that cell's production of protein. Viruses are very good at penetrating human cells, and some common viral-derived vectors for gene delivery are adenovirus (AV), adeno-associated virus (AAV), herpes simplex virus (HSV), all of which are DNA viruses, and retroviruses, which are RNA viruses. Each of these vectors, as well as new and different vectors in development, has its advantages and disadvantages and specific uses or potential uses [21]. Needless to say, to be useful and safe these viruses must be unable to divide, multiply ("replication deficient"), or harm the recipient, and this hazard is a very important consideration with viral vectors.

Another type of gene therapy is to prevent or reduce or downregulate the production of a harmful protein with genetic material that interferes with gene expression. This type of gene therapy is known as "antisense", and it consists of the introduction of exogenously manufactured short sequences of nucleic acid, oligonucleotides (ODNs), with a base sequence complementary to that of a chosen and normal "sense" mRNA [7]. These exogenous strands will then bind to the normal message used by the cell for translation into a polypeptide, thus preventing protein synthesis and blocking expression of the target gene.

Gene Therapy for Vascular Disease

Gene therapy has been applied experimentally to prevent and treat a number of different vascular and cerebrovascular conditions (Table 1), although to my knowledge none has yet been applied clinically to treat human vascular disease at the time of this writing.

While most familial predispositions to stroke are polygenic and multifactorial, some specific conditions are associated with a single gene defect and a resulting stroke risk, and they are potential candidates for gene therapy. Examples include sickle cell disease, protein S and C deficiencies, homocystinuria, neurofibromatosis and some of the hyperlipidemias [27]. Since many of these have multi-organ involvement cure or palliation would require diffuse or germ line gene therapy – introducing the correct gene into a zygote which could then populate the growing organism, providing it and its tissues with the correct and functional enzyme or structural protein.

Table 1. *Gene Therapy for Vascular Diseases*

Potential cerebrovascular applications:
– Correct a defined mutation causing a hereditary predisposition to stroke, *i.e. sickle cell disease, protein S and C deficiencies, homocystinuria, NF-1, hyperlipidemias, etc.*
– Prevent cell proliferation and arterial stenosis/restenosis, *i.e. eNOS, HSV thymidine kinase-ganciclovir system, VEGF production, antiapoptotic gene products, etc.*
– Reduce ischemic neuronal damage, *i.e. SOD, HSPs, IEGs (c-FOS, c-JUN), nNOS, trophic factors, (FGF) etc.*

Another area that has received great interest for genetic intervention is vascular stenosis, and especially restenosis following endarterectomy or bypass or angioplasty, often due to myointimal or smooth muscle cell proliferation – processes related to the pathogenesis of atherosclerosis. Genetically modifying a segment of arterial wall in vivo requires penetrating the wall with gene, and transfecting the vessel from the luminal side, the commonest approach considered, requires a temporary blockage of blood flow. A number of different arterial catheters which can cause temporary occlusion and release vector at the same time for penetration in the proximal arterial segment, have been designed [6, 22, 27]. Genes used in this approach in experimental models include those coding for endothelial nitric oxide synthase (eNOS), since NO relaxes arteries and reduces cell proliferation, and thymidine kinase which renders proliferating cells sensitive to ganciclovir killing much like in the more common application of this same system for tumors. Antisense ODNs directed at genes involved in cell cycle regulation have also been used to reduce cell proliferation and neointimal formation.

There is also interest in trying to ameliorate ischemic damage by altering the expression of proteins in threatened brain tissue, perhaps in the ischemic penumbra, and examples here include the upregulation of neuroprotective proteins, such as free-radical scavengers, heat-shock proteins, immediate early gene products, and trophic factors, or downregulating neuronal NOS, the activity of which appears to generate excessive free radicals [27].

Gene Therapy for Cerebral Vasospasm

The pathogenesis of cerebral vasospasm may lie in part or in whole in an over or underexpression of specific proteins within the vessel wall, or a combination of both. Increased levels of the vasoconstrictor endothelin (ET) and downregulation of eNOS, which synthesizes vasodilator NO, are several possibilities [4]. Supporting these hypotheses has been the demonstration in animal experiments that either supplying NO donors or antagonizing ET can prevent or reduce vasospasm [1–3, 5, 8, 10, 11, 13, 20, 23, 24, 28, 29]. The genes for these proteins might, therefore, be suitable targets for vasospasm prevention or treatment.

Vasospasm is potentially quite suitable for gene therapy approaches. It is a relatively short-lived disease process, lasting several weeks at the most, which is therefore consistent with the generally transient nature of somatic gene therapy. Cerebral arteries are also unique in that they travel through a liquid environment in the subarachnoid space, making at least the larger conducting vessels at or near the circle of Willis (the arteries generally most affected by vasospasm) accessible to gene delivery on their abluminal or adventitial side simply by injecting vector or genetic material directly into the CSF.

Muhonen *et al.* used an AV vector to transfer the reporter gene β-galactosidase to cerebral arteries, which when expressed in tissue can be easily detected with histochemical staining [12]. The virus was injected into the cisterna magna of dogs two days following experimental subarachnoid hemorrhage (SAH). They found efficient transfer of the gene to the leptomeninges on the basal surface of the brain for up to a week, and the gene also penetrated the adventitial but not the tunica media or intima of the cerebral vessels in contact with the subarachnoid space. They speculated that if genes encoding enzymes with vasodilator functions could be transferred to arteries in this way, this might be a useful way of treating vasospasm.

Onoue *et al.* successfully transferred the eNOS gene into both normal and vasospastic canine basilar artery strips ex vivo using an AV vector, and demonstrated partial restoration of NO-mediated relaxations in the transfected arteries [19].

The first study to examine the effects of eNOS gene transfer in vivo following SAH also used an AV vector, bearing either the eNOS or reporter β-galactosidase gene, injected into the cisterna magna of dogs along with the first of two blood injections a day apart [25]. Seven days later β-galactosidase was expressed in both leptomeninges and adventitial layer of the cerebral arteries, just as Muhonen *et al.* found. There was also good evidence that eNOS was expressed in the dogs that received it, with increased NO metabolites detected in the CSF on day 2, greater in vitro sensitivity to L-arginine (the substrate for eNOS) when arteries were studied in vitro after harvesting on day 7, and mRNA for eNOS detectable in the leptomeninges of only those animals given the eNOS gene. However, despite this evidence of increased eNOS activity and therefore greater vasorelaxant production in treated animals, angiographic vasospasm was not prevented in this experiment, and the authors speculated that this might be due to either inadequate amounts of eNOS, or perhaps the powerful scavenging effect of free hemoglobin in the subarachnoid space destroying the NO as it was being generated.

Another approach to vasospasm prevention has been to use antisense technologies to try to suppress synthesis of the powerful vasoconstrictor polypeptide, endothelin. Onoda *et al.* administered prepro-endothelin-1 (the longer polypeptide chain precursor to ET-1) antisense ODNs into the cisterna magna of rats and found histopathological evidence that they penetrated the basilar artery wall, a reduction in arterial levels of preproET-1 mRNA (good evidence of gene suppression), and finally an inhibitory effect of antisense treatment on vasoconstrictor responses to blood hemolysate when the arteries were observed in vivo [16].

This same approach was examined in a large animal model by Ohkuma *et al.* [14]. In the canine double-hemorrhage model of vasospasm, these investigators used antisense preproET-1 alone or in combination with the fibrinolytic agent recombinant tissue plasminogen activator (rt-PA). Once again, immunohistochemical staining of the arteries indicated on ODN penetration of the cerebral artery walls. In this model, vasospasm on day 7 was mildly reduced by antisense treatment alone ($64 \pm 13\%$ of baseline caliber, compared to $51 \pm 8\%$ baseline caliber for controls, NS), and rt-PA alone resulted in moderate reduction ($81 \pm 5\%$ baseline caliber, $p < 0.01$). The combination of antisense treatment with rt-PA, however, almost completely prevented vasospasm ($95 \pm 6\%$ baseline caliber, $p < 0.01$). The antisense treatment combined with rt-PA resulted in reduced preproET-1 expression, as demonstrated by immunohistochemical staining of the arteries, and reduced preproET-1 mRNA levels on day 4, as measured by reverse transcription-polymerase chain reaction. Nonsense DNA sequences had no effect on the vessels. The results of this experiment supported a causative role for ET-1 early in the course of vasospasm development in dogs. The apparent additive therapeutic effects of antisense and fibrinolytic treatments could be due to clot lysis allowing better delivery of ODNs to arteries within the subarachnoid space.

The preproET-1 antisense approach has also been used in a monkey model of vasospasm, again with results suggesting an inhibition of the vasospastic response of cerebral arteries to blood [17]. Antisense has also been directed at a mediator of inflammation,

Table 2. *Possible Gene Therapy Strategies for Cerebral Vasospasm*

- Add or augment gene for free radical scavenging enzyme or protein (*free radical generation may initiate the vasospasm cascade*)
- Add or augment gene for vasorelaxant production (*i.e. nitric oxide*)
- Inhibit expression of phospholipase (*phospholipid hydrolysis may lead to diacylglycerol generation and protein kinase C activation*)
- Inhibit gene expression of proinflammatory proteins (*inflammation may play a role in the structural changes found in the vasospastic vessel wall*)
- Inhibit gene expression of vasoconstrictor (*i.e. endothelin*)
- Inhibit gene expression of receptor or G protein (*endothelin may trigger vasospasm through this interaction*)
- Inhibit gene expression of protein kinase C (*may mediate the vasospastic cascade*)
- Add or augment gene for contractile regulatory proteins (*i.e. calponin, caldesmon, the degradation of which may result in unrestricted chronic vasospasm*)
- Inhibit gene expression for contractile protein (*i.e. alpha actin, necessary for actin-myosin sliding and smooth muscle contraction*)

nuclear factor KB, in a rabbit model of SAH [15], as well as procollagen in the rat femoral artery model of vasospasm [18], both studies reporting positive results in terms of vasospasm reduction.

The Future of Gene Therapy for Cerebral Vasospasm

As one surveys the number of cellular mechanisms possibly or probably involved in the induction of vasospasm, it becomes apparent that there are a number of potential targets for gene therapy in this condition. Up-regulation of free radical scavengers or contraction regulatory proteins (i.e. calponin and caldesmon), or conversely down-regulation of contractile enzymes or proteins (i.e. protein kinase C, alpha actin) are just several examples, and some of these have already been tested (Table 2). Perhaps the very complexity of the vasospastic process, involving multiple mediators and several pathways activated either simultaneously or sequentially over time, will be the undoing of this particular application of gene therapy. A single protein target may just not be sufficient. Other concerns include vector-induced inflammation and of course disturbance of normal cellular functions. Finally, the size and complexity of the clot-laden human subarachnoid space might provide a greater obstacle to gene therapy delivery via CSF in man than has been seen in most experimental models.

Still, the transient nature of vasospasm and gene therapy alike, and its at least potential simplicity and safety when delivered into the CSF, make it an attractive area of research, where more work is sure to follow.

References

1. Afshar JKB, Pluta RM, Boock RJ, Thompson BG, Oldfield ED (1995) Effect of intracarotid nitric oxide on primate cerebral vasospasm after aneurysm subarachnoid hemorrhage. J Neurosurg 83: 118–122
2. Clozel M, Watanabe H (1993) BQ-123 a peptidic endothelin ETA receptor antagonist, prevents the early cerebral vasospasm following subarachnoid hemorrhage after intracisternal but not intravenous injection. Life Sci 52: 825–834
3. Cosentino F, McMahon EG, Carter JS, Katušic ZS (1993) Effect of endothelinA-receptor antagonist B1-123 and phosphoramidon on cerebral vasospasm. J Cardiovasc Pharmacol 22: S332–335
4. Dietrich HH, Dacey Jr. RG (2000) Molecular keys to the problems of cerebral vasospasm. Neurosurgery 46: 517–530
5. Foley PL, Caner HH, Kassell NF, Lee KS (1994) Reversal of subarachnoid hemorrhage-induced vasoconstriction with an endothelin receptor antagonist. Neurosurgery 34: 108–112
6. Heistad DD, Faraci FM (1996) Gene therapy for cerebral vascular disease. Stroke 27: 1688–1693
7. Helene C, Toulme JJ (1990) Specific regulation of gene expression by antisense, sense, and antigene nucleic acids. Biochim Biophys Acta 1049: 99–125
8. Hino A, Weir BKA, Macdonald RL, Thisted RA, Kim C, Johns LM (1995) Prospective, randomized, double-blind trial of BQ-123 and bosentan for prevention of vasospasm following subarachnoid hemorrhage in monkeys. J Neurosurg 83: 503–509
9. Itoh S, Sasaki T, Ide K, Ishikawa K, Nishikibe M, Yano M (1993) A novel endothelin ET_A receptor antagonist, BQ-485, and its preventative effect on experimental cerebral vasospasm in dogs. Biochem Biophys Res Comm 195: 969–975
10. Kwan A, Bavbek M, Jeng AY, Maniara W, Toyoda T, Lappe RW, Kassell NF, Lee KS (1997) Prevention and reversal of cerebral vasospasm by an endothelin-converting enzyme inhibitor, CGS 26303, in an experimental model of subarachnoid hemorrhage. J Neurosurg 87: 281–286
11. Matsumura Y, Ikegawa R, Suzuki Y, Takaoka M, Uchida T, Kido H, Shinyama H, Hayashi K, Watanabe M, Morimoto S (1991) Phosphoramidon prevents cerebral vasospasm following subarachnoid hemorrhage in dogs: the relationship to endothelin-1 levels in the cerebrospinal fluid. Life Sci 49: 841–848
12. Muhonen MG, Ooboshi H, Welsh MJ, Davidson BL, Heistad DD (1997) Gene transfer for cerebral blood vessels after subarachnoid hemorrhage. Stroke 28: 822–829
13. Nirei H, Hamanda K, Shoubo M, Sogabe K, Notsu Y, Ono T (1993) An endothelin ETA receptor antagonist, FR139317, ameliorates cerebral vasospasm in dogs. Life Sci 52: 1869–1874
14. Ohkuna H, Parney I, Megyesi J, Ghahary A, Findlay JM (1999) Antisense preproendothelin-oligoDNA therapy for vasospasm in a canine model of subarachnoid hemorrhage. J Neurosurg 85: 846–852
15. Ono S, Date I, Onoda K, Shiota T, Ohmoto T, Ninomiya Y, Asari S, Morishita R (1998) Decoy administration of NF-KB into the subarachnoid space for cerebral angiopathy. Human Gene Ther 9: 1003–1011
16. Onoda K, Ono S, Ogihara K, Shiota T, Asari S, Ohmoto T, Ninomiya Y (1996) Inhibition of vascular contraction by intracisternal administration of preproendothelin-1 mRNA antisense

oligoDNA in a rat experimental vasospasm model. J Neurosurg 85: 846–852
17. Onoda K, Ohmoto T, Yasuda T, Ninomiya Y, Mayberg M (1997) Attempted gene therapy for a monkey vasospasm model. Proceedings of the Fith International Conference on Cerebral Vasospasm – Sydney pp 144–146
18. Onodo K, Ono S, Ogihara K, Shiota T, Asari S, Ohmoto T, Ninomiya Y (1996) Role of extracellular matrix in experimental vasospasm. Inhibitory effect of antisense oligonucleotide on collagen induction. Stroke 27: 2102–2109
19. Onoue H, Tsutsui M, Smith L, Stelter A, O'Brien T, Katusic ZS (1998) Expression and function of recombinant endothelial nitric oxide synthase gene in canine basilar artery after experimental subarachnoid hemorrhage. Stroke 28: 822–828
20. Pluta RM, Oldfield EH, Boock RJ (1997) Reversal and prevention of cerebral vasospasm by intracarotid infusions of nitric oxide donors in a primate model of subarachnoid hemorrhage. J Neurosurg 87: 746–751
21. Robbins PD, Ghivizzani SC (1998) Viral vectors for gene therapy. Pharmacol Ther 80: 35–47
22. Shafron DH, Frizzel RT, Day AL (1997) Gene therapy for cerebrovascular disease. Lippincott-Raven Publishers, Philadelphia, pp 127–138
23. Shigeno T, Mima T, Yanagisawa M, Saito A, Goto K, Yamashita K, Takenouchi T, Matsuura N, Yamasaki Y, Yamada K, Masaki T, Takakura K (1991) Prevention of cerebral vasospasm by actinomycin D. J Neurosurg 74: 940–943
24. Shigeno T, Clozel M, Sakai S, Saito A, Goto K (1995) The effect of bosentan, a new potent endothelin receptor antagonist, on the pathogenesis of cerebral vasospasm. Neurosurgery 37: 87–90
25. Stoodley M, Weihl CC, Zhang Z, Lin G, Johns LM, Kowalczuk, Ghadge G, Roos RP, Macdonald RL (2000) Effect of adenovirus-mediated nitric oxide synthase gene transfer on vasospasm after experimental subarachnoid hemorrhage. Neurosurgery 46: 1193–1203
26. Watson JD, Crick FHC (1953) Molecular structure of nucleic acids: A structure for deoxyribose nucleic acid. Nature 171: 737–738
27. Weihl C, Macdonald RL, Stoodley M, Lüders J, Lin G (1999) Gene therapy for cerebrovascular disease. Neurosurgery 44: 239–253
28. Zimmermann M, Seifert V, Löffler BM, Stolke D, Stenzel W (1996) Prevention of cerebral vasospasm after experimental subarachnoid hemorrhage by RO 47-0203, a newly developed orally active endothelin receptor antagonist. Neurosurgery 38: 115–120
29. Zuccarello M, Boccaletti R, Romano A, Rapoport RM (1998) Endothelin B receptor antagonists attenuate subarachnoid hemorrhage – induced cerebral vasospasm. Stroke 29: 1924–1929

Correspondence: J. Max Findlay, M.D., Ph.D., Division of Neurosurgery, University of Alberta, 2D1.02 WMC, 8440-112 Street, Edmonton, AB T6G 2B7.

Acta Neurochir (2001) [Suppl] 77: 89–91

The Functional Significance of Heme Oxygenase-1 Gene Induction in a Rat Vasospasm Model

H. Suzuki[1,2,3], **K. Kanamaru**[2], **H. Tsunoda**[1], **H. Inada**[1], **M. Kuroki**[2], **H. Sun**[2], **S. Waga**[2], and **T. Tanaka**[1]

[1] Department of Molecular and Cellular Pharmacology, Mie University School of Medicine, Japan
[2] Department of Neurosurgery, Mie University School of Medicine, Japan
[3] Department of Neurosurgery, Mie Prefectural General Medical Center, Japan

Introduction

Many investigators have tried to clarify the pathogenesis of vasospasm and to treat or to prevent vasospasm by its reversal [4]. However, the mechanism of spontaneous resolution, one of the crucial features of vasospasm, has not been sufficiently investigated [10]. We studied the intrinsic mechanism of spasmolysis and report the possible role of heme oxygenase (HO)-1 gene induction against vasospasm.

Keywords: Subarachnoid hemorrhage; cerebral artery; vasospasm; heme oxygenase.

Material and Methods

The following rat vasospasm model was produced by cisternal blood injection [3, 10]: one-hemorrhage rats received either 0.3 or 0.5 ml of fresh whole autologous arterial blood, and two-hemorrhage rats received two injections of 0.3 ml of blood, 48 hours apart. Control rats received saline instead of blood. Vertebral angiography was performed on Day 0 (at pre-injection, 10 minutes, 1 and 3 hours after the injection), Day 1, Day 2 (at pre-injection, 10 minutes, 1 and 3 hours after the injection) and Days 3 to 14.

Fluorescent differential display (FDD) analyses were performed on the basilar arteries with no, early, and delayed vasospasms, and the results were confirmed using quantitative reverse transcriptase – PCR (RT-PCR) analyses [10].

Antisense HO-1 oligodeoxynucleotide (ODN), sense HO-1 ODN, or scrambled ODN treatment was performed on the one-hemorrhage rats receiving 0.3 ml of blood [10]. Vertebral angiography, determination of HO-1 mRNA and protein levels in both basilar arteries and brains, and the measurement of cisternal levels of hemoglobins were performed prior to the injection of each ODN and after the injections on Days 1 to 7.

All data were expressed as mean ± S.E.M. Intergroup comparisons between the two groups or among the three groups were determined by unpaired t-test or one-way ANOVA, respectively. $p < 0.05$ was considered statistically significant.

Results

The one- and two-hemorrhage rats showed biphasic vasospasms occurring at 10 minutes (early vasospasm) and on Day 2 and Day 7 (delayed vasospasm) after blood injections. By using FDD and quantitative RT-PCR, we found that HO-1 mRNA was markedly induced in the basilar artery and modestly induced in brain tissue after blood injections.

Early Vasospasm

HO-1 mRNA was not induced in the basilar artery with early vasospasm nor in the brain 10 minutes after the injection of blood on Day 0 (Figs. 1 and 2). On the other hand, in the two-hemorrhage rats, early vasospasm did not occur after the second blood injection on Day 2, when HO-1 had been already induced (Figs. 1 and 2).

Delayed Vasospasm

In the rats receiving a larger amount of blood, more severe vasospasm and higher levels of HO-1 mRNA expression were observed (Figs. 1 and 2). A significant linear correlation was observed between the degree of delayed vasospasm and HO-1 mRNA levels in the basilar arteries exhibiting vasospasm. However, the degree and the time course of HO-1 induction in the brain did not correlate with that of delayed vasospasm. Furthermore, antisense HO-1 ODN significantly delayed the clearance of oxyhemoglobin (oxyHb) and deoxyhemoglobin (deoxyHb) from the subarachnoid space, and aggravated and prolonged delayed vaso-

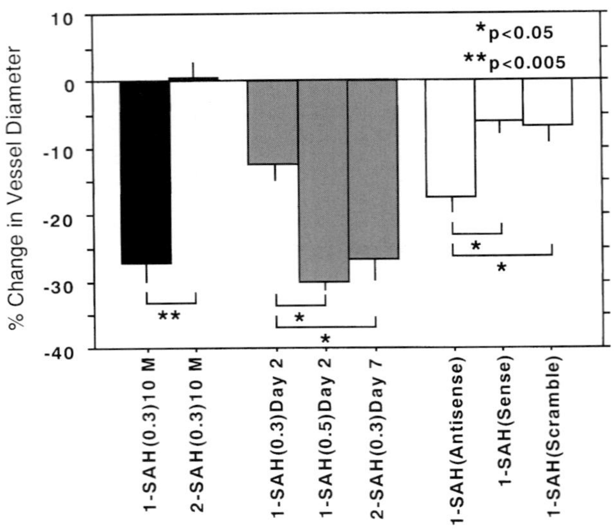

Fig. 1. The percent change from the baseline of the basilar artery diameter. 1-SAH(0.3)10 M, early vasospasm occurring 10 minutes after blood injection on Day 0 in one-hemorrhage rats receiving 0.3 ml of blood (n = 18); 2-SAH(0.3)10 M, early vasospasm occurring 10 minutes after the second blood injection on Day 2 in two-hemorrhage rats receiving two injections of 0.3 ml of blood 48 hours apart (n = 9); 1-SAH(0.3)Day 2 and 1-SAH(0.5)Day 2, delayed vasospasm occurring on Day 2 in one-hemorrhage rats receiving 0.3 (n = 15) and 0.5 (n = 3) ml of blood, respectively; 2-SAH(0.3)Day 7, delayed vasospasm occurring on Day 7 in two-hemorrhage rats (n = 12); 1-SAH(Antisense), 1-SAH(Sense) and 1-SAH(Scramble), delayed vasospasm occurring on Day 4 in one-hemorrhage rats receiving 0.3 ml of blood after the treatment with antisense HO-1 ODN (n = 10), sense HO-1 ODN (n = 8) and scrambled ODN (n = 8), respectively. The peak time of delayed vasospasm was delayed from Day 2 to Day 4 after the antisense treatment

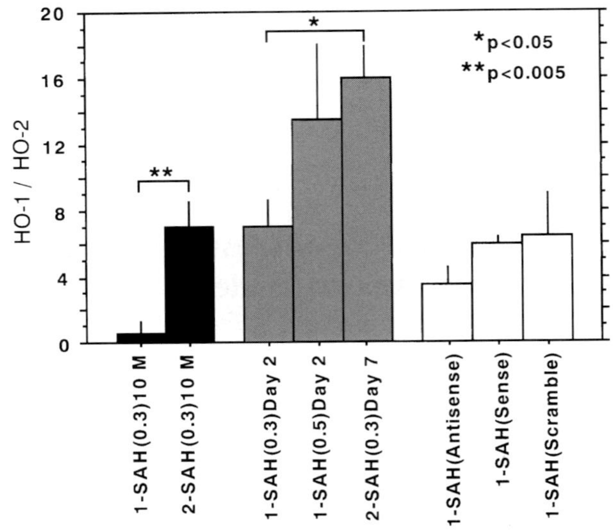

Fig. 2. The HO-1 mRNA level in the basilar artery. HO-1 mRNA levels are expressed as a ratio of HO-1 mRNA to HO-2 mRNA, since HO-2 mRNA levels were unchanged (a ratio of HO-1 mRNA to HO-2 mRNA at the baseline is 1). The abbreviations used in this figure are the same as used in figure 1. 1-SAH(0.3)10 M, 1-SAH(0.5)Day 2, 2-SAH(0.3)Day 7, 1-SAH(Antisense), 1-SAH-(Sense) and 1-SAH(Scramble), n = 3, respectively; 2-SAH(0.3)10 M and 1-SAH(0.3)Day 2, n = 6, respectively

spasm by selective HO-1 inhibition in the basilar arteries (Figs. 1 and 2).

Discussion

This study showed that subarachnoid hemorrhage (SAH) caused both vasospasm and HO-1 induction, and that HO-1 induction in the spastic artery had antivasospastic effects on early and delayed vasospasms. HO-2 in the artery wall, which may be involved in vascular tone, was unchanged after SAH.

HO is the rate-limiting enzyme in the heme degradative pathway [1, 5]. All isozymes of HO, HO-1, HO-2 and HO-3, metabolize hemin and generate carbon monoxide (CO), free iron and biliverdin (subsequently reduced to bilirubin) (Fig. 3) [1, 5, 6]. In the artery wall, HO-1 expression has been observed in the endothelial cells, smooth muscle cells, fibroblasts and inflammatory cells [1, 5, 8]. Possible mechanisms of

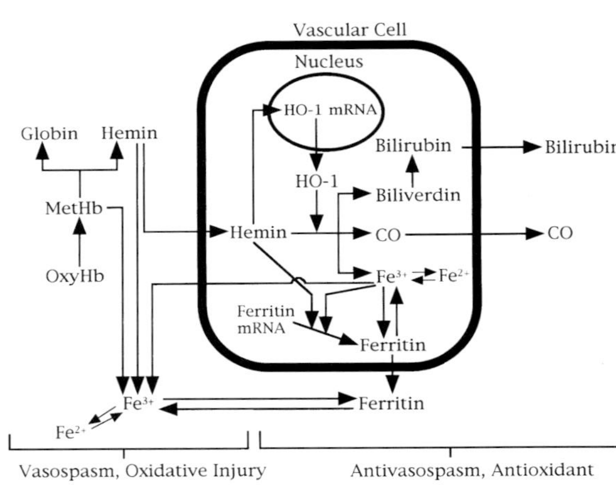

Fig. 3. Biological activities of hemoglobin, its derivatives, and HO-1. OxyHb, metHb, hemin and free iron all act as oxidants, but oxyHb has most pro-oxidant activity [2]. OxyHb may cause delayed vasospasm through multiple mechanisms including inhibition of NO and guanylate cyclase, activation of ET-1, oxidative injury (lipid peroxidation, inflammation) and proliferative angiopathy [4]. On the other hand, bilirubin and ferritin act as antioxidants, and CO may activate guanylate cyclase and inhibit ET-1 and PDGF mRNA [1, 5]. The interaction between CO and NO is also known [5]

antivasospastic effects of HO-1 induction are follows: 1) Removal of oxyHb and deoxyHb, a major factor of vasospasm, in the perivascular space as shown in this study [9, 10]; 2) Protection of vascular cells from oxidative injury by metabolizing heme which is in itself cytotoxic, by synthesizing the antioxidant bilirubin, and by sequestering catalytically active iron with ferritin [1, 2, 8]; 3) Vascular relaxation by CO (via cGMP production as nitric oxide [NO] and/or via inhibition of endothelin-1 [ET-1] production) [5]; and 4) Inhibition of proliferative angiopathy by CO (via prevention of platelet-derived growth factor [PDGF] production) [7]. OxyHb and deoxyHb may cause delayed vasospasm through multiple mechanisms [4, 9], which may be reversed by the intriguing biological activities of HO-1 and its catalytic by-products (Fig. 3). HO-1 may be induced intracellularly by hemin, which is released after oxyHb and deoxyHb possibly cause delayed vasospasm and are oxidized to methemoglobins (metHbs) (Fig. 3) [1, 2]. Therefore, a level of HO-1 upregulation in the artery may be closely correlated with the occurrence of delayed vasospasm. The development or resolution of vasospasm may be determined by the balance between the spasmogens including oxyHb and deoxyHb and the HO-1 system as the antivasospastic mechanism.

Conclusion

Not only does SAH cause delayed vasospasm, but SAH also causes HO-1 induction in the artery wall, which is an intrinsic regulatory mechanism that acts against delayed vasospasm. Therapeutic gene induction of HO-1 may prove to be a novel approach for the prevention and treatment of delayed vasospasm.

References

1. Choi AMK, Alam J (1996) Heme oxygenase-1: function, regulation, and implication of a novel stress-inducible protein in oxidant-induced lung injury. Am J Respir Cell Mol Biol 15: 9–19
2. Everse J, Hsia N (1997) The toxicities of native and modified hemoglobins. Free Radic Biol Med 22: 1075–1099
3. Kuroki M, Kanamaru K, Suzuki H, Waga S, Semba R (1998) Effect of vasospasm on heme oxygenases in a rat model of subarachnoid hemorrhage. Stroke 29: 683–689
4. Macdonald RL, Weir BKA (1991) A review of hemoglobin and the pathogenesis of cerebral vasospasm. Stroke 22: 971–982
5. Maines MD (1997) The heme oxygenase system: a regulator of second messenger gases. Annu Rev Pharmacol Toxicol 37: 517–554
6. Mccoubrey Jr. WK, Huang TJ, Maines MD (1997) Isolation and characterization of a cDNA from the rat brain that encodes hemoprotein heme oxygenase-3. Eur J Biochem 247: 725–732
7. Morita T, Kourembanas S (1995) Endothelial cell expression of vasoconstrictors and growth factors is regulated by smooth muscle cell-derived carbon monoxide. J Clin Invest 96: 2676–2682
8. Ono S, Zhang ZD, Marton LS, Yamini B, Windmeyer E, Johns L, Kowalczuk A, Lin G, Macdonald RL (2000) Heme oxygenase-1 and ferritin are increased in cerebral arteries after subarachnoid hemorrhage in monkeys. J Cereb Blood Flow Metab 20: 1066–1076
9. Pluta RM, Afshar JKB, Boock RJ, Oldfield EH (1998) Temporal changes in perivascular concentration of oxyhemoglobin, deoxyhemoglobin, and methemoglobin after subarachnoid hemorrhage. J Neurosurg 88: 557–561
10. Suzuki H, Kanamaru K, Tsunoda H, Inada H, Kuroki M, Sun H, Waga S, Tanaka T (1999) Heme oxygenase-1 gene induction as an intrinsic regulation against delayed cerebral vasospasm in rats. J Clin Invest 104: 59–66

Correspondence: Hidenori Suzuki, M.D., Department of Neurosurgery, Mie Prefectural General Medical Center, 5450-132 Hinaga, Yokkaichi, Mie 510-0885, Japan.

Acta Neurochir (2001) [Suppl] 77: 93–96

Adenovirus-Mediated Heme Oxygenase-1 Gene Transfection Prevents Hemoglobin-Induced Contraction of Rat Basilar Artery

S. Ono, T. Komuro, and **R. L. Macdonald**

Section of Neurosurgery, Department of Surgery, Pritzker School of Medicine, University of Chicago Medical Center, Chicago, Illinois, USA

Introduction

Vasospasm is a consequence of erythrocyte lysis in the subarachnoid space that releases hemoglobin and possibly other spasmogenic substances. Removing the blood clot early after SAH, either surgically or by intracisternal fibrinolysis with tissue plasminogen activator or urokinase, may prevent vasospasm [1]. In view of the critical role that hemoglobin appears to play in the pathogenesis of vasospasm, modification of the metabolism of hemoglobin and heme may be important to preventing vasospasm. Oxidation of ferrous iron in oxy- or deoxyhemoglobin produces methemoglobin that more readily releases its heme groups from the globin chains. Globin chains probably are degraded by intra- and extracellular proteases. The heme group is metabolized to biliverdin, carbon monoxide (CO) and iron by heme oxygenases (HO) that consist of at least 3 isozymes including the oxidative stress-inducible protein HO-1 [2]. Induction of HO-1 after SAH in rats was suggested to have neuroprotective effects in brain [3] and inhibition of HO-1 expression in cerebral arteries was reported to increase vasospasm [4]. It remains unknown, however, whether induction of HO-1 may be used to modify cerebral vasospasm. A first step, which was undertaken in this experiment, would be demonstration that increased HO-1 expression decreases cerebrovascular contractions to hemoglobin.

Keywords: Subarachnoid hemorrhage; vasospasm; heme oxygenase; gene therapy.

Materials and Methods

Procedures on animals were approved by the Institutional Animal Care and Use Committee. Replication-defective adenoviruses expressing β-galactosidase (Ad-βGal) or rat HO-1 (Ad5HO-1) were grown and purified [5]. Animals were anesthetized with intraperitoneal ketamine (80 mg/kg) and xylazine (15 mg/kg) and allowed to breathe spontaneously. Under sterile microsurgical conditions, a midline scalp incision was made over the suboccipital area and a 26-gauge needle was inserted into the cisterna magna. Purified adenovirus (0.1 ml Ad5HO-1 [n = 6] or Ad-βGal [n = 6] containing 10^{10} plaque-forming units [pfu]) or 0.1 ml of 10% glycerol in saline (vehicle, n = 5) were injected into the cisterna magna. The needle was withdrawn and the hole in the arachnoid membrane and dura mater was sealed with cyanoacrylate glue. One day later, rats were reanesthetized and placed supine. A cranial window was made over the basilar artery by microsurgical removal of the clivus under controlled ventilation with monitoring of blood pressure, blood gases, temperature and heart rate. Diameter of the basilar artery was monitored using a calibrated optical measuring device (Fisher Scientific, Pittsburgh, PA). Measurements were at baseline and in response to application of pure human ferrous hemoglobin A_0 (Hemosol, Toronto, Canada). Applications were made so that the final concentration in window was 10^{-7} to 10^{-4} mol/l oxyhemoglobin based on a volume of the rat subarachnoid space of 0.3 ml. Brain stem blood flow was measured by laser Doppler flow meter (Transonic Systems, Ithaca, NY) 1 mm lateral to the basilar artery. In separate groups of rats, the same doses of Ad5HO-1, Ad-βGal or vehicle were injected into the cisterna magna and 24 hours later the animals were euthanized and transgene expression was assessed by reverse transcriptase polymerase chain reaction (RT-PCR) and Western blotting to detect HO-1 messenger ribonucleic acid (mRNA) and protein in the basilar arteries and to measure HO-1 activity in arterial homogenates by bilirubin production assay. Bands on gels were quantified by densitometry. Data are given as means ± standard errors with significance as $P < 0.05$ for comparisons between groups by analysis of variance (ANOVA) followed by pairwise comparisons if significant variance occurred.

Results

Basilar arteries removed 1 day after injection of Ad5HO-1 into the cisterna magna contained increased amounts of HO-1 mRNA whereas injection of Ad-βGal or vehicle did not result in substantial expression of HO-1 mRNA. There was minimal expression of

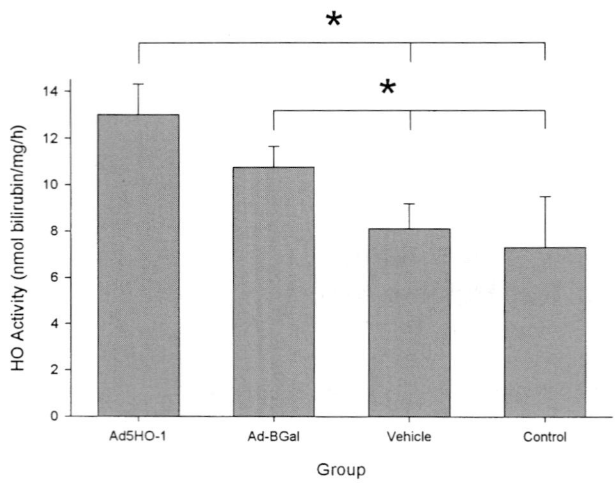

Fig. 1. Heme oxygenase activity in rats receiving intracisternal injections 1 day earlier of Ad5HO-1 (n = 6), Ad-βGal (n = 6), vehicle (n = 5) or non-treated control rats (n = 4). Heme oxygenase activity was increased significantly in the Ad5HO-1 group compared to the vehicle and non-treated control groups ($P < 0.001$, ANOVA) and compared to the Ad-βGal group ($P < 0.05$, unpaired t-test)

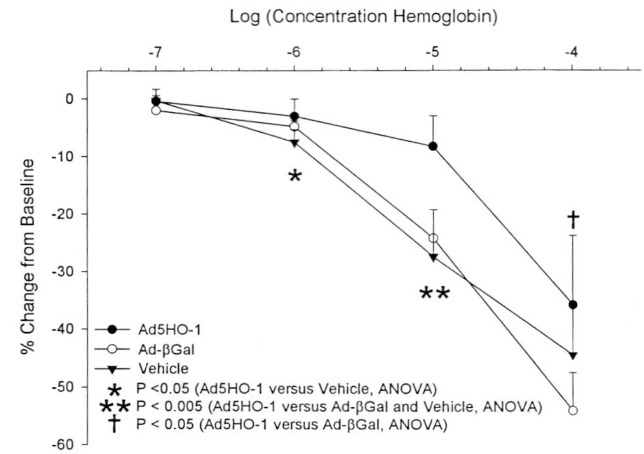

Fig. 2. Concentration-contraction curves generated by application of pure hemoglobin to the basilar artery of rats that had Ad5HO-1, Ad-βGal or vehicle injected into the cisterna magna 1 day earlier. Data are expressed as per cent change from baseline. Injection of Ad5HO-1 was associated with less contraction to hemoglobin (10^{-6} and 10^{-5} mol/l hemoglobin, $P < 0.05$, ANOVA) compared to the other groups

HO-1 mRNA in basilar arteries of rats injected with Ad-βGal although it was significantly less than in the basilar arteries of rats injected with Ad5HO-1 ($P < 0.05$, ANOVA). Significantly increased HO-1 protein, as determined by immunoblot analysis, also was observed in the basilar artery 1 day after intracisternal injection of Ad5HO-1 ($P < 0.05$ compared to other groups, ANOVA). Injection of Ad-βGal resulted in a low level of expression of HO-1 protein in the basilar artery whereas injection of vehicle did not. HO activity was measured in non-treated control rats (n = 4) and in rats 1 day after injection of Ad5HO-1 (n = 6), Ad-βGal (n = 6) or vehicle (n = 5) into the cisterna magna. HO activity was increased significantly in the Ad5HO-1 group compared to the vehicle and non-treated control groups ($P < 0.001$, ANOVA, Fig. 1). Activity was higher in the Ad5HO-1 group than in the Ad-βGal group although this was significant only by unpaired t-test ($P < 0.05$).

The diameter of the basilar artery at baseline was significantly greater in the Ad5HO-1 (423 ± 17 mm) and Ad-βGal (419 ± 13 mm) groups compared to vehicle (367 ± 11 mm, $P < 0.001$, ANOVA) although there was no significant difference in diameter between Ad5HO-1 and Ad-βGal groups. Application of pure hemoglobin led to contraction that started within minutes and that reached a maximum in 10 minutes. Washout of the hemoglobin with phosphate-buffered saline reversed the contraction to baseline diameter in 50 minutes. Hemoglobin caused a concentration-dependent contraction of the basilar artery in each group. To correct for differences in baseline diameter between groups, the contractions to hemoglobin were expressed as a percent of baseline diameter. This did not change the overall pattern, however, which was that contractions of arteries from animals transfected with Ad5HO-1 were always less. Maximal per cent contraction (Fig. 2) was significantly less ($P < 0.05$, ANOVA) in the group injected with Ad5HO-1 compared to Ad-βGal. For laser Doppler blood flow, baseline flow and flow after application of hemoglobin, 10^{-7} to 10^{-5} mol/l was significantly higher in both groups injected with virus than in vehicle-injected controls ($P < 0.001$, ANOVA, Fig. 3). For hemoglobin, 10^{-4} mol/l, flow was significantly higher in the Ad5HO-1 group compared to the other groups ($P < 0.001$, ANOVA).

Discussion

Prior investigations have shown that injection of replication-defective adenoviruses expressing β-galactosidase [6], nitric oxide synthase [7] or calcitonin gene-related peptide [8] into the cisterna magna can be used to transfect cells in the adventitia and arachnoid membrane of dogs, rats and mice. Injection of nitric

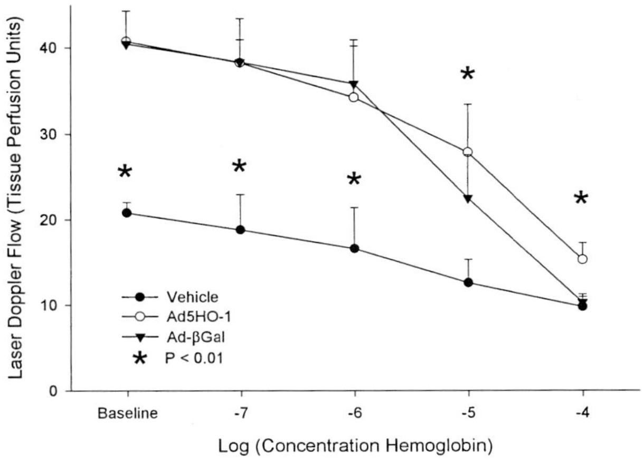

Fig. 3. Bar graph of baseline laser Doppler brainstem blood flow 1 day after injection of Ad5HO-1 (n = 5), Ad-βGal (n = 5) or vehicle (n = 6). Baseline flow and flow after application of hemoglobin, 10^{-7} to 10^{-5} mol/l was significantly higher in both groups injected with virus than in vehicle-injected controls ($P < 0.001$, ANOVA). For hemoglobin, 10^{-4} mol/l, flow was significantly higher in the Ad5HO-1 group compared to the other groups ($P < 0.001$, ANOVA)

oxide synthase and calcitonin gene-related peptide were associated with alteration of vascular function when the arteries were removed and studied in vitro [7, 8]. Most of these studies did not assess vascular function, arterial diameters at baseline or cerebral blood flow in vivo. The present study showed that injection of both control adenovirus expressing β-galactosidase and HO-1 increased basilar diameter and brainstem blood flow 1 day later. This may be because injection of virus was associated with acute inflammation and inflammation is known to increase cerebral blood flow acutely [9]. The increase in cerebral blood flow may be due to expression of inducible nitric oxide synthase in inflammatory cells with vasodilation due to the production of NO. The finding that inhibition of inflammation after SAH by intracisternal administration of antisense oligonucleotides to NF-κB, however, prevented vascular contraction 7 days after SAH argues against this mechanism [10]. Another explanation is that both viruses were associated with HO-1 expression and that CO produced by HO-1 led to vasodilation. There is evidence that CO dilates systemic arteries. CO increased cerebral blood flow in rats [11] although this also could be due to reduced oxygen-carrying capacity of carboxyhemoglobin. Brian, *et al.*, reported that CO did not dilate cerebral arteries but this finding is at variance with accepted opinion that CO is a vasodilator [12]. It is unlikely that HO-1 expression was a nonspecific response to the inflammation in the Ad5HO-1 group since the virus is known to produce HO-1 in rats [5] and there was greater HO-1 expression after injection of this virus than after injection of Ad-βGal. HO-1 may suppress inflammation so it would be expected that nonspecific induction of HO-1 due to inflammation would be less in this group. The dilation of the basilar artery at baseline that was observed could be due to nonspecific effects of inflammation. On the other hand, the specific significant increase in HO activity associated with Ad5HO-1 suggests that increased production of CO may be involved. This also would be consistent with the selective reduction in hemoglobin-induced contraction of the basilar artery and reduction in brainstem blood flow that was observed. These experiments show that overexpression of HO-1 can reduce the contractile effect of hemoglobin. Numerous mechanisms are possible. Overproduction of CO could mediate vascular relaxation or could bind to hemoglobin, preventing hemoglobin from scavenging NO. The HO could metabolize hemoglobin, producing even more CO that would have the same effects and reducing the amount of vasoactive hemoglobin. Induction of HO-1 may mediate similar effects in the systemic vasculature. Infusion of hemoglobin into rats elevates blood pressure although this does not occur 1 day after animals are stressed and at a time when HO-1 is induced in the vasculature [13]. HO-1 induction often is associated with increased expression of ferritin. Iron uptake by ferritin could theoretically be involved in preventing hemoglobin contraction since iron compounds may contract cerebral arteries and iron chelators may prevent experimental vasospasm.

Acknowledgments

Supported by a grant from the National Institutes of Health to Dr. Macdonald (K08 NS01831) and from the Brain Research Foundation. An American College of Surgeons Faculty Fellowship supports Dr. Macdonald. We thank Hemosol for supplying hemoglobin.

References

1. Findlay JM, Weir BK, Steinke D, Tanabe T, Gordon P, Grace M (1988) Effect of intrathecal thrombolytic therapy on subarachnoid clot and chronic vasospasm in a primate model of SAH. J Neurosurg 69: 723–735
2. Maines MD (1997) The heme oxygenase system: a regulator of second messenger gases. Ann Rev Pharmacol Toxicol 37: 514–554
3. Matz PG, Massa SM, Weinstein PR, Turner C, Panter SS, Sharp FR (1996) Focal hyperexpression of hemeoxygenase-1

protein and messenger RNA in rat brain caused by cellular stress following subarachnoid injections of lysed blood. J Neurosurg 85: 892–900

4. Suzuki H, Kanamaru K, Tsunoda H, Inada H, Kuroki M, Sun H, Waga S, Tanaka T (1999) Heme oxygenase-1 gene induction as an intrinsic regulation against delayed cerebral vasospasm in rats. J Clin Invest 104: 59–66
5. Otterbein LE, Kolls JK, Mantell LL, Cook JL, Alam J, Choi AMK (1999) Exogenous administration of heme oxygenase-1 by gene transfer provide protection against hyperoxia-induced lung injury. J Clin Invest 103: 1047–1054
6. Christenson SD, Lake KD, Ooboshi H, Faraci FM, Davidson BL, Heistad DD (1998) Adenovirus-mediated gene transfer in vivo to cerebral blood vessels and perivascular tissue in mice. Stroke 29: 1411–1416
7. Chen AF, O'Brien T, Tsutsui M, Kinoshita H, Pompili VJ, Crotty TB, Spector DJ, Katusic ZS (1997) Expression and function of recombinant endothelial nitric oxide synthase gene in canine basilar artery. Circ Res 80: 327–335
8. Toyoda K, Faraci FM, Russo AF, Davidson BL, Heistad DD (2000) Gene transfer of calcitonin gene-related peptide to cerebral arteries. Am J Physiol 278: H586–H594
9. Koedel U, Bernatowicz A, Paul R, Frei K, Fontana A, Pfister HW (1995) Experimental pneumococcal meningitis: cerebrovascular alterations, brain edema, and meningeal inflammation are linked to the production of nitric oxide. Ann Neurol 37: 313–323
10. Ono S, Date I, Onoda K, Shiota T, Ohmoto T, Ninomiya Y, Asari S, Morishita R (1998) Decoy administration of NF-kappaB into the subarachnoid space for cerebral angiopathy. Hum Gene Ther 9: 1003–1011
11. Koehler RC, Jones MDJr, Traystman RJ (1982) Cerebral circulatory response to carbon monoxide and hypoxic hypoxia in the lamb. Am J Physiol 235: H27–H32
12. Brian JEJr, Heistad DD, Faraci FM (1994) Effect of carbon monoxide on rabbit cerebral arteries. Stroke 25: 639–644
13. Motterlini R, Gonzales A, Foresti R, Clark JE, Green CJ, Winslow RM (1998) Heme oxygenase-1-derived carbon monoxide contributes to the suppression of acute hypertensive responses in vivo. Circ Res 83: 568–577

Correspondence: R. L. Macdonald, M.D., Ph.D., Section of Neurosurgery, MC3026, University of Chicago Medical Center, 5841 South Maryland Avenue, Chicago, Illinois, USA, 60637.

Experimental Vasospasm

Acta Neurochir (2001) [Suppl] 77: 99–102

In Vivo Animal Models of Cerebral Vasospasm: A Review

J. F. Megyesi and **J. M. Findlay**

Division of Neurosurgery, University of Western Ontario, London Health Sciences Centre, London, Ontario, Canada

Introduction

In vitro studies of subarachnoid hemorrhage (SAH) and vasospasm in animals involve the removal of the artery to be tested immediately after the animal has been killed [3]. The artery is then held in a fixation device and subjected to various test substances, which may include autologous blood. The artery is observed to determine whether contraction or relaxation occurs. Physiological, pharmacological, and morphological properties can be studied depending on the focus of the experiment. With the use of in vitro techniques, putative spasmogens have been studied, as well as potential vasospasm therapies [3].

Because in vitro experiments require the removal of arteries from their natural environment, as well as artificial manipulation, there are limitations as to the amount of information that may be obtained from such studies. For example, long-term experiments are not possible using in vitro systems. Accordingly, in vivo models of SAH and vasospasm have been developed and proposals for ideal experimental models have been put forth [8]. At a minimum, an in vivo model should have as its fundamental component a blood clot surrounding a vessel in a living animal. This blood clot should result in consistent and reproducible delayed vasoconstriction lasting several days. In better models, the vasoconstriction should be detectable angiographically, the time course of vasospasm development and resolution should be similar to that observed in humans, and animal survival should be such that efficacy and toxicity studies of therapeutic modalities are possible. In the ideal model, the experimental animal should be as similar to humans as possible and the SAH should be created in a manner that most closely resembles an aneurysmal rupture. Other desirable features of in vivo models are that they be relatively easy to produce and cost effective.

Because there are no naturally occurring animal models of vasospasm, a number of techniques have been used to deliberately produce SAH in animals, which leads to the development of delayed-onset sustained arterial narrowing. These techniques generally fall into one of three categories: 1) an artery is punctured allowing blood to escape and collect around the artery and its neighbors; 2) an artery is surgically exposed, and autologous blood obtained from another site is placed around the artery; or 3) blood from another site is injected into the subarachnoid space and is allowed to collect around arteries. Each of these techniques has its advantages and disadvantages. One common feature to all animal models of SAH and vasospasm is that the animals very rarely develop a vasospasm-related ischemic neurological deficit [4]. This is probably because the brains of animals have an abundance of collateral blood flow. Because most vasospasm experiments study vessel constriction and how it can be reversed, rather than vasospasm-related ischemia, the absence of ischemic neurological deficits in experimental animals is probably of little significance.

Keywords: Vasospasm; animal models; review.

Materials and Methods

The literature was searched to find all references to in vivo animal models of SAH and vasospasm. An online search of the medical database MEDLINE was initially performed using the key words "cerebral," "vasospasm," "subarachnoid," "hemorrhage," "animal," and "model." References were checked to determine the first description of each in vivo animal model.

Results

Fifty-seven models of SAH and vasospasm were identified in the MEDLINE search. In those models 28% use a technique in which the vessel is punctured or torn to induce SAH (and vasospasm), whereas 72% use a technique in which blood is placed or injected around blood vessels to induce vasospasm. Most models used intracranial arteries. The main advantage of these models is the presence of a cisternal space into which autologous blood can be introduced and retained. Hence, comparisons with human SAH and vasospasm are probably more valid. In vivo models using intracranial arteries have been developed in rats, rabbits, cats, pigs, dogs, and primates.

A number of in vivo animal models of vasospasm that use extracranial arteries have been developed. These use rats, rabbits, and dogs. The advantages of these models include the following: 1) the application and maintenance of blood clot around the arteries is less demanding technically; 2) the arteries are generally more accessible for endovascular procedures such as transluminal balloon angioplasty; and 3) operative morbidity and mortality are lower, animal handling is simpler, and the overall cost of experiments is lower, especially when small-animal models are used. The principal disadvantage is that the arteries under study are noncerebral.

Discussion

There is evidence that the degree of vasospasm that develops after SAH secondary to aneurysmal rupture is related to the volume and location of the blood in the subarachnoid cisterns [5]. However, the importance of the arterial rupture and the immediate pressure effects of the ejected blood to vasospasm development are unclear. Older studies performed in primates concluded that the vessel puncture technique was superior in the degree and the morphological appearance of subsequent vasospasm [1]. Nevertheless, as demonstrated in numerous models, placement or injection of blood around arteries in the basal cisterns results in consistent and significant vasospasm. Furthermore, these techniques are generally easier to perform and are associated with less animal morbidity and mortality, which may explain their greater popularity.

The use of extracranial arteries in the study of cerebral vasospasm remains controversial. There is evidence that smooth muscle vascular spasm is a general phenomenon. It probably becomes a clinical problem after aneurysmal SAH because: 1) large volumes of blood remain entrapped in the basal cisterns around intracranial vessels (and such circumferential and thick periarterial clots are unlikely to form around systemic arteries traveling in soft tissues outside of the cranium); 2) there are fewer mechanisms in the cerebrospinal fluid to dissipate and phagocytize blood breakdown products than in the soft tissues around systemic vessels; and 3) the brain is a more sensitive organ to even slight oxygen and nutrient deprivation. Experiments continue to demonstrate that under some circumstances extracranial arteries develop vasospasm that follows the same time course and has angiographic, morphological, and pharmacological features similar to those of intracranial vasospasm [7]. Such models are less costly and technically easier to perform than intracranial models. Furthermore, some extracranial models may be particularly suited to studies not readily performed using intracranial arteries.

It is interesting that so many different in vivo animal models of vasospasm have been developed in so many different species. In vivo experimental models have been used to investigate diverse aspects of vasospasm, including its natural history, pathogenesis, pathology, diagnosis, and treatment. A model used to investigate one aspect may not be suitable for another. In addition, some models require specialized equipment, facilities, and personnel that may not be available in all laboratories. Some models are considerably more costly than others. Clearly, no one model meets all the criteria as laid out by previous authors [8] or in the introduction to this paper. Some models are probably unnecessarily complex or, more importantly, do not consistently and reproducibly produce vasospasm; most of these models were used only once or twice and then abandoned.

The end point most commonly measured in animal models of vasospasm is angiographic vessel diameter. In rat models, decreased cerebral perfusion pressure (which reflects vessel constriction) is also a popular end point [10]. Morphometric determination of vessel diameter is also a precise and reproducible indicator of vasospasm [6]. Animal models have allowed authors to study the pathophysiology of vasospasm using immunohistochemical and molecular biological techniques.

Because of the relative cost advantage in using rats and rabbits, large numbers of these animals are more readily used in studies involving these models. How-

Table 1. *Animal Models of Vasospasm: Comparisons to Human Vasospasm and Suggested Best Uses*

Model	Overall correlation with human vasospasm	Best use: pathogenesis	Best use: treatment
Rat, intracranial	fair	fair	screening for pharmacological prevention and reversal
Rabbit, intracranial	good	good	screening for pharmacological prevention and reversal
Cat, intracranial	fair	fair	screening for pharmacological prevention and reversal
Pig, intracranial	good	good	screening for pharmacological/angioplasty prevention and reversal
Dog, intracranial	very good	very good	screening and preclinical trials for pharmacological/angioplasty prevention and reversal
Primate, intracranial	excellent	excellent	preclinical trials for pharmacological/angioplasty prevention and reversal
Rat, femoral	good	good	screening for pharmacological prevention and reversal
Rabbit, extracranial carotid	fair	fair	screening for pharmacological/angioplasty prevention and reversal
Dog, extracranial carotid	good	good	screening for pharmacological/angioplasty prevention and reversal

ever, the small vessel size in these species makes it more difficult to perform angiography and angioplasty, and greater leap is required to apply results from these models to human vasospasm. These models may be ideal for initially screening new pharmacological therapies in high numbers of animals before moving to more expensive large animal models.

Cat, pig, and dog models of SAH and vasospasm are generally more costly than rat or rabbit models. However, these species' cerebral vessels are larger, they are more easily subjected to angiography and angioplasty, and the results of experiments are more readily extrapolated to human vasospasm. If the number of studies using a model is any sign of its merit, the canine model of Varsos *et al.* [9] has gained the widest acceptance in vasospasm research. This model, which involves a double injection of blood into the dog's basal cistern, is the most popular vasospasm model, and its use facilitates comparison among studies at different centers.

Because primates are phylogenetically closest to humans, it may be that models using primates provide results that are most applicable to vasospasm in humans. The primate model of Espinosa *et al.* [2], developed in the laboratory of Bryce Weir in Edmonton, Alberta, Canada, has been particularly useful in this regard and is probably the best model of SAH and vasospasm available. Many of the most significant contributions to vasospasm research have been made using this model, including observations on the pathological changes that occur in vasospasm and the determinations that hemoglobin is the principal spasmogen in vasospasm, that surgical or fibrinolytic clot removal will decrease vasospasm, and that nimodipine and tirilazad mesylate may be efficacious in the treatment of vasospasm. See Table 1 for a summary of the suggested best uses for different animal models.

Conclusion

Over the past 40 years, our understanding of the pathogenesis of vasospasm and our ability to treat it have improved. Concomitantly, there has been a continual effort to develop a model that is most suitable for vasospasm study. Many models have proven to be good, some have found specific roles in vasospasm research, and a few have become mainstays, although others have fallen by the wayside. The pursuit of a better model will doubtless continue.

References

1. Clower BR, Smith RR, Haining JL, Lockard J (1981) Constrictive endarteropathy following experimental subarachnoid hemorrhage. Stroke 12: 501–508
2. Espinosa F, Weir B, Overton T, Castor W, Grace M, Boisvert D (1984) A randomized placebo-controlled double-blind trial of nimodipine after SAH in monkeys: part I – clinical and radiological findings. J Neurosurg 60: 1167–1175
3. Hongo K, Kobayashi S, Kassell NF (1990) In vitro perfusion system for the study of cerebral vasospasm. In: Sano K, Takakura K, Kassell NF, Sasaki T (eds) Cerebral vasospasm: Proceedings of the IVth International Conference on cerebral vasospasm. University of Tokyo Press, Tokyo, pp 203–206
4. Kaoutzanis M, Yokota M, Shibilia R, Peterson JW (1993) Neurologic evaluation in a canine model of single and double subarachnoid hemorrhage. J Neurosci Method 50: 301–307
5. Kistler JP, Crowell RM, Davis KR, Heros R, Ojemann RG, Zervas T, Fisher CM (1983) The relation of cerebral vasospasm to the extent and location of subarachnoid blood visualized by CT scan: a prospective study. Neurology 33: 424–436
6. Mayberg MR, Okada T, Bark DH (1990) The significance of morphological changes in cerebral arteries after subarachnoid hemorrhage. J Neurosurg 72: 626–633
7. Megyesi JF, Vollrath B, Cook DA, Chen MH, Findlay JM

(1999) Long-term effects of in vivo angioplasty in normal and vasospastic canine carotid arteries: pharmacological and morphological analyses. J Neurosurg 91: 100–108
8. Simeone FA, Vinall PE (1980) Evaluation of animal models of cerebral vasospasm. In: Wilkins RH (ed) Cerebral arterial spasm: Proceedings of the Second International Workshop. Williams and Wilkins, Baltimore, pp 284–286
9. Varsos VG, Liszczak TM, Han DH, Kistler JP, Vielma J, Black PMcL, Heros RC, Zervas NT (1983) Delayed cerebral vasospasm is not reversible by aminophylline, nifedipine, or papaverine in a "two-hemorrhage" canine model. J Neurosurg 58: 11–17
10. Veelken JA, Laing RJC, Jakubowski J (1995) The Sheffield model of subarachnoid hemorrhage in rats. Stroke 26: 1279–1284

Correspondence: Dr. J. F. Megyesi, Division of Neurosurgery, London Health Sciences, Centre – University Campus, Room 10GE-8, 339 Windermere, Road, London, Ontario, Canada, N6A 5A5.

Acta Neurochir (2001) [Suppl] 77: 103–105

Functional Characteristics of the Spasm Model by the Polystyrene Latex Bead

S. Kang

Department of Neurosurgery and Institute of Wonkwang Medical Science, School of Medicine, Wonkwang University, Iksan, Korea

Introduction

Many different and innovative approaches to prevention and treatment of cerebral vasospasm have been made, most of them promising in the laboratory but unsuccessful in clinical usage. This has been due in part to a lack of understanding of the pathogenesis of vasospasm. Furthermore, there is no animal model that duplicates all of the key aspects of human cerebral vasospasm.

Several investigators have reported that chronic cerebral vasospasm may be related to inflammatory processes [6, 9], and there are some studies which have shown that inflammatory reactions by foreign bodies such as talc [6] or polystyrene latex beads [9] cause arterial narrowing in subarachnoid space.

Currently known vasodilatory drugs that primarily influence the intracellular second messenger system were administered topically in the vasospasm models, which were created by injection of polystyrene latex beads into rabbit cisterna magna. Cyclo(D-Asp-L-Pro-D-Val-L-Leu-D-Trp) which is an endothelin receptor A antagonist (ETant) [1], nicardipine (nicar, Ca^{2+} channel blocker) [2], H7 (protein kinase C antagonist) [5], dibutyryl-cAMP and 8-bromo-cGMP (membrane permeable cyclic nucleotides) [4], nitroglycerine (NG, agents that elevate cGMP) [4], forskolin (forsk, agents that elevate cAMP levels) [7], and cromakalim (cromak, ATP-sensitive K^+ channel activators) [10] were selected. The others were papaverine (PPV) [3] classified as a phosphodiesterase inhibitor and calcitonin gene-related peptide (CGRP) as a vasodilatory transmitter [8]. This in vivo study was undertaken to determine the effects of these vasodilatory drugs on bead-induced constriction and additionally to characterize its vascular reactivity.

Keywords: Vasospasm; latex bead; vasodilators.

Materials and Methods

Uniform sterile spherical polystyrene latex beads (1.11 μm diameter) were obtained from Duke Scientific Corporation (Palo Alto, CA), and ETant from Peptides International Inc. (Louisville, KY). Thirty-one male white New Zealand rabbits weighing 3.0–3.5 kg were assigned to one of the three groups described below. In 22 animals, 1.0 ml doses of artificial cerebrospinal fluid (ACSF) containing latex beads (5 or 10 volume%) were injected into the cisterna magna 2 days before transclival exposure of basilar artery. The animals were then positioned with their head down for a minimum of 40 minutes to insure stable bead formation around the basilar artery. Two days later, rabbits were anesthetized by intramuscular injection of ketamine (50 mg/kg) and xylazine (8 mg/kg). A transclival approach was utilized to expose the basilar artery. Before opening the dura and arachnoid membrane, bleeding was controlled meticulously by bipolar coagulator. The basilar artery was visualized by stereomicroscope (Wild M8 Bunton Instrument Co., Rockville, MD) with a CCD camera (World Video Inc., Boyerton, PA) attachment. The image was projected into a videomonitor and arterial diameter was measured using a digital caliper system. Arterial diameter, blood pressure and heart rate were recorded every five minutes to insure physiological environment. Blood gas analyses were obtained every 30 minutes and blood gases were maintained within accepted tolerance levels by modulation of respiration rate and volume when necessary. Fluid level over the basilar artery was maintained at a constant level by suction and a superfusion rate of 0.9 ml/minute with ACSF. First, ACSF alone was superfused continuously for 20 minutes in order to establish a baseline arterial diameter. The superfusing solution was then changed to ACSF containing each of the following vasodilators: PPV (100 μM), H7 (100 μM), nicar (10 μM), cromak (10 μM), NG (100 μM), dibutyryl-cAMP (1 mM), 8-bromo-cGMP (1 mM), forsk (10 μM), ETant (10 nM), and CGRP (30 nM). The basilar artery was exposed to each drug for 15 to 20 minutes. Prior to application of a new drug, the artery was washed with ACSF and then allowed to stabilize for at least 15 minutes. It was not possible to administer all the different drugs to any one rabbit due to the subsequent deterioration of the rabbit's condition over time, and thus only 4 to 8 drugs could be used for one animal. Animals were divided into three groups: 1) control (non-bead) rabbits (n = 9), 2) 5 volume% bead rabbits receiving vasodilators (n = 11), 3) 10 volume% bead rabbits receiving vasodilators (n = 11). After all, the number of 5 volume% bead

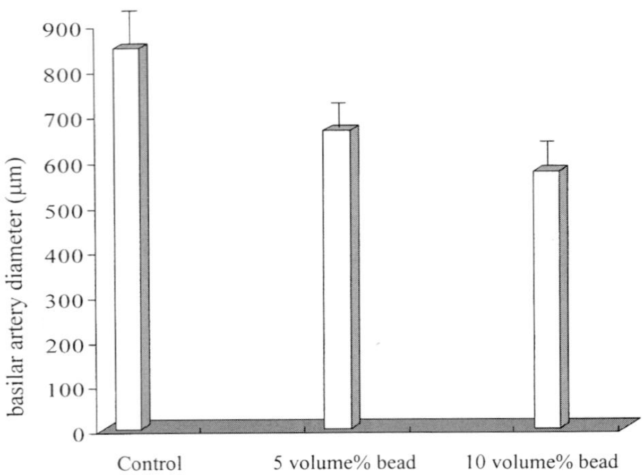

Fig. 1. Effect of bead on normal basilar artery

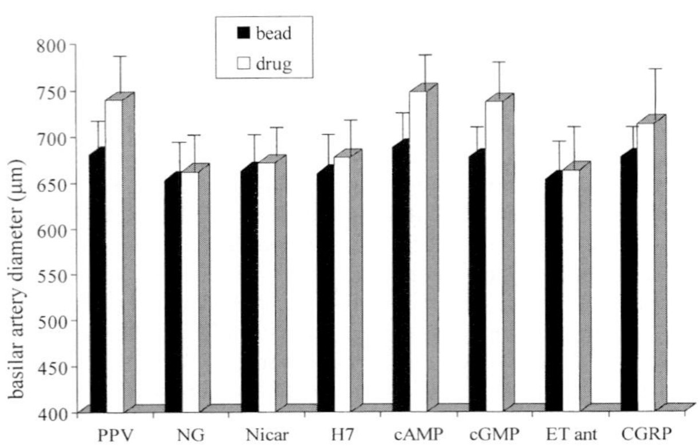

Fig. 2. Effect of vasodilators on bead (5 volume%) induced constriction

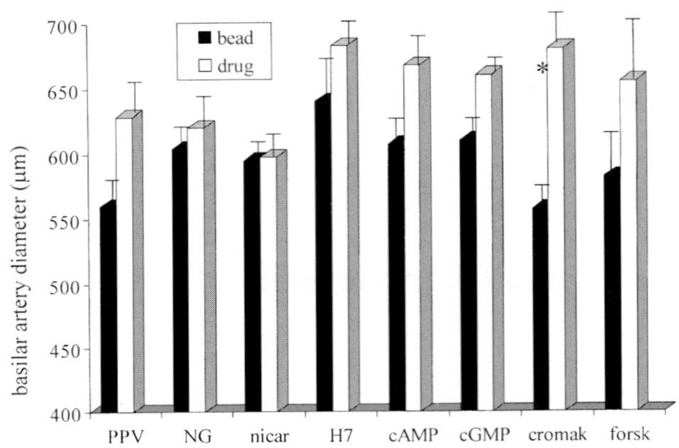

Fig. 3. Effect of vasodilators on bead (10 volume%) induced constriction. *Mann-Whitney test, $p < 0.05$

rabbits for each drug was six, and 10 volume% bead rabbits was five.

Results

The bead elicited an arterial constriction, reducing arterial diameter to 78.5% of resting tone in 5 volume% and 67.7% in 10 volume% (Fig. 1). PPV, NG, nicar, H7, dibutyryl-cAMP, 8-bromo-cGMP, ETant, and CGRP did not make a significant vasodilation of 5 volume% bead-induced constriction (Fig. 2). Moreover, PPV, nicar, H7, dibutyryl-cAMP, 8-bromo-cGMP, NG, and forsk also failed to dilate 10 volume% bead-induced constriction. Cromak alone reversed bead-induced constriction by a mean value of 89.3% of resting tone at a concentration of 10 μM (Mann-Whitney test, $p < 0.05$) (Fig. 3). Physiological parameters were not significantly different in the treated groups.

Discussion

Polystyrene latex beads are chemically stable and negatively charged in a living organism but not vasoactive. Additionally, they are recognized as foreign by the host defense mechanism [9]. Yanamoto *et al.* [9] observed maximum narrowing of the basilar artery on day two following cisternal injection of the beads in rabbits and histologically found phagocytosis of beads by macrophages in the subarachnoid space, representing the terminal phase of a non-specific immune reaction. In their experiments, 10 volume% beads provoked more severe and persistent vasospasm angiographically when compared with the model of subarachnoid haemorrhage (SAH) and vasospasm, a finding consistent with the present in vivo study.

Although the most common experimental approach for vasospasm is still to induce SAH by autologous blood injection, this has led to some of the discrepancies between results in experimental and clinical settings. In the present study, all drugs could not be administered to one rabbit with subarachnoid beads due to the high mortality rate during video monitoring, and known vasodilators that were effective in vasospasm models using autologous blood did not make a significant vasodilation. Both SAH-induced vasospasm and bead-induced spasms have advantages and disadvantages. Ultimately, refractoriness to vasodilator therapy resulting in morbidity and mortality is the hallmark of arterial narrowing that is of clinical concern, rather than reversible mild to moderate vasospasm. On the basis of this fact, drugs that reverse bead-induced spasms will have a higher probability of clinical effectiveness.

In the present results, at a concentration that selectively activates ATP-sensitive K^+ channels, only cromak relaxed vessels with latex bead-induced vasospasms. Zuccarello *et al.* [10] demonstrated that smooth muscle cells from spastic basilar arteries are depolarized and that this depolarization can be overcome by cromak. These results suggest that inactivation of ATP-sensitive K^+ channels by inflammation is possibly responsible for the bead-induced vasospasm.

Conclusion

Latex beads spasm models seem to be more similar to clinical vasospasm than models which use subarachnoid blood injection, because spastic cerebral vessels clinically tend to be rather resistant to dilation by most vasodilatory drugs. This supports the concept that targeting vascular potassium channels can be of benefit in preventing vasospasm. Further investigation is necessary to clarify the functional characteristics of vasospasm resulting from inflammation by latex beads.

Acknowledgments

This paper was supported by Wonkwang University in 2000.

References

1. Foley PL, Caner HH, Kassell NF, Lee KS (1994) Reversal of subarachnoid hemorrhage-induced vasoconstriction with an endothelin receptor antagonist. Neurosurgery 34: 108–113
2. Haley EC Jr, Kassell NF, Torner JC (1993) A randomized controlled trial of high-dose intravenous nicardipine in aneurysmal subarachnoid hemorrhage. A report of the cooperative aneurysm study. J Neurosurg 78: 537–547
3. Kazan S (1998) Effects of intra-arterial papaverine on the chronic period of cerebral arterial vasopasm in rats. Acta Neurol Scand 98: 354–359
4. Kroeger EA (1983) Roles of cyclic nucleotides in modulating smooth muscle function. In: Stephens NL (ed) The biochemistry of smooth muscle, vol 3. CRC Press, Broca Raton, Fla., pp 129–139
5. Matsui T, Sugawa M, Johshita H, Takuwa Y, Asano T (1991) Activation of the protein kinase c-mediated contractile system in canine basilar artery undergoing chronic vasospasm. Stroke 22: 1183–1187
6. Nagata K, Sasaki T, Mori T, Nikaido H, Kobayashi E, Kim P, Kirino T (1996) Cisternal talc injection can induce delayed and prolonged arterial constriction resembling vasospasm morphologically and pharmacologically. Surg Neurol 45: 442–447
7. Sasaki T, Enta A, Nozaki T, Ishii S, Senda M (1993) Carbon-11-forskolin: A ligand for visualization of the adenylate cyclase-related second messenger system. J Nucl Med 34: 1944–1948
8. Toshima M, Kassell NF, Tanaka Y, Dougherty DA (1992) Effect of intracisternal and intravenous calcitonin gene-related peptide on experimental cerebral vasospasm in rabbits. Acta Neurochir (Wien) 119: 134–138
9. Yanamoto H, Kikuchi H, Okamoto S, Nozaki K (1994) Cerebral vasospasm caused by cisternal injection of polystyrene latex bead in rabbits is inhibited by a serine protease inhibitor. Surg Neurol 42: 374–381
10. Zuccarello M, Bonasso CL, Lewis AL, Sperelakis N, Rapoport RM (1996) Relaxation of subarachnoid hemorrhage-induced spasm of rabbit basilar artery by the potassium channel activator cromakalim. Stroke 27: 311–316

Correspondence: Sung-Don Kang, M.D., Department of Neurosurgery, Wonkwang University Hospital, Sinyong-dong, Iksan, 570-711, Republic of Korea.

Acta Neurochir (2001) [Suppl] 77: 107–109

The Effect of Sympathetic Nervous System Exclusion on Cerebral Vasospasm Following Subarachnoid Hemorrhage in Rabbits

G. Bunc[1], **S. Kovačič**[2], and **S. Strnad**[3]

[1] Department of Neurosurgery, Maribor Teaching Hospital, Maribor, Slovenia
[2] Department of Pathologic Morphology, Maribor Teaching Hospital, Maribor, Slovenia
[3] Institute of Textile Chemistry, Faculty of Mechanical Engineering at Maribor University, Maribor, Slovenia

Introduction

The mechanisms of vasospasm after subarachnoid hemorrhage (SAH) are still not fully known. Most likely, local factors mediated by blood extravasation from the ruptured aneurysm under arterial pressure into the subarachnoid space are involved [10]. However, evidence that vasospasm is manifested both in extra- and intracranial arteries after SAH indicates that other factors might be involved in the patophysiology of vasospasm [3]. It is certain that, in the majority of cases, the most intensive vasospasm occurs near the largest blood collection in the subarachnoid space. However, it may also develop in cerebral vessels in other parts of the subarachnoid space in which CT reveals no blood, and even in extracranial arteries. Thus, local as well as systemic mechanisms appear to exist. Such a mechanism could be the stimulation of the sympathetic nervous system (SNS) that occurs in conjunction with SAH. The hypothesis that the SNS could be involved in vasospasm is not new and has never been thoroughly refuted [1, 4, 5]. In the present study we intended to reconsider this theory in the light of a possible further clinical applicability of SNS exclusion to prevent or mitigate vasospasm. The first aim of this study was to test the hypothesis that SNS is involved in the development of chronic vasospasm after SAH. The second aim was to explore whether the SNS acted as a mediator of vasospasm under research conditions simulating as closely as possible those seen in SAH in humans. This was achieved by the following: 1. The SNS was excluded 60–120 minutes after experimental SAH, since therapeutic measures in humans are instituted only after SAH has occurred. 2. Animals (New Zealand rabbits) whose chronological course of vasospasm is similar to that seen in humans were studied [9]. 3. Single experimental SAH was studied [13], as clinical practice also usually involves a single event of SAH.

Keywords: Cerebral vasospasm; subarachnoid hemorrhage; sympathetic nervous system; intimal corrugation.

Material and Methods

The effect of sympathetic exclusion on vasospasm was studied in 29 New Zealand rabbits under conditions similar to human subarachnoid hemorrhage divided into four protocol groups: 1. Group A: Five rabbits without SAH, which served as the control group for comparing morphologic changes in the vessel walls. 2. Group B: Eight rabbits with only experimental SAH. 3. Group C: Nine rabbits in which, immediately after experimental SAH, peroral administration of the alpha-blocking agent phenoxybenzamine hydrochloride (PBZ) at a dose of 6 mg/kg BW daily was initiated [7, 8]. 4. Group D: Seven rabbits in which, immediately after experimental SAH, a bilateral upper cervical postganglionic sympathectomy was performed. The anesthetic ketamine hydrochloride (Ketamin 10%, Veyx-Pharma GmbH, Schwarzenborn, BRD) 50 mg/kg BW administered IM was used for general anesthesia [12]. Changes in the basilar arteries of rabbits were evaluated by computer image analysis (KS 300 by Kontron Electronik), using histologic preparations of vessel walls obtained by the method of intracardial perfusion fixation (on 8th day) and stained by the H.E. method. A new measuring procedure was developed to assess changes in intimal corrugation per unit of measured vessel wall length in the form of the corrugation coefficient (CC). For each rabbit the mean value of measurements was calculated from slices of BA cut at three locations (upper, middle and inferior third of BA). CC is the coefficient between the length of intimal corrugations measured by computer image analysis and the length of the vessel section on which the measurements of corrugation length were carried out.

$$CC = \frac{\text{length of intimal corrugations } (\mu m)}{\text{length of the vessel section } (\mu m)}$$

The researchers performing these measurements were blinded for different protocol groups of animals.

Table 1. *The Results of Measurements of Corrugation Coefficient (CC) on the Basilar Arteries (BA) as well as the Basic Statistics*

	Group A (control group without SAH and treatment)	Group B (SAH-only group)	Group C (SAH plus α-blocker PBZ)	Group D (SAH plus cervical gangliectomy)
Mean CC of rabbit 1	1.188	1.544	1.124	1.19
Mean CC of rabbit 2	1.32	1.38	1.15	1.162
Mean CC of rabbit 3	1.206	1.444	1.138	1.099
Mean CC of rabbit 4	1.142	1.352	1.174	1.298
Mean CC of rabbit 5	1.104	1.312	1.126	1.272
Mean CC of rabbit 6		1.348	1.104	1.283
Mean CC of rabbit 7		1.29	1.158	1.166
Mean CC of rabbit 8		1.278	1.134	
Mean CC of rabbit 9			1.172	
n	5	8	9	7
x_{mean}	1.192	1.3685	1.142222	1.21
Stdev	0.081915	0.088536	0.023312	0.075142
Var	0.00671	0.007839	0.000543	0.005646

n The number of all rabbits in a group, x_{mean} the arithmetic mean of CC in a group, *Stdev* the standard deviation of CC in a group, *Var* the variance of CC in a group.

The study included only the vascular specimens of those rabbits in which the procedure of internal fixation was flawless. We excluded those in which in close proximity of the vessel no subarachnoid blood clot was found. The data were analyzed with the two-tailed Student t-test with Bonferroni correction. $P < 0.017$ was considered statistically significant.

Results

The results of CC measurements on the BA as well as the basic statistics are summarized in Table 1. The results of comparisons of mean arithmetic values of CC between groups A, C and D on the one hand and group B on the other using Student t-test, are presented in Fig. 1. The statistical analysis revealed intimas which were significantly less corrugated (less vasospastic) after pharmacological exclusion of the SNS by means of the α-blocker PBZ in group C, in comparison with the SAH-only group B ($P = 0.00012$). Comparison of CC values between operatively excluded SNS by means of bilateral upper cervical gangliectomy in group D, and SAH-only group B, demonstrated corrugations which were less expressed (less vasospastic) to a statistically significant degree in vessels of group D relative to group B, as well ($P = 0.0026$). The difference in CC values between control group A (without SAH and without treatment) and SAH-only group B showed that intimas were significantly smoother in group A ($P = 0.0042$). The differences in CC values among groups A, C and D revealed no statistical significance.

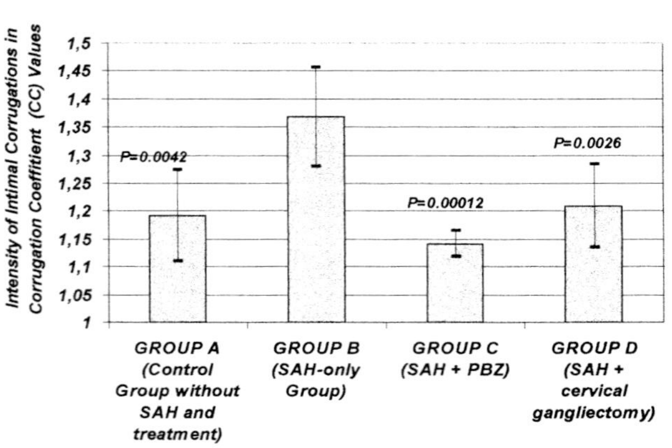

Fig. 1. Effect of SNS exclusion on intensity of rabbit basilar artery vasospastic response, demonstrated as intimal corrugation (in the form of CC) after SAH

Discussion

To our knowledge this study is the first to investigate the effect of long-term experimental SNS exclusion [4]. The results of pharmacological exclusion of SNS after SAH in group C (by the alpha-blocking agent PBZ), and of surgical exclusion of SNS after SAH in group D (by bilateral upper cervical gangliectomy) suggested that vasospasm in rabbits could also be prevented in conditions which resembled SAH in human circumstances. In fact, Vorkapic's study concerning chronic vasospasm in rabbits, which demonstrated a very similar time course in comparison with human vasospasm prompted us to perform the present study [9]. We developed a new method to measure the intensity of vasospasm. In similar histologic studies conducted thus far, researchers have compared the real luminal areas with the areas of the control animals (in angiographic studies the diameters of vessels are compared [9]) – a method which may be less accurate because of inter-specimen variability. In our method, the secondary manifestation of cerebral vasospasm, i.e. the intensity of intimal folding or corrugation per length of the same vessel section, is evaluated. Accordingly, there is no need to compare it with that of control animals. In fact, we did not compare intimal corrugations of our groups with those in the control group A, but rather ascertained significant differences, if any, in intimal corrugations between the untreated SAH group B and the treated groups C and D. In fact, the control group A merely served only as an illustration of what happens in normal vessels during the experiment. Aided by this concept of expressing intimal corrugation in the form of CC, it was possible to assess the circumference of the vessel lumen in the completely relaxed state, in which case CC is expected to equal one – a possibility which provided insight into some aspects of the physiologic behavior of rabbit cerebral arteries. Surprisingly the results of our measurements revealed that the vessels in group A were more corrugated than the vessels in group C, a finding which meant that CC was higher for the vessels of group A than in those of C. These differences were not statistically significant, yet consistent. This finding stressed again how effective SNS exclusion by PBZ was at the location of α-receptors in group C, a conclusion which is well in accordance with Fraser's research work [5]. An interesting finding was the slightly (but not statistically significant) higher CC in group D in comparison with group C. In other words, the intimas of the arteries of group D were slightly more corrugated than in group C, although SNS was excluded in both groups. A possible explanation for this difference in CC values could be that the vessels of group D are innervated not only by the excluded peripheral SNS, but also by another adrenergic innervation which had been effectively excluded by the systemic α-blocking drug PBZ in group C. Based on previous findings from research work by Csillik, Urbanski, Solomon and others, we assumed that this might be the central SNS with its humoral or direct innervational influence on the arteries under investigation [2, 6, 8]. It would be very interesting to ascertain why, after a period of intense research and clinical application some decades ago, sympathectomy became obsolete and has been nearly abandoned. Perhaps the presence of merely short-term effects in the management of migraine and other peripheral sympathetic diseases is the reason. Peripheral SNS is, in fact, known as a vital structure, and its fibers regrow relatively early after sympathectomy, which makes this treatment ineffective in the long term. As vasospasm, in these terms, is a disease of short duration, we assumed that upper cervical sympathectomy might be useful in preventing or treating vasospasm in humans as well, as Suzuki established some decades ago [7].

Conclusion

The results of the present study confirm the effectiveness of SNS exclusion in preventing vasospasm after experimental SAH in rabbits, surgically by upper cervical sympathectomy, and/or pharmacologically by the α-blocking agent PBZ. Based on these results and the potential therapeutic implications thereof, the hypothesis of a critical role of SNS in pathophysiology of vasospasm after SAH should be reevaluated.

References

1. Alksne JF, Greenhoot JH (1974) Experimental catecholamine-induced chronic cerebral vasospasm. J Neurosurg 41: 440–445
2. Csillik B, Jancso G, Toth L, Kozma M, Kalman G, Karcsu S (1971) Adrenergic innervation of hypothalamic blood vessels. A contribution to the problem of central thermodetectors. Acta Anat 80: 142–151
3. Endo S, Hori S, Suzuki J (1975) Vasoconstriction of external carotid arteries after rupture of intracranial aneurysm. Acta Neurochir (Wien) 50: 281–287
4. Flamm ES, Yasargil MG, Ransohoff J (1972) Alteration of experimental cerebral vasospasm by adrenergic blockade. J Neurosurg 37: 294–301
5. Fraser RAR, Stein BM, Barrett RE, Pool JL (1970) Noradrenergic mediation of experimental cerebrovascular spasm. Stroke 1: 356–362
6. Solomon RA, Mc Cormack BM, Lovitz RN, Swift DM, Hagemann MT (1986) Elevation of brain norepinephrine concentration after experimental subarachnoid haemorrhage. Neurosurgery 19: 363–366
7. Suzuki J, Iwabuchi T, Hori S (1975) Cervical sympathectomy for cerebral vasospasm after aneurysm rupture. Neurol Med Chir (Tokyo) 15: 41–50
8. Urbanski RW, Sapru HN (1988) Evidence for a sympathoexcitatory pathway from the nucleus tractus solitarii to the ventrolateral medullary pressor area. J Auton Nerv Syst 23: 161–174
9. Vorkapic P, Bevan RD, Bevan JA (1991) Longitudinal time course of reversible and irreversible components of chronic cerebrovasospasm of the rabbit basilar artery. J Neurosurg 74: 951–955
10. Willkins RH (1986) Attempts at prevention or treatment of intracranial arterial spasm: an update. Neurosurgery 18: 808–825

Correspondence: Gorazd Bunc, M.D., M.Sc., Department of Neurosurgery, Maribor Teaching Hospital, Ljubljanska 5, SI-2000 Maribor, Slovenia.

Acta Neurochir (2001) [Suppl] 77: 111–114

Comparison of Cerebral Vasospasm Between Young and Old Animals: Preliminary Report

I. Date[1], **M. Nakajima**[1], **K. Takahashi**[1], **S. Ono**[1], **M. Satoh**[1], **K. Iseda**[1], **H. Manabe**[1], **Y. Ninomiya**[2], **S. Asari**[3], and **T. Ohmoto**[1]

[1] Department of Neurological Surgery, Okayama University Medical School, Okayama, Japan
[2] Department of Molecular Biology and Biochemistry, Okayama University Medical School, Okayama, Japan
[3] Faculty of Health Sciences, Okayama University Medical School, Okayama, Japan

Introduction

There have been controversies regarding the influence of aging on the degree of vasospasm after subarachnoid hemorrhage. Most of the previous reports are studies based upon clinical data and there have not been detailed experimental studies. Contractile responses of cerebral arteries to vasoconstricting agents have been demonstrated to be increased with age, athelosclerosis and hypertension [4]. The cause of vasospasm is considered multifactorial, thus aging might influence the degree of vasospasm. Issues related to intraarterial infusion of papaverine for the treatment of vasospasm have often been discussed [3]. However, vasodilating responses induced by papaverine in young and in old arteries have not been compared. The present study was conducted to clarify age-related differences in vasospasm and the efficacy of papaverine.

Keywords: Cerebral vasospasm; age; papaverine; rabbit.

Materials and Methods

In the present study male New Zealand White rabbits were used. Rabbits were classified as young (2 to 3 months old) and old (20 to 40 months old). All animals underwent baseline cerebral angiography before induction of SAH and received injection of autologous arterial blood into the cisterna magna. On Days 1, 2, 4 and 7, cerebral angiography was repeated to assess the degree of vasospasm. For papaverine infusion, day 2 was selected because maximal constriction was observed on day 2 in this animal model of SAH. 5 mg/kg of papaverine was infused via the left vertebral artery and serial angiography was repeated over the subsequent 2 hours.

As for the induction of SAH, the cisterna magna was punctured by a 24-gauge butterfly needle and 1 mg/kg of fresh autologous arterial blood was injected over 5 minutes. The animals were then placed in a head down position for more than 20 minutes to facilitate blood settling around the basilar artery.

Regarding the analysis of angiograms, the basilar artery diameter was measured on a digital subtraction film with an optical micrometer scale at three points. The averages of each artery diameter at three points were obtained. The basilar artery diameter on each day post-SAH and after papaverine infusion on day 2 was expressed as a percentage of that of pre-SAH.

After the rabbits were euthanized by administration of a lethal dose of pentobarbital, perfusion fixation was performed with phosphate buffer solution followed by a solution of paraformaldehyde and glutaraldehyde in phosphate buffer. Sections of 4.5 micrometer thickness were cut and mounted on glass slides and stained with Elastica van Gieson for light microscopic examination.

All values are expressed by mean ± SEM. To compare the degree of vasospasm within groups overtime and between groups at each time, ANOVA was performed followed by post hoc Scheffe's F test. A value of $P < 0.05$ was considered significant.

Results

The magnitude of vasospasm showed maximal constriction of the basilar artery on day 2 in both young and old animals (61% in young and 44% in old). Although the arterial diameter returned to the baseline level of pre-SAH on day 7 in young animals, such a recovery was not observed in old animals (Fig. 1). Representative angiograms in young animals and old animals are shown in Fig. 2.

Although the magnitude of vasospasm demonstrated significant relaxation after injection of papaverine both in young and old animals, the effect was more prominent and prolonged in young animals than in old animals. The vessel diameter returned to the preinfusion level in about 90 minutes in young animals whereas in about 30 minutes in old animals (Fig. 3).

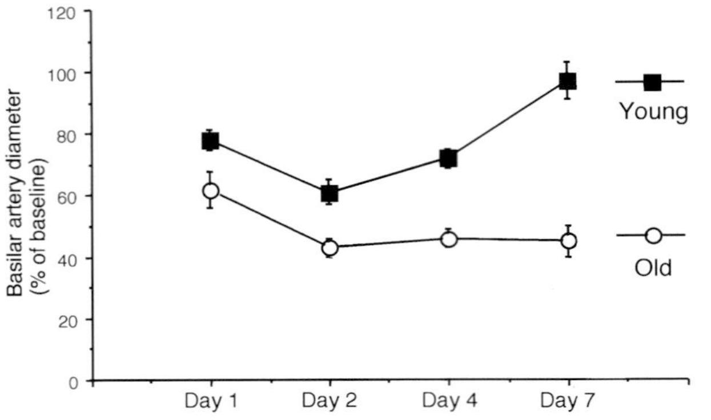

Fig. 1. Basilar artery diameter after SAH. The graph shows percent change of the basilar artery diameter compared with pre-SAH. Maximum constriction is observed on day 2 both in young and old animals. The degree of vasospasm is more prominent at all time points investigated in old animals than in young animals

Histological analysis showed that corrugation of the internal elastica lamina was observed on day 2 and resolved on day 7 in young animals. However, in old animals, corrugation of the internal elastica lamina was observed on day 1 and also on day 7. Thus, the corrugation appeared earlier and persisted longer in old animals than in young animals. Corrugation of internal elastica lamina was observed in small arteries and intraparenchymal arterioles in old animals but not in young animals. Regarding the changes after papaverine infusion, corrugation decreased in 10 minutes after infusion and disappeared in 30 minutes in young animals. In old animals, however, persistence of corrugation was observed in 10 minutes as well as in 30 minutes after infusion of papaverine.

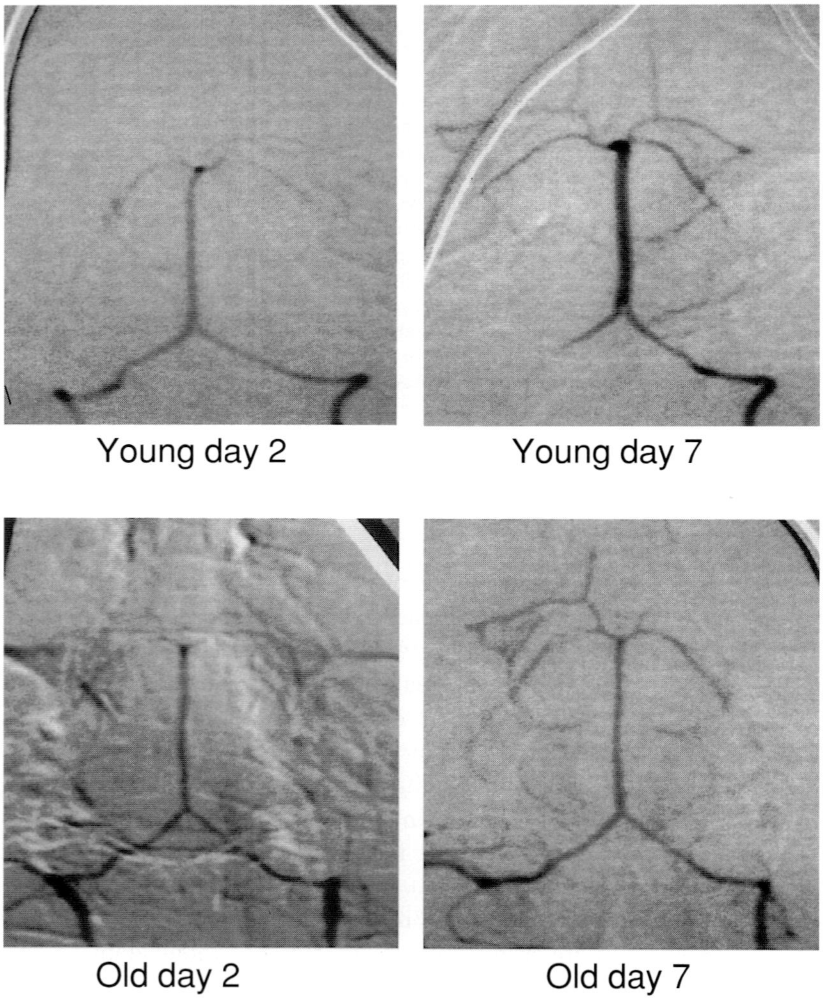

Fig. 2. Angiograms in young and old animals after SAH. Although the recovery of vasospasm is observed on day 7 in young animals, such a recovery is not seen on day 7 in old animals

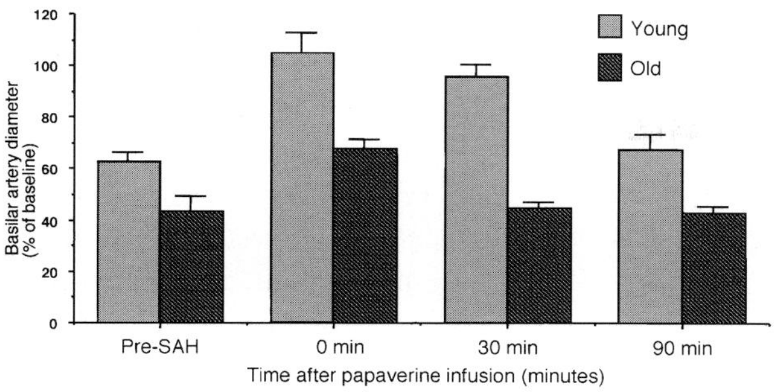

Fig. 3. Change of basilar artery diameter after papaverine infusion. The effect of papaverine in old animals is less and shorter than that in young animals

Discussion

The present study demonstrated that the degree of vasospasm was augmented and the resolution of vasospasm after maximal constriction was impaired more strongly with advancing age. Also, the vasodilating responses to intraarterial infusion of papaverine was impaired with aging.

Previous clinical studies have suggested that the incidence of symptomatic vasospasm is higher with advancing age [1, 6]. Although a rabbit model of SAH with single injection of arterial blood into the cisterna magna usually represents a mild to moderate vasospasm of the basilar artery, old rabbits in the present study showed the severe vasospasm which lasted even on day 7. This pattern in old rabbits is similar to that observed in a canine double-SAH model which is considered as an established SAH model with severe vasospasm which lasts for 14 days, suggesting that the rabbit basilar arteries are vulnerable to vasospasm with aging.

It has been reported that the efficacy of papaverine to reverse vasospasm depends on the time after SAH [5]. In the present study, the relaxation response of young basilar artery to papaverine on day 2 was significant as previously reported [2]. However, this effect was less prominent in old animals. Vorcapic *et al.* [5] reported that there are two phases regarding the arterial narrowing based on the in vivo relaxation responses to papaverine: an early pharmacologically reversible phase and a later irreversible phase and that a papaverine-resistant phase emerges on day 3 after SAH. We speculate that basilar artery in old animals had already become a papaverine-resistant phase on day 2 and that aging process may accelerate the earlier transition of the vessel after SAH to papaverine-resistant chronic stage.

We have to consider the duration of papaverine effect according to the age of the patient and the severity of angiographic vasospasm in the clinical situation.

Previous studies have shown that vasoactive agents such as serotonin, endothelin-1, thromboxane, histamine and prostaglandin E2, all of which have been considered as spasmogens, increased the direct contractile effect with aging. This may explain the part of the reasons why the aging arteries in the present study showed more prominent vasospasm than young arteries.

Conclusion

This study demonstrated that aging renders the brain vulnerable to SAH and leads to increased constricting responses of basilar arteries and intraparenchymal arterioles. Impaired reactivity to papaverine with increasing age might be a consequence of the early transition of the vessel to papaverine-resistant chronic stage. This in vivo study may explain part of the reasons why the prognosis of elderly patients suffering from cerebral vasospasm after SAH was poorer than that of young patients.

Acknowledgment

This work was supported in part by Grants-in-Aid for Scientific Research from the Ministry of Education, Science, Sports and Culture, Japan, Special Coordination Funds (SPSBS) of the Science and Technology Agency of the Japanese Government, and Health Sciences Research Grants for Research on Brain Science.

References

1. Lanzino G, Kassell NF, Kongable GL, Truskowski LL, Tomer JC, Jane JA (1996) Age and outcome after aneurysmal subarachnoid hemorrhage: why do older patients fare worse? J Neurosurg 85: 410–418
2. Macdonald RL, Zhang J, Sima B, Johns L (1995) Papaverine-sensitive vasospasm and arterial contractility and compliance after subarachnoid hemorrhage in dogs, Neurosurgery 37: 962–968
3. Marks MP, Steinberg GK, Lane B (1993) Intraarterial papaverine for the treatment of vasospasm. Am J Neuroradiol 14: 822–826
4. Mayhan WG, Faraci FM, Baumbach GL, Heistad DD (1990) Effects of aging on responses of cerebral arterioles, Am J Physiol 258: H1138–H1143
5. Vorkapic P, Bevan RD, Bevan JA (1991) Longitudinal time course of reversible and irreversible components of chronic cerebrovasospasm of the rabbit basilar artery. J Neurosurg 74: 951–955

6. Yoshimoto Y, Kwak S (1995) Age-related multifactorial causes of neurological deterioration after early surgery for aneurysmal subarachnoid hemorrhage. J Neurosurg 83: 984–988

Correspondence: Isao Date, M.D., Department of Neurological Surgery, Okayama University Medical School, 2-5-1 Shikata-cho, Okayama 700-8558, Japan.

Acta Neurochir (2001) [Suppl] 77: 115–117

Molecular Weight Interactions in Experimental Vasospasm

R. Loch Macdonald, S. Ono, L. Johns, L. S. Marton, B. Weir, Z.-D. Zhang, B. Yamini, T. Komuro, I. Ahmed, and M. Stoodley

Section of Neurosurgery, Department of Surgery, Pritzker School of Medicine, University of Chicago Medical Center, Chicago, Illinois, USA

Introduction

Vasospasm is believed to be primarily due to the release of substances from the subarachnoid clot that act upon the arterial wall to contract the artery initially and then produce pharmacological and morphological changes in the artery [2]. Numerous questions remain. For example, hemoglobin is an important spasmogen but how it causes vasospasm is not clearly understood. Whether other interactions between the brain and cerebral arteries are involved for the complete manifestations of vasospasm to occur is also unknown. In this experiment dialysis membranes of differing molecular weight cutoffs were placed between subarachnoid blood clot and the middle cerebral artery and brain of cynomolgus monkeys in order to study the molecular weight of the interaction required between clot and brain/artery to produce vasospasm.

Keywords: Subarachnoid hemorrhage; vasospasm.

Materials and Methods

14 cynomolgus monkeys underwent cerebral angiography and unilateral right subarachnoid haemorrhage (SAH) on day 0 using methods described previously [1, 4]. The procedure was modified, however, in that a dialysis membrane of differing molecular weight cutoff was placed between the clot and the middle cerebral artery (MCA). The MCA remained in contact with the brain of the Sylvian fissure. Animals were randomly allocated to have the following membranes placed: 1. 500 D cellulose ester membrane (Spectra/Por® CE sterile membrane, Spectrum, Houston, TX), 2. 300 kD cellulose ester membrane (Spectrum, Houston, TX), or 3. 100 μm nylon mesh filter (Spectrum, Houston, TX). For control measurements, each animal had left craniectomy and arachnoid dissection on day 0 under the same anesthetic. A piece of the same dialysis membrane was placed on the left side but without clot. The membrane was several centimeters wide and folded over in the depths of the exposure at the intradural entrance of the internal carotid artery so as to contain to some extent the blood clot and prevent diffusion around the edges and back to the artery. Angiography was repeated on day 7 and the animals were euthanized. Vasospasm was assessed by measuring intracranial artery diameters on angiograms. Brains and clots were studied histologically. The weight of all blood clots placed and removed was determined. Procedures on animals were approved by the Animal Care and Use Committee of the University of Chicago. Significance was taken at $p < 0.05$. All values are means $\pm$ standard deviation.

Results

There were no differences between groups at baseline. Comparisons within groups showed significant vasospasm of the right MCA in all groups (500 D: $-30 \pm 9\%$ [x $\pm$ sem] reduction in diameter, 300 kD: $-33 \pm 10\%$, 100 μm: $-36 \pm 4\%$, $p < 0.05$, paired t-tests, Fig. 1). The 100 μm membrane caused mild but significant arterial narrowing on the left side ($-10 \pm 3\%$, $p < 0.05$) but significant vasospasm was present even when this was corrected for by comparing the right and left side arteries at day 7 (500 D: $-26 \pm 9\%$ [x $\pm$ sem] reduction in diameter, 300 kD: $-31 \pm 11\%$, 100 μm: $-28 \pm 5\%$, $p < 0.05$, paired t-tests). Histopathology showed vasospasm of right-sided arteries as evidenced by reduced lumen area, corrugation of the internal elastic lamina and contraction of the medial smooth muscle cells. The magnitude of these changes was similar and not qualitatively different in the 3 groups. The left MCAs were histologically normal. There was a similar degree of inflammatory cell infiltration in the subarachnoid space around the right MCAs in each group which was mild and appeared to consist of mononuclear inflammatory cells and proliferated arachnoid cells. Very similar changes were noted on the left side and the degree of these changes

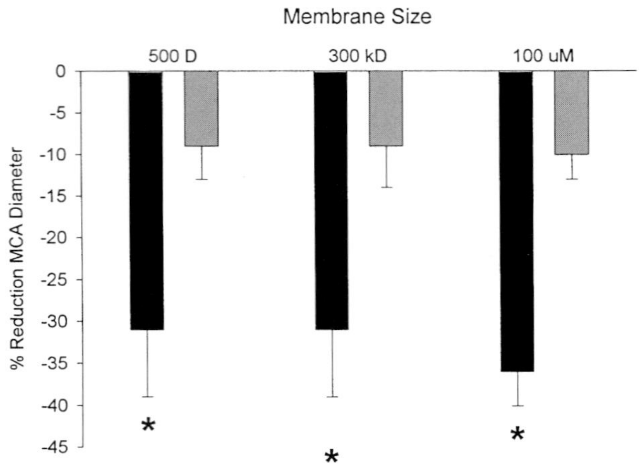

Fig. 1. Bar graph of per cent reduction in right (solid bars) and left (shaded bars) MCA between day 0 and 7 days after (day 7) placement of clot separated from the artery by 500 D, 300 kD or 100 μm molecular weight cut-off membranes (right) or membranes alone (left). There is significant reduction in right MCA diameter in all 3 groups. ▬ Right MCA, ▭ Left MCA, * $p < 0.05$

was only minimally more severe on the right. Histology of the clots in all 3 groups also was very similar and not distinguishable. There was minimal inflammatory infiltrate in the clots consisting of areas of macrophages. The most prominent change was formation of a capsule around the clot composed of spindle-shaped cells with features of fibroblasts.

Discussion

This study found that vasospasm could not be prevented by a dialysis membrane with a molecular weight cutoff of 500 D. Vasospasm that occurred was not as severe as that produced by whole blood, however, which usually causes an average of 40 to 50% reduction in MCA diameter 7 days after clot placement. Therefore, these results suggest that a substantial portion of vasospasm is mediated by an interaction that requires only low molecular weight substances to be transmitted from the clot to the artery plus brain. The limitations of the present findings need to be considered and they include the observation that no membrane completely prevented vasospasm. This study was undertaken with the idea that the 500 D membrane would constitute such a "negative" control. Further experiments are required with placement of an impermeable membrane to show that vasospasm does not occur under such circumstances. This would rule out the possibility that substances diffused around the membrane to interact with the brain and/or artery to produce vasospasm. This would seem unlikely, however, since this diffusion distance is longer than that from the edge of the membrane to the contralateral anterior cerebral artery of which the arachnoid had also been dissected. This artery did not develop vasospasm and indeed in our standard clot placement experiments, it did not, suggesting that vasospasm is a local phenomenon in this model occurring only in arteries in close proximity to the clot. It also raises the possibility that some of the reduced severity of vasospasm seen in this experiment could be due to the increased distance between the clot and artery imposed by the interposition of a dialysis membrane. The mild mononuclear inflammatory infiltrate and proliferation of arachnoid cells bilaterally suggests that at least a portion of this response is secondary to surgical dissection. There was mild, statistically insignificant narrowing of the left MCA.

We did not observe a great number of macrophages in the subarachnoid space while the clot did contain some macrophages. This does not rule out the possibility that such inflammatory cells mediate or are important in vasospasm. Peterson *et al.* noted that inflammation was necessary for vasospasm in dogs since it seemed to mediate clot lysis and release of spasmogens [4]. These results do suggest that vasospasm does not require a cellular interaction between the clot and cerebral artery. It was noted that the clot was covered with a layer of cells that have not yet been definitively identified but which resemble fibroblasts. Their role in vasospasm in this model also remains to be determined.

Acknowledgments

Supported by grants from the National Institutes of Health to Dr. Macdonald (K08 NS01831) and Dr. Weir (RO1 NS25946) and from the Brain Research Foundation. An American College of Surgeons Faculty Fellowship supports Dr. Macdonald.

References

1. Kim CJ, Bassiouny M, Macdonald RL, Weir B, Johns LM (1996) Effect of BQ-123 and tissue plasminogen activator on vasospasm after subarachnoid hemorrhage in monkeys. Stroke 27: 1629–1633
2. Macdonald RL, Zhang J, Sima B, Johns L (1995) Papaverine-sensitive vasospasm and arterial contractility and compliance after subarachnoid hemorrhage in dogs. Neurosurgery 37: 962–967
3. Peterson JW, Kwun BD, Teramura A, Hackett JD, Morgan JA,

Nishizawa S, Bun T, Zervas NT (1989) Immunological reaction against the aging human subarachnoid erythrocyte. A model for the onset of cerebral vasospasm after subarachnoid hemorrhage. J Neurosurg 71: 718–726
4. Stoodley M, Macdonald RL, Weir BK, Marton LS, Johns LM, Zhang ZD, Kowalczuk A (2000) Subarachnoid hemorrhage causes an adaptive response in cerebral arteries. J Neurosurg (in press)

Correspondence: R. L. Macdonald, M.D., Ph.D., Section of Neurosurgery, MC3026, University of Chicago Medical Center, 5841 South Maryland Avenue, Chicago, Illinois, USA, 60637.

Part 2: Diagnosis and Therapy of Clinical Vasospasm

Diagnosis of Vasospasm

Acta Neurochir (2001) [Suppl] 77: 121–126

Diffusion-Weighted and Perfusion-Weighted MR of Cerebral Vasospasm

K.-O. Lövblad[1], **M. El-Koussy**[1], **R. Guzman**[2], **C. Kiefer**[1], **L. Remonda**[1], **M. Taleb**[1], **M. Reinert**[2], **T. Wels**[3], **A. Barth**[2], **G. Schroth**[1], and **R. W. Seiler**[2]

[1] Department of Neuroradiology, Inselspital, University of Bern, Switzerland
[2] Department of Neurosurgery, Inselspital, University of Bern, Switzerland
[3] Schering Diagnostics, Berlin, Germany

Introduction

With the development of acute efficacious means of treatment of subarachnoid haemorrhage by operative or endovascular means, it is important to prevent and monitor the occurrence of late events such as vasospasm. Indeed, cerebral vasospasm is the cause of delayed ischemic deterioration in a subset of patients with subarachnoid haemorrhage. Methods such as cerebral angiography or transcranial doppler sonography [15] have been used to demonstrate its presence. Functional studies have been performed with SPECT and PET [9] and MRI was primarily used as an anatomical correlate [10, 11] for late cerebral dysfunction. In order to be able to acutely assess and select the patients suspected of suffering from vasospasm ischemia, it is necessary to dispose of a sensitive and specific modality that is able to both detect acutely ischemia and to exclude other causes of brain dysfunction. Until recently, computed tomography was the modality of choice in acute ischemia: indeed not only were there initial concerns about the safety of performing MRI in patients with intracranial clips, but CT has been shown to be very reliable for the demonstration of acute bleeding (not only in cases of SAH, but also in cases of subdural and epidural hematomas). Conventional T2-weighted imaging of the brain, which is indeed very sensitive to edema, has also been shown to not be very capable of demonstrating ischemia in the hyperacute setting; the new modality should also be able to demonstrate changes within a therapeutic window beyond which therapeutic measures would be unsuccessful. However, new generations of aneurysm clips are allowed for use in MR imaging, making the investigation of vasospasm possible.

Keywords: Magnetic resonance imaging; subarachnoid haemorrhage; vasospasm; diffusion imaging; echo; planar.

Diffusion-Weighted Imaging

Diffusion-weighted imaging, developed by Le Bihan [4], is a relatively new method that allows to image the motion of tissular protons. It consists of a so-called Stejskal-Tanner modification of a spin-echo where a pair of diffusion-sensitizing gradients are applied on both sides of the 180° pulse (Fig. 1). In this model, protons that have moved, such as water (or CSF intracranially), show high diffusion values, therefore give back no signal on diffusion images, whereas protons that have stayed in place will give back a higher signal; this will be the case with cytotoxic edema that is encountered classically in acute stroke. Indeed, it is believed that a dysfunction of the membrane-bound $Na^{+-}K^{+}$ ATPase might cause an entry of water into the cells therefore minimizing diffusion [8].

Isotropy and Anisotropy Phenomena

Since diffusion occurs in all directions, it is very important to take all information about anatomical structures into account when performing imaging; indeed structures such as the myelin fibers of the long tracts are known to induce different diffusion effects and values [3]: diffusion is freer along the longitudinal direction of the fiber whereas in the perpendicular plane it is restricted; therefore if imaging is done with

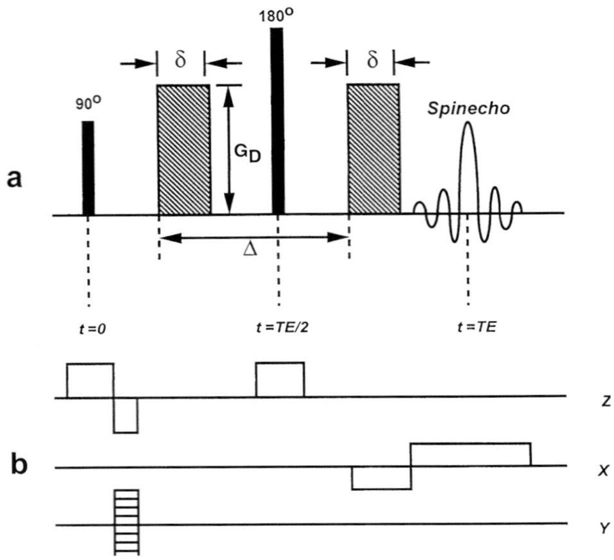

Fig. 1. Schematic representation of a PGSE sequence for diffusion-weighted imaging. It consists of a conventional spin echo sequence with identical gradient pulses before and after the 180 refocussing pulse. The diffusion weighting is dependent on the gradient strength (*GD*), the duration and the distance between the pulses

the diffusion gradient only switched in one plane, this natural restriction might be misleading and cause a false interpretation of images by untrained eyes: an infarct might be lost in the internal capsule which is bright when the gradient is switched in the corresponding direction. It is therefore important to acquire images with the gradients switched in at least 3 directions: along the phase, read and slice directions (corresponding to the x, y and z directions); one might then either look sequentially at all three image sets or from these images a so-called trace image may be calculated which contains no more information about fiber direction; direct isotropic imaging may also be performed with the correct sequence.

Apparent Diffusion Coefficient (ADC)

Since diffusion is measured in tissue, it is very susceptible to the presence of natural obstacles such as membranes. Thus the diffusion we are now measuring is not free but apparent. The apparent diffusion coefficient can be calculated by measuring at least two identical images at different b values; this b value corresponds to the diffusion sensitivity of an image. Usually the b0 (corresponding to a T2-weighted image) and the maximum b value, which is close to 1000 (which is the diffusion-weighted image itself) are used. So-called ADC maps can then be calculated and values can be determined on-line: on these images there is a signal drop (hypointensity) in an area of decreased diffusion (corresponding to ischemia), which is bright (hyperintense) on diffusion-weighted images obtained at the maximum b value, which might not be seen on T2-weighted images at the same acute moment. The ADC has initially a low value in stroke and tends to pseudo-normalize and to be elevated lately [14]. When one has gathered knowledge about the dynamics of the ADC, measuring the ADC should allow to obtain an indication not only about the objective quantity of diffusion but also about the age of certain strokes. In some cases, e.g. when the T2 effects (chronic strokes or tumors) are very important, a so-called shine-through effect might give the false impression of hyperintensity on diffusion-weighted images (since they also contain some amount of T2 information). By itself, diffusion-weighted imaging is very motion sensitive; therefore it was initially quite difficult to implement in a clinical setting. Echo-planar imaging, which allows to collect the data necessary to the formation of an image in a few milliseconds, has changed this: indeed it is now possible to acquire images that are less prone to bulk motion or to physiological artifacts (CSF, cardiac pulsations). This led to first clinical studies of whole-brain diffusion-weighted imaging [1, 6, 7, 14, 16, 17]. EPI is however associated with severe anatomic distortions and susceptibility artifacts; this renders imaging of structures in the posterior fossa and close to the skull base difficult.

Studies of the Sensibility and Specificity of DWI in Acute Stroke

Retrospective studies have shown that DWI has a high sensitivity and specificity for the detection of ischemia [7] and to correlate with clinical signs and eventual outcome [6]. Also, in addition to the information about tissue damage given by diffusion-weighted MRI, it is important to be able to assess the state of perfusion in both the areas of normal and abnormal perfusion. Indeed, we have seen that infarcts have a tendency to grow, especially if the so-called diffusion/perfusion mismatch was large. When looking at a series of patients with acute stroke that had undergone both DWI and PWI, Sorensen found that the DWI volume was generally smaller and the PWI larger than the final infarct, indicating that both methods are necessary complements to determine the exact extent of the underlying ischemia [16]. This should allow to better select and follow-up patients for studies of stroke, whether only for the investigation of the natural history (if a patient declines treatment or arrives at our institution well beyond the therapeutic window). This explains why perfusion imaging is an important adjunct to the assessment of patients with cerebrovascular diseases.

Perfusion-Weighted MR Techniques

With the advent of echo-planar imaging techniques, it was also possible to implement studies of cerebral perfusion done with MR [13]: Indeed by repeatedly acquiring a whole-brain data set of susceptibility-sensitive MR sequences, it is possible to demonstrate the susceptibility effects caused by the arrival of Gd-DTPA in the vessels. A power injector is to be used in order to obtain a reproducible high rate of injection.

Vasospasm Following SAH

Rordorf *et al.* sought to identify tissue ischemia and early ischemic injury with combined diffusion-weighted (DW) and hemodynamically weighted (HW) MRI in patients with vasospasm after SAH. They hypothesized that large HW imaging (HWI) abnormalities would be present in treated patients at the time they develop neurological deficit due to vasospasm without matching DW imaging (DWI) abnormalities. They found that small, sometimes multiple, ischemic lesions on DWI were seen encircled by a large area of decreased rCBF and increased MTT in all patients with symptomatic vasospasm. Decreases in rCBV were not prominent. MRI hemodynamic abnormalities occurred in regions supplied by vessels with angiographic vasospasm or in their watershed territories. All patients with neurological deficit showed an area of abnormal tMTT much larger than the area of DWI abnormality. MRI images were normal in the asymptomatic patient with angiographic vasospasm and the patient with normal angiogram and no clinical signs of vasospasm. They concluded that DW/HW MRI in symptomatic vasospasm can detect widespread changes in tissue hemodynamics that encircle early foci of ischemic injury [12]. Bracard *et al.* further reported the case of a patient presenting an asymptomatic vasospasm with a focal, reversible apparent diffusion coefficient (ADC) decrease after a middle cerebral artery aneurysm rupture [2]: the decrease was found to be localized in the MCA territory. Two further patients were imaged with multimodality MRI during spasm in another study [5] and in one case a hyperintensity could be detected by DWI.

Bern fMRI Vasospasm Study

Patients with clinical and CT signs of SAH admitted to the Neurosurgical department of the University of Bern were included in this study. MRI of the brain was performed on a 1.5 T Magnetom Vision system (Siemens, Erlangen), equipped with a head coil, capable of echo-planar imaging and which also has a three-axis gradient booster, gradient amplitude of 35 mT/m, rise-time of 150 milliseconds and a slew rate of 170 T/m. For DWI, an isotropic multi-slice single-shot spin-echo echo-planar sequence is used (TR = 4000 ms, TE = 133 ms, FOV = 210 mm, matrix 128 × 128, NEX = 4 with a total imaging time of 24 seconds), which generates eighteen 5 mm thick axial slices with b values of 0 and 972 s/mm2. Apparent diffusion coefficient (ADC) values were subsequently calculated from pixel-by-pixel ADC maps generated with the MR console software: the slices with b values of 0 and 972 were matched and ADC maps were obtained for each slice: ADC values are obtained corresponding to the Stejskal and Tanner equation; normal values established on this system on 30 volunteers previously were: 0.92×10^{-3} mm^2/s for grey matter, 0.93×10^{-3} mm^2/s for white matter and 3.3×10^{-3} mm^2/s for cerebrospinal fluid.

Using the same methodology, regions of interest were determined using the console software as circles in the small areas of disturbed signal on the ADC maps. Then spin-echo T1 (TE = 12 ms, TR = 528 ms, twenty-four 5 mm thick slices, matrix 96 × 200, NEX = 2) – and turbo-spin-echo T2/PD (TE = 98/16 ms, TR = 3176, 24 5 mm thick slices, matrix 180 × 256, 5 mm thick slices, NEX = 2)-weighted imaging in the axial plane was performed. Currently the imaging protocol we perform for patients with proven SAH also comprises: T2*-weighteed susceptibility sensitive sequences (TR: 640 ms; TE: 15 ms, flip angle 20°; twenty 5 mm thick slices, matrix: 180 × 256), as well as a dynamic perfusion sequence: twelve images being acquired repeatedly every two seconds forty times (for a total of 80 seconds). Parameters currently used are: TR: 2000 ms, TE: 60 ms, 12 slices 5 MM thick, axial, 40 acquisitions, FOV: 240 × 240, Matrix: 128 × 128, with a total acquisition time of 01 : 20 (80 sec). Contrast is administered at a rate of 5 ml/sec through a cubital vein with a total of 15 ml of Gadovist 1.0 (gadobutrol, Schering AG, Berlin, Germany). A power injector is currently being used to guarantee an optimal bolus (Spectris, Medrad)

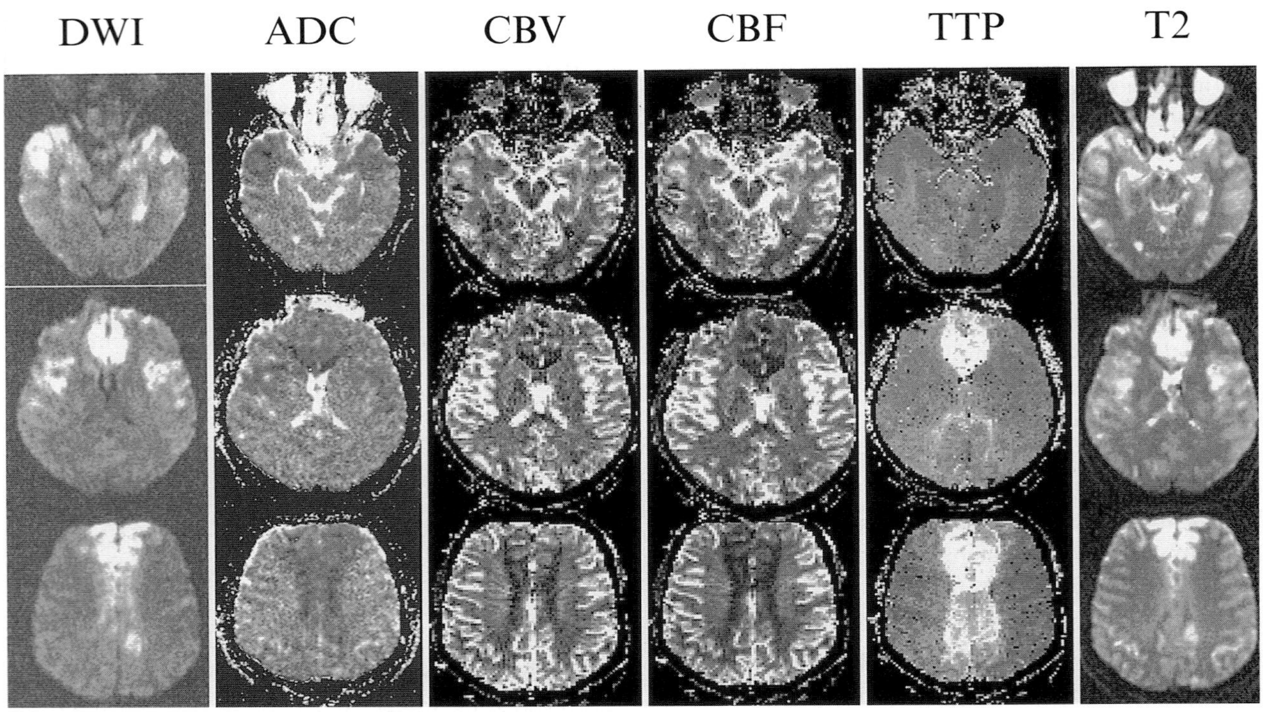

Fig. 2. Multimodality MR of a 32 year-old patient presenting with SAH and signs of delayed ischemic dysfunction. The images from left to right are diffusion-weighted images (*DWI*), apparent diffusion coefficient maps (*ADC*), parametric images of cerebral blood volume (*CBV*), cerebral blood flow (*CBF*), time-to peak (*TTP*) and T2-weighted images, all acquired at the three same levels in the axial projection. DWI at a high b value shows diffuse hyperintense areas in mainly both areas supplied by the anterior cerebral arteries bilaterally as well as slightly in the middle cerebral artery circulation. ADC values were lowered and parametric images show reduced perfusion accordingly

with a speed of 5 ml/second followed by 20 ml of a saline solution. Conventional T2/PD weighted MR imaging is also performed. An Angio MR sequence (with long and short echo times) is optional but often performed on scientific grounds (TR: 35 ms; TE: 6 ms; flip angle: 20°, 40 partitions, matrix: 192 × 256).

The current MR software package generates automatically maps of TTP and blood volume images, but the images are then transferred to a separate workstation where they are again postprocessed and maps of cerebral blood flow, blood volume and mean transit time are generated for final interpretation.

The imaging protocol corresponds to a modified MR stroke protocol which lasts in total less than 20 minutes. We have currently studied 8 patients with SAH. There were no complications related to safety. The artifacts caused by the clips were more important on echo-planar DWI or PWI sequences than on conventional spin-echo MR imaging, as expected. One patient with signs of delayed ischemic dysfunction showed large areas of DWI hyperintensities with decreased ADC values in the regions perfused by the anterior and middle cerebral arteries bilaterally. Perfusion-weighted imaging confirmed slightly larger areas of hypoperfused cerebral tissue on parametric images of cerebral blood volume and flow (Fig. 2).

Conclusions

Not only is DWI a reliable, sensitive and specific method for the detection of acute ischemia, it is also now becoming relatively widely available, in part due to the development of non-echo-planar techniques. Indeed, only when this promising technique leaves the laboratories and research centers, its full impact on patient management will be felt. A few select studies, including our own have shown its potential interest in the investigation of the delayed ischemic dysfunction associated with vasospam following SAH. While cerebral angiography remains the gold standard method to demonstrate the spastic vessel itself and Doppler ultrasound is an easily available bedside non-invasive technique, new less invasive methods such as DWI and PWI will allow to visualize the presence of hypoperfusion and possible ischemia. The light bulb effect, described in ischemic stroke, of an acute lesion could indeed be likened to an early ECG sign of stroke which could herald a new era in the management of stroke. Whether the treatment available is going to be neuroprotective or thrombolytic (local or systemic) or a combination, it is clear that in order to be effective, it should be started as soon as possible with as certain a diagnosis as possible. Now that more and more medical metallic objects are becoming MR-compatible, MRI seems to become the method of choice for the future for investigating patients with SAH (whether they have been coiled, clipped or not), since it now allows not only to show edema and structural damage to the tissues by conventional T1 and T2 weighted imaging, but also allows to determine hemorrhage by susceptibility imaging and can investigate the state of the vasculature by MRA; MRA can be done both intracranially and extracranially, where the carotids can be very quickly imaged in toto from the aortic arch to the circle of Willis by using the first pass gadolinium enhanced technique. Some issues that still need to be cleared are what the diffusion changes we see really do correspond to: are they truly a marker of membrane dysfunction, cytotoxic edema or are they simply another unspecific sign of tissular damage (some sort of ultra-early T2-weighted effect?) When isotropic imaging is performed, and when the trace is calculated DWI can also give an idea of the underlying structure, whether it be pathological or not; this could be of special interest in the study of myelination itself (in children) or diseases of myelin (e.g. Multiple sclerosis).

The addition of perfusion-weighted imaging to the method should allow us to investigate the areas that most interest us: the cerebral tissue that is hypoperfused but not necrotic, and which is therefore at risk for further infarction: this potential penumbra might most benefit from any intervention or neuroprotection. Such areas can be demonstrated as areas of DWI/PWI mismatches or decreases of the ADC that do not evolve into infarction. The implementation of the combination of DWI and PWI techniques should therefore allow us to non-invasively investigate changes due to vasospasm: DWI can demonstrate changes due to ischemia whereas perfusion imaging can demonstrate the possibly affected cerebral blood flow.

References

1. Baird AE, Benfield A, Schlaug G, Siewert B, Lövblad KO, Edelman RR, Warach S (1997) Enlargement of human cerebral ischemic lesion volumes measured by diffusion-weighted magnetic resonance imaging. Ann Neurol 41: 581–589
2. Bracard S, Auliac S, Anxionnat R, Lacour JC, Ducrocq X, Braun M, Moret C, Picard L (1999) Imagerie de diffusion dans le vasospasme focalisé asymptomatique. J Neuroradiol 26(4): 269–272
3. Chenevert TL, Brunberg JA, Pipe JG (1990) Anisotropic diffusion in human white matter: demonstration with MR techniques in vivo. Radiology 177: 401–405
4. Le Bihan D, Breton E, Lallemand D, Grenier P, Cabanis E, Laval-Jeantet M (1986) MR Imaging of intravoxel incoherent motions: application to diffusion and perfusion in neurologic disorders. Radiology 161: 401–407
5. Liot P, Oppenheim C, Dormont D, Sahel M, Casaco A, Marro B, Clémenceau S, Philippon J, Marsault C (1999) Intérêt de l' IRM pour le diagnostic d' hémorragie méningée en période de spasme. J Neuroradiol 26: 249–256
6. Lövblad KO, Baird AE, Schlaug G, Benfield A, Siewert B, Voetsch B, Connor A, Burzynski C, Edelman RR, Warach S (1997) Ischemic lesion volumes in acute stroke by diffusion-weighted magnetic resonance imaging correlate with clinical outcome. Ann Neurol 42: 164–170
7. Lövblad KO, Laubach HJ, Baird AE, Curtin F, Schlaug G, Edelman RR, Warach S (1998) Clinical experience with diffusion-weighted MR in patients with acute stroke. AJNR 19: 1061–1066
8. Moseley ME, Cohen Y, Mintorovitch J, Chileuitt L, Shimizu H, Kucharczyk J, Wendland MF, Weinstein PR (1990) Early detection of regional cerebral ischemia in cats: Comparison of diffusion- and T2-weighted MRI and spectroscopy. Mag Res Med 14: 330–346
9. Nakagawara J, Nakamura JI, Matsuzaki T, Takeda R, Wada K, Toshima M, Suematsu K (1988) Assessment of hemodynamic changes due to delayed cerebral vasospasm in subarachnoid hemorrhage using SPECT and 123I-IMP. In: Wilkins RH (ed) Cerebral vasospasm. New York, Raven Press
10. Romner B, Olsson M, Ljunggren B, Holtas S, Säveland H, Brandt L, Persson B (1989) Magnetic resonance imaging and aneurysm clips. J Neurosurg 70: 426–431
11. Romner B, Sonesson B, Ljunggren B, Brandt L, Säveland H, Holtas S (1989) Late magnetic resonance imaging related to neurobehavioral functioning after aneurysmal subarachnoid hemorrhage. Neurosurgery 25: 83–89
12. Rordorf G, Koroshetz WJ, Copen WA, Gonzalez G, Yamada K, Schaefer PW, Schwamm LH, Ogilvy CS, Sorensen AG (1999) Diffusion- and perfusion-weighted imaging in vasospasm after subarachnoid hemorrhage. Stroke 30(3): 599–605
13. Rosen BR, Belliveau JW, Vevea JM, Brady TJ (1990) Perfusion Imaging with NMR contrast agents. Mag Res Med 14: 249–265
14. Schlaug G, Siewert B, Benfield A, Edelman RR, Warach S (1997) Time course of the apparent diffusion coefficient (ADC) abnormality in human stroke. Neurology 49: 113–119
15. Seiler RW, Grolimund P, Aaslid R, Huber P, Nornes (1986) Cerebral vasospasm evaluated by transcranial ultrasound with clinical grade and CT-visualized subarachnoid haemorrhage. J Neurosurg 64: 594–600
16. Sorensen AG, Buonano FS, Gonzalez RG, Schwamm LH, Lev MH Huang-Hellinger FR, Reese TG, Weisskoff RM, Davis TL, Suwnwela N, Can U, Moreira JA, Copen WA, Look RB,

Finkelstein SP, Rosen BR, Koroshetz WJ (1996) Hyperacute stroke: Evaluation with combined multisection diffusion-weighted and hemodynamically-weighted echo-planar MR imaging. Radiology 199: 391–401

17. Warach S, Gaa J, Siewert B, Wielopolski P, Edelman RR (1995) Acute human stroke studies by whole brain echo planar diffusion-weighted magnetic resonance imaging. Ann Neurol 37: 231–241

Correspondence: Karl-Olof Lövblad, M.D., Department of Neuroradiology, C212 DRNN, Inselspital, Freiburgstrasse, CH-3010 Bern, Switzerland.

Acta Neurochir (2001) [Suppl] 77: 127–130

Assessment of Cerebral Microcirculatory Changes During Cerebral Vasospasm by Analyzing Cerebral Circulation Time on DSA Images

H. Ohkuma, K. Ogane, M. Tanaka, and **S. Suzuki**

Department of Neurosurgery, Hirosaki University School of Medicine, Hirosaki, Japan

Introduction

Cerebral microcirculation is disturbed during cerebral vasospasm, however, its influence on cerebral blood flow (CBF) and delayed ischemic neurological deficits (DIND) has not been determined, since there has been no easy method to evaluate microcirculatory changes. Cerebral microcirculation is regulated by regional cerebral blood flow (rCBF), cerebral circulation time (CCT), and regional cerebral blood volume (rCBV). In order to evaluate microcirculatory changes, CCT was measured on digital subtraction angiography (DSA).

Keywords: Subarachnoid hemorrhage; cerebral aneurysm; cerebral vasospasm; microcirculation.

Subjects and Methods

In 96 patients with aneurysmal SAH, 5 to 7 days after SAH, digital subtraction angiography (DSA) and ^{123}I-N-isopropyl-p-iodoamphetamine single photon emission tomography (^{123}I-IMP SPECT) were routinely carried out on the same day. In addition to these routine examinations, if DIND occurred, ^{123}I-IMP SPECT followed by DSA was carried out again. Out of 96 patients, the 24 patients who fulfilled the following criteria were included as the subjects of this study: 1) CT scan on admission showed group 3 in Fisher classification; 2) intracranial pressure was controlled by ventricular drainage or lumber drainage; 3) age was under 70 years old; 4) no brain damage was caused during aneurysm surgery; 5) atherosclerotic stenosis was not seen in either the cervical carotid artery or in the intracranial large arteries on angiography; 6) arterial pH value, partial pressure of oxygen in arterial blood, $PaCO_2$, and hematocrit were confirmed to be within the physiological range during the examination; 8) mean arterial blood pressure during the examination was maintained between 105 and 120 mmHg.

DSA was performed by injecting 6 ml of the contrast agent into the internal carotid artery, and serial images were obtained. The degree of angiographic vasospasm was defined as follows: a reduction in arterial diameter exceeding 50% was categorized as severe vasospasm group, a reduction between 25% and 50% was categorized as moderate vasospasm group, and a reduction of less than 25% was categorized as none or mild vasospasm group. In order to estimate the cerebral circulation time, the regions of interest (ROI) were set in the vertical intracavernous portion of the internal carotid artery (C_5), the cortical segment of the rolandic artery (M_4), and the rolandic vein (V_R) on the images of lateral projection (Fig. 1a,b). The time-density curve of the contrast media in each ROI was obtained from the series of DSA images and was fitted to a gamma variate function, and mean transit time (MTT) in each ROI was determined. Cerebral circulation time (CCT) was divided into proximal CCT, which was the circulation time in the extraparenchymal large arteries and was defined as the difference between MTT in C_5 and MTT in M_4, and peripheral CCT, which was the circulation time in the intraparenchymal small vessels and was defined as the difference between MTT in M_4 and MTT in V_R.

The rCBF was estimated by the ^{123}I-IMP autoradiographic (ARG) method. ROI consisting of 15×30 mm along the cerebral cortex were drawn around the rolandic artery on the two consecutive slices 20 to 30 mm above the slice showing the foramina of Monro so that the rolandic artery became the center of this ROI (Fig. 1c).

Results

Examinations were performed 31 times in 24 patients, and 62 sides were obtained for this study. Out of 24 cases, 8 cases showed symptomatic vasospasm.

Angiographic Vasospasm and CCT

Arterial diameter correlated well with proximal CCT ($r = 0.681$, $p < 0.0001$; Spearman's rank correlation coefficient), however, there was no correlation between arterial diameter and peripheral CCT.

Angiographic Vasospasm and rCBF

In the severe angiographic vasospasm group, rCBF statistically decreased compared with that in the moderate vasospasm group ($p < 0.05$) and none/mild

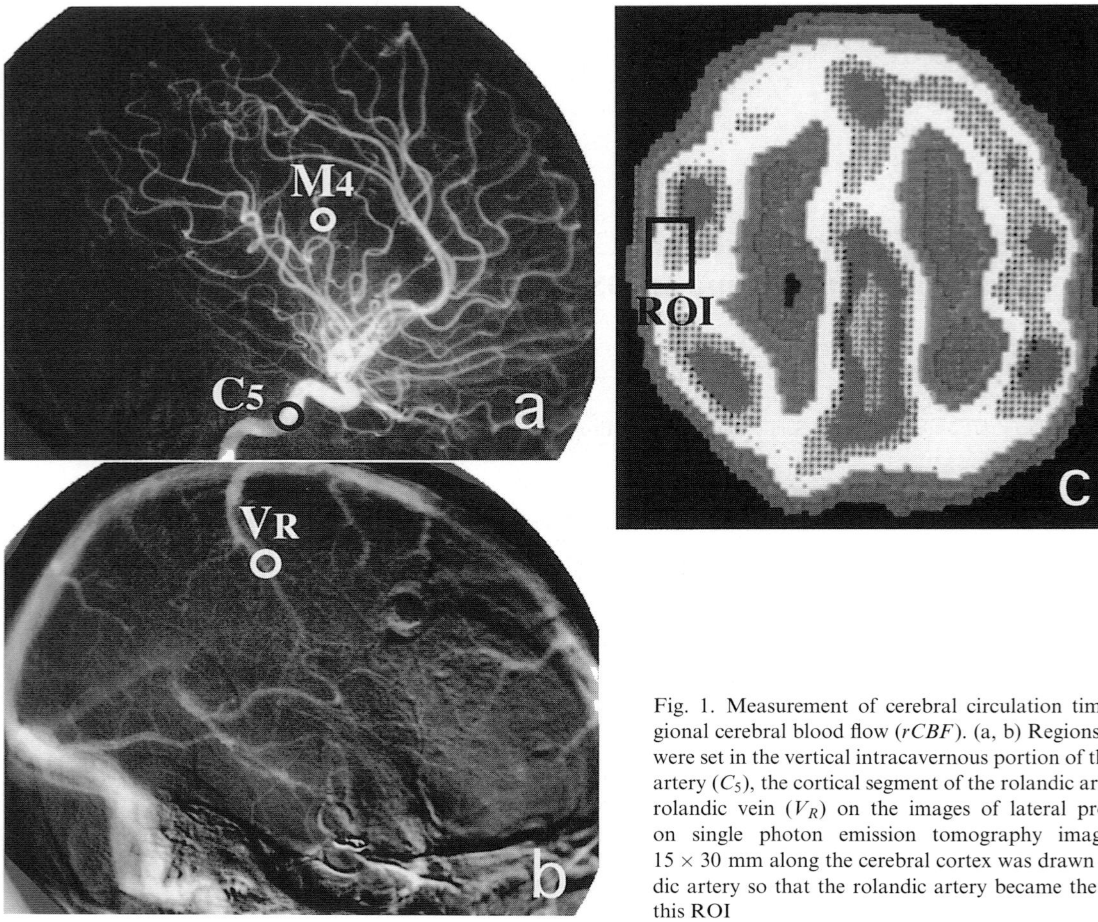

Fig. 1. Measurement of cerebral circulation time (*CCT*) and regional cerebral blood flow (*rCBF*). (a, b) Regions of interest (*ROI*) were set in the vertical intracavernous portion of the internal carotid artery (C_5), the cortical segment of the rolandic artery (M_4), and the rolandic vein (V_R) on the images of lateral projection. (c) ROI on single photon emission tomography images consisting of 15×30 mm along the cerebral cortex was drawn around the rolandic artery so that the rolandic artery became the cortical center of this ROI

vasospasm group ($p < 0.01$) (Fig. 2). There was no statistical difference between the moderate vasospasm group and none/mild vasospasm group. Overall, there was correlation between arterial diameter and rCBF ($r = 0.429$, $p = 0.0006$; Spearman's rank correlation coefficient).

CCT and rCBF

Statistical correlation was not seen between proximal CCT and rCBF ($r = 0.367$, $p = 0.0042$; Spearman's rank correlation coefficient). Peripheral CCT showed strong inverse correlation with rCBF ($r = -0.767$, $p < 0.0001$; Spearman's rank correlation coefficient) (Fig. 3). When correlation between peripheral CCT and rCBF was evaluated in each angiographic vasospasm group, strong inverse correlation between peripheral CCT and rCBF were seen in each and every angiographic vasospasm group ($r = -0.660$, $p = 0.0002$ in the none/mild vasospasm group; Fig. 3a, $r = -0.848$, $p < 0.0001$ in the moderate vasospasm group; Fig. 3b, and $r = -0.929$, $p < 0.0229$ in the severe vasospasm group; Fig. 3c; Spearman's rank correlation coefficient).

Effects of Intraarterial Papaverine Injection. In the 4 cases with symptomatic vasospasm who received intraarterial papaverine infusion, CCT just after papaverine infusion was compared with those just before papaverine infusion. In the 2 cases who had neurological improvement immediately after papaverine infusion, peripheral CCT were 4.26 and 3.84 seconds before papaverine infusion, which decreased to 3.72 and 3.28 seconds after papaverine infusion, respectively. In the 2 cases without neurological improvement after papaverine infusion, peripheral CCT before papaverine infusion were 4.17 and 4.88 seconds, and those after papaverine infusion were 4.22 and 4.79 seconds, respectively.

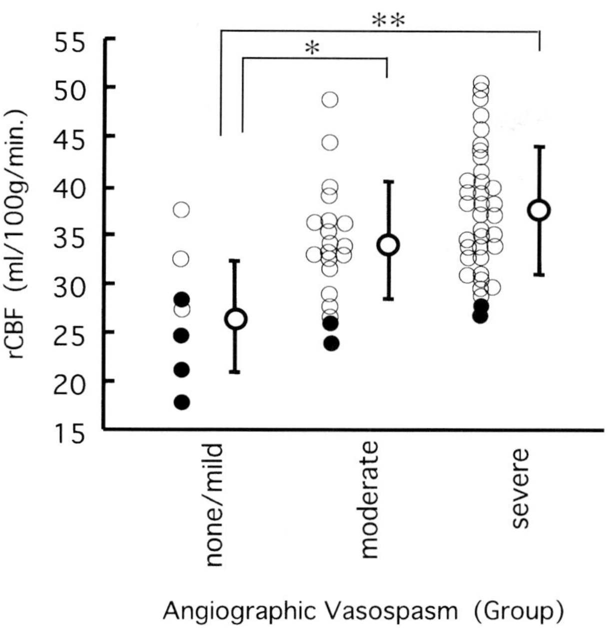

Fig. 2. Angiographic vasospasm and rCBF. rCBFs were compared among the three different angiographic vasospasm groups. * $p < 0.05$, ** $p < 0.01$. Closed circles indicate the cases with symptomatic vasospasm

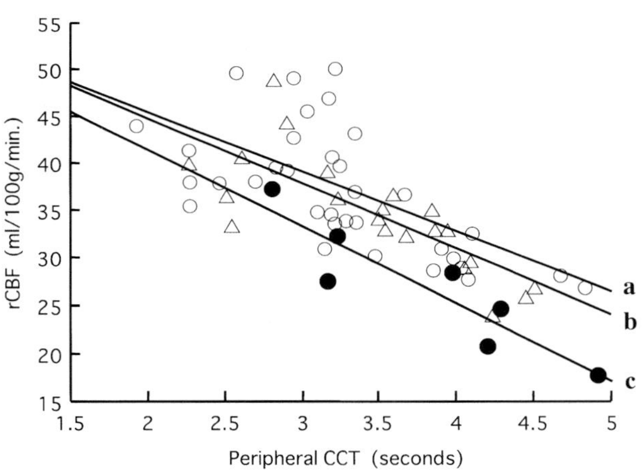

Fig. 3. Correlation between peripheral CCT and rCBF, ○: none/mild angiographic vasospasm, △: moderate angiographic vasospasm, ●: severe angiographic vasospasm

Discussion

Cerebral vasospasm associated with aneurysmal subarachnoid hemorrhage (SAH), which is angiographically characterized as the persistent luminal narrowing of the major extraparenchymal cerebral arteries, affects cerebral microcirculation and causes decreased cerebral blood flow (CBF) and delayed ischemic neurological deficits (DIND). Microcirculatory changes after SAH have been investigated especially in association with autoregulation of CBF. Several reports have indicated that autoregulation is impaired during vasospasm, since autoregulatory response to the changes of arterial carbon dioxide pressure ($PaCO_2$) or acetazolamide administration is reduced and CBF is vulnerable to change by the changes of systemic arterial blood pressure. The weak response to the $PaCO_2$ or acetazolamide administration have been attributed to maximal dilation in the peripheral arterioles in an attempt to maintain sufficient CBF in the face of decreased cerebral perfusion pressure (CPP) due to vasospasm. Increased cerebral blood volume (CBV) after SAH detected by positron emission tomography (PET) or radioisotope tracer method could explain this maximal dilation of peripheral arterioles [1].

Contrary to this, however, recent PET studies have shown decreased CBV during cerebral vasospasm, which suggests that the appropriate vasodilating capacity of distal vessels in response to reductions in local CPP is impaired after SAH [5]. Furthermore, our recent histopathological studies have revealed that intraparenchymal small arteries or arterioles show luminal narrowing rather than dilation during cerebral vasospasm after experimental SAH [2, 3].

Therefore, the changes of microcirculation, especially whether microcirculatory vessels dilate or not during vasospasm, are controversial and still uncertain. CBV measured by PET has been used clinically for estimating the changes of microcirculatory blood volume, however, it is difficult to determine which type of peripheral vessels out of arterioles, capillaries, and venuoles play a main part in the changes of CBV. Furthermore, PET is not feasible for routine clinical use. The aim of this study was to investigate the role of microcirculatory changes in cerebral ischemia during cerebral vasospasm after SAH by analyzing CCT and rCBF.

The results of this study showed that a major factor affecting cerebral ischemia during cerebral vasospasm was the luminal narrowing of the large extraparenchymal arteries, which was detected as angiographic vasospasm. Severe angiographic vasospasm, which was defined as over 50% narrowing, induced statistically significant reduced rCBF, however, there was no statistically significant difference between rCBF in the none/mild vasospasm group and that in the moderate vasospasm group. These results are consistent with the results of experimental and clinical studies showing that rCBF was significantly reduced only when vessel caliber decreased under 50%. However, even in the none/mild or moderate angiographic vasospasm groups, some of the cases showed decreased rCBF and/or DIND, which indicated that factors other than angiographic vasospasm might affect cerebral ischemia.

Microcirculatory changes detected as prolonged peripheral CCT is thought to be another factor inducing cerebral ischemia during cerebral vasospasm, since rCBF decreased in statistically significant correlation with prolonged peripheral CCT in any of the angiographic vasospasm groups. Prolonged CCT has been thought to reflect microvascular rarefaction or increased small-vessel resistence. Touho H [4] indicated that prolonged CCT during cerebral vasospasm was improved by injecting sodium papaverine and suggested that the dilation of small arteries induced by papaverine administration was attributable to shortening of prolonged CCT. Therefore, prolonged peripheral CCT seen in this study is thought to represent increased small vessel resistance or narrowing of small vessel caliber.

The therapy for cerebral vasospasm should be reconsidered by taking into account the microcirculatory changes. Induced hypertension and hypervolemia might improve rCBF by affecting small vessels with increased resistance; the effectiveness of calcium blockers for cerebral vasospasm, despite the absence of apparent effect on angiographic vasospasm, may partially depend on dilating the contractile arterioles; and intraarterial injection of papaverine may have an influence on intraparenchymal small vessels in addition to large extraparenchymal arteries.

Conclusion

The results indicated two factors, which are the marked luminal narrowing of large arteries and microcirculatory changes detected as prolonged CCT, independently affect cerebral ischemia during cerebral vasospasm. Prolonged CCT could be caused by impaired autoregulatory vasodilation of parenchymal vessels or contraction of intraparenchymal small arteries. CCT was easily measured and useful to determine the therapy with considering the microcirculatory disturbance.

References

1. Grubb RL Jr, Raichle ME, Eichling JO, Gado MH (1977) Effects of subarachnoid hemorrhage on cerebral blood volume, blood flow, and oxygen utilization in humans. J Neurosurg 46: 446–453
2. Ohkuma H, Itoh K, Shibata S, Suzuki S (1997) Morphological changes of intraparenchymal arterioles after experimental subarachnoid hemorrhage in dogs. Neurosurgery 41: 230–236
3. Ohkuma H, Suzuki S (1999) Histological dissociation between intra- and extraparenchymal portion of perforating small arteries after experimental subarachnoid hemorrhage in dogs. Acta Neuropathol 98: 374–382
4. Touho H (1995) Hemodynamic evaluation with dynamic DSA during the treatment of cerebral vasospasm: a retrospective study. Surg Neurol 44: 63–74
5. Yundt KD, Grubb RLJr, Diringer MN, Powers WJ (1998) Autoregulatory vasodilation of parenchymal vessels is impaired during cerebral vasospasm. J Cereb Blood Flow Metab 18: 419–424

Correspondence: Hiroki Ohkuma, M.D., Department of Neurosurgery, Hirosaki University School of Medicine, 5 Zaifu-cho, Hirosaki, 036-8216 Japan.

Acta Neurochir (2001) [Suppl] 77: 131–134

Bedside Monitoring of Cerebral Blood Flow in Patients with Subarachnoid Hemorrhage

T. Hegner, N. Krayenbühl, M. Hefti, Y. Yonekawa, and **E. Keller**

Department of Neurosurgery, University Hospital Zurich, Switzerland

Introduction

Changes of cerebral hemodynamics and oxygenation in patients with cerebral vasospasm (CVS) after subarachnoid hemorrhage (SAH) might be underestimated if transcranial Doppler sonography (TCD) and angiography findings are considered singularly [1]. Low cerebral blood flow (CBF) has been identified as independent predictor of poor outcome after SAH [7]. Nevertheless the established methods for bedside measurement of CBF with inert tracers, such as the nitrous oxide or the ^{133}Xenon dilution technique are technically difficult and time consuming [6, 9]. Stable xenon-enhanced computed tomography, positron emission tomography and magnetic resonance spectroscopy are powerful research tools [1], but require that the patient be transported, which carries a potentially high risk. Recently a new double indicator dilution technique for bedside monitoring of CBF became available [5].

The purpose of the present study was to establish the new double indicator dilution technique for CBF measurement in patients with SAH and to estimate its clinical value in detection and treatment of CVS.

Keywords: Subarachnoid hemorrhage; vasospasm; cerebral blood flow; double indicator dilution method.

Material and Methods

Patient Population

17 patients with severe aneurysmal SAH Hunt & Hess Grade 3–5 (14 patients) or with secondary deterioration from CVS (three patients) were prospectively studied. Surgery to clip the ruptured aneurysm was performed as soon as scheduling permitted (mean day 2). CBF monitoring was installed if the patient's GCS was 9 or lower after aneurysm surgery or if he deteriorated secondary from CVS. The study was approved by the Ethics Committee of the University of Zurich (E-015/99). Patients with peripheral occlusive arterial disease or coagulation disorders were excluded. Hemoglobin and systemic oxygen saturation were maintained constant during the course of illness.

Measurements

Jugular bulb saturation ($SjvO_2$) values (calibrated by blood gas analysis), arteriovenous difference of oxygen lactate (avDL) and CBF measurements were obtained every 12 hours by routine. The cerebral metabolic rate of oxygen ($CMRO_2$) was calculated by multiplying the CBF value by the arteriovenous difference of oxygen content ($avDO_2$). The measurement period was limited, either by the patient recovering from CVS or by his death. Additional measurements were performed before and within 30 mins after specific treatment of CVS with triple-H therapy (hypertensive, hypervolemic, hemodilution) or superselective intraarterial papaverine infusion. Paired studies before and after CVS treatment were excluded from analysis if arterial pCO_2 changed more than 10% between the measurements. According to our standardized treatment regimen triple-H therapy was induced if TCD blood flow velocities increased (middle cerebral artery mean blood flow velocities >120 cm/sec or increased >30 cm/sec within 24 hours) and/or if the patient developed delayed ischemic deficits (DID) from CVS. If patients with DID didn't improve or worsened in spite of triple-H therapy, after exclusion of hypoxia, electrolyte imbalance and hydrocephalus, angiography and treatment with superselective papaverine infusion into the vasospastic vessels were performed. Symptomatic CVS, resistant or reoccurring after papaverine infusion were treated with barbiturate coma and/or hypothermia. With each CBF measurement blood gas analysis from the arterial site and the jugular bulb were performed (ABL 700 Radiometer, Copenhagen, Denmark).

CBF values were estimated by a new double indicator dilution method [5]. Two fiberoptic thermistor catheters 5F (PV-2024, Pulsion-Medizintechnik, Munich, Germany) were placed in the thoracic aorta via a femoral artery port, and in the jugular bulb by retrograde cannulation of the dominant internal jugular vein. To avoid extracerebral contamination correct positioning of the jugular bulb catheter tip was verified by x-ray after injection of 1 ml Omnipaque^R. Bolus injections of ice-cold indocyanine green (ICG) (20 mg, 40 ml, <5 °C) were given using a 12 Gauge central venous line. The resulting thermodilution and dyedilution curves were recorded digitally (Pulsion COLD Medical Systems Z 021 and IVH5, Munich, Germany). CBF was measured by calculating the mean transit times of the cold bolus and dye. Thermodilution and dye-dilution curves were rejected if the following artifacts were identified: thermal drift in the baseline, wall artifacts by the jugular bulb catheter, or insufficient result of curve fitting because of respiratory artifacts induced by mechanical ventilation.

Statistical Analysis

Patient characteristics, $SjvO_2$, CBF and $CMRO_2$ are expressed as mean ($\pm$SD). Comparisons of measurements before and after specific treatment of CVS are performed using two-tailed t-tests. Significance was judged at the $P < 0.05$ level.

Results

In 17 patients 151 valuable measurements were obtained. Patient characteristics are listed in Table 1. No complications related to the measurement method were observed. The mean value of the 151 measurements in all 17 patients was 72% ($\pm$10) for $SjvO_2$, 60 ml/100g/min ($\pm$26) for CBF and 2.25 mlO_2/100 g/min ($\pm$1.48) for $CMRO_2$.

16 measurements were obtained with the occurrence of CVS. Eight pairs of measurements were performed immediately before and within 30 minutes after specific treatment of CVS (three studies before and after initiation of triple-H therapy and five studies before and after superselective intraarterial papaverine infusion). Absolute values in these eight studies for $SjvO_2$ varied between 55 and 85%. No episode of jugular desaturation ($SjvO_2$ values <50%) was identified and confirmed by blood gas sampling. From 16 avDL measurements six values were −0.2 umol/dl or below. CBF before and after triple-H therapy/papaverine varied between 25 and 117 ml/100g/min and $CMRO_2$ between 0.87 to 6.95 ml O_2/100g/min. The measurements obtained immediately before and after specific treatment of CVS are given for every single patient separately in Fig. 1a–c. There was no significant difference between $SjvO_{2mean}$ before (71%) and after triple-H therapy/papaverine (70%). Five $SjvO_2$ values increased after specific treatment of CVS, whereas three values remained unchanged or decreased (Fig. 1a). CBF after treatment increased in all patients (Fig. 1b). CBF_{mean} increased significantly after triple-H therapy/papaverine (51 to 79 ml/100 g/min; $P = 0.015$). $CMRO_{2mean}$ tended to increase after treatment of CVS (1.95 to 3.21 ml O_2/100 g/min), but without significance because of the high interindividual variability ($P = 0.055$). In all but one patient $CMRO_2$ increased after triple-H therapy/papaverine treatment (Fig. 1c). In three of eight studies with varying $CMRO_2$, changes of $SjvO_2$ didn't reflect CBF: $SjvO_2$ remained unchanged or decreased before and after treatment whereas CBF increased more than 10%.

Table 1. *Patient Characteristics*

Gender	
Number of patients	17
– Male	1
– Female	16
Age mean (range)	65 (40–73)
Hunt & Hess Grade	
Number of patients	
II*	3
III	2
IV	9
V	3
Localisation of ruptured aneurysm	
Number of patients	
– ICA	1
– AcoA	4
– Pericallosal artery	1
– MCA	6
– Basilar artery	2
– PcoA	3
Number of measurements	
– All patients	151
– Per patient, mean (SD)	8 ($\pm$4.5)
Measurement period	
– Number of days, mean (SD)	6.5 ($\pm$2.5)

ICA Internal carotid artery; *ACoA* anterior communicating artery; *MCA* middle cerebral artery; *PcoA* posterior communicating artery; * patients with secondary deterioration from CVS.

Discussion

In patients with severe SAH symptomatic CVS are difficult to detect. Radiographic CVS do not reflect cerebral hemodynamics and oxygenation, and may occur in the absence of clinical deficit and vice-versa [8]. TCD [1] and jugular bulb oximetry [10] give indices that can be related to CBF, but do not measure true flows. The relationship between CBF and metabolism can only be examined if the flow is measured directly.

Recently, a new double indicator dilution technique for CBF measurement, which is easy to perform on the ICU, became available [5]. In contrast to the established time consuming methods for CBF measurement, the new technique allows CBF measurements at the bedside repeatable within 20 mins. With increasing TCD blood flow velocities or new ischemic deficits, additional measurements may be rapidly performed to guide clinical management of CVS. In 17 patients with SAH 135 measurements were obtained routinely every

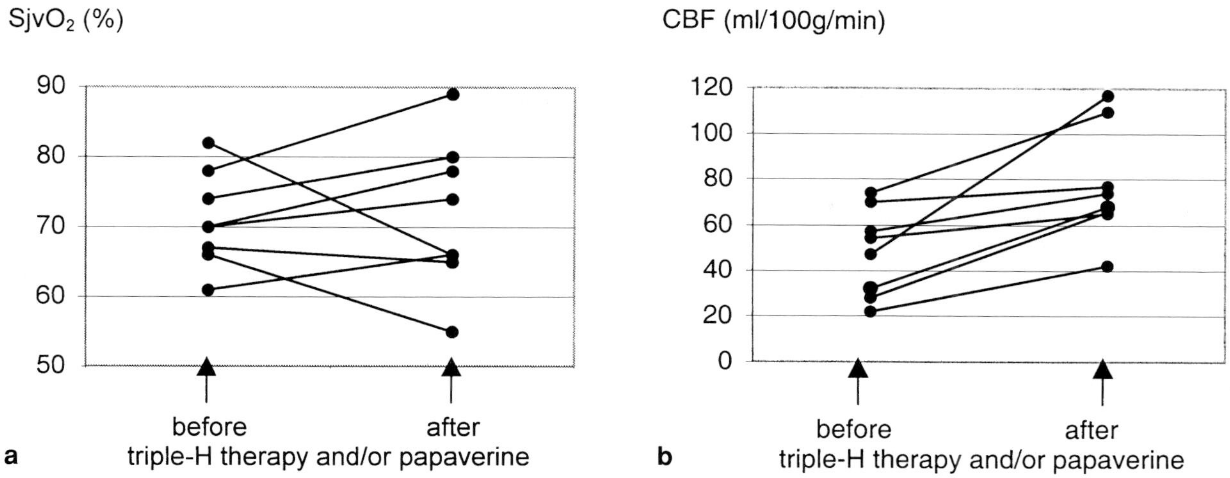

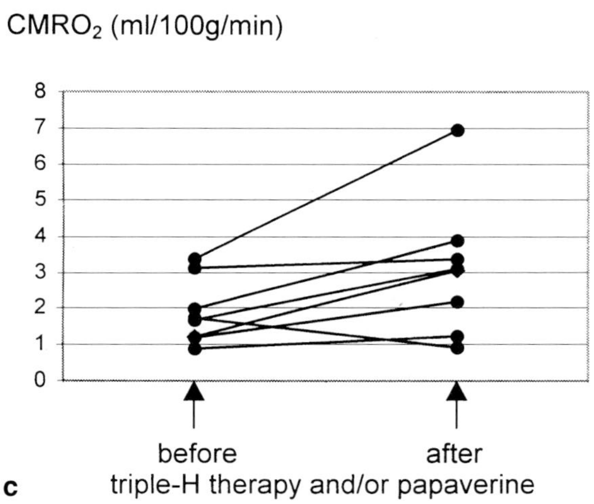

Fig. 1. Graphs showing $SjvO_2$ (jugular bulb saturation) (a), CBF (cerebral blood flow) (b) and $CMRO_2$ (cerebral metabolic rate of oxygen) (c) before and after initiation of triple-H therapy or superselective infusion of papaverine

12 hours and 16 measurements were additionally performed immediately before and after specific treatment of CVS. CBF_{mean} in all our studies significantly increased after triple-H therapy or superselective intraarterial papaverine infusion. Recently, Lennihan *et al.* showed that prophylactic hypervolemia doesn't increase CBF [7]. Nevertheless patients with symptomatic CVS were excluded in this study and treated with triple-H therapy. Using the ^{133}Xenon dilution method with multiple collimators, CBF measurements were performed only once a day on day 0, 1 and thereafter every three days. With the time consuming measurement method there was no attempt to measure CBF immediately before and after the start of therapeutic triple-H therapy [7].

In all our patients CBF increased after treatment of CVS, whereas $SjvO_2$ increased in only five studies, remained unchanged in one study and decreased in two paired measurements. In the two studies with decreasing $SjvO_2$ after CVS treatment, avDL was −0.2 umol/l or below, showing the pattern of definitive infarction [10]. In our patients $CMRO_2$ showed a high variation, between 0.87 and 6.95 ml O_2/100g/min, and $CMRO_2$ recovered in all but one patient parallel to the increasing CBF after treatment of CVS. Under these circumstances with varying $CMRO_2$, $SjvO_2$ can not be assumed to reflect CBF. Nevertheless therapeutic interventions in patients with CVS may be most successful in the early stage of ischemia with compensated hypoperfusion before brain lactic acidosis and irreversible infarction occur [2]. Therefore the dynamic relationship between cerebral oxygen supply and metabolism in CVS can only be observed if CBF is measured directly and if $CMRO_2$ can be calculated in short time intervals at the bedside.

Critical thresholds for $SjvO_2$ and avDL to detect

secondary ischemia, defined in severe head injury [4, 11], may not be extrapolated to ischemic events related to CVS. In our study population no $SjvO_2$ value was below the critical level of 50% and only 6 avDL measurements were −0.2 umol/dl or below. The localization of the jugular bulb catheter in relation to the site of ischemia may cover typical patterns of the hemodynamic values induced by CVS. In this study the right internal jugular vein, in most individuals being dominant, was cannulated in all patients. Measurements from one internal jugular bulb may not be representative of truly mixed bihemispheric cerebral venous blood. Furthermore secondary ischemic events may occur in a part of the brain being drained by the opposite jugular vein. These limitations of the method have to be considered especially in patients with regional ischemia and may influence the sensitivity of a global CBF measurement method and jugular bulb oximetry to detect CVS [2]. Reductions in CBF with symptomatic CVS are usually focal and topographically heterogeneous [7, 8]. The limitation of $SjvO_2$ monitoring and the new double indicator dilution technique for CBF measurement to detect smaller areas of ischemia encourage to combine global measurement techniques with methods to evaluate focal cerebral oxygenation. Monitoring of partial pressure of brain tissue oxygen ($PbtO_2$) may be suitable to be combined with $SjvO_2$ monitoring to detect focal as well as global changes in cerebral oxygenation patterns [3].

Conclusion

The new double indicator dilution method for CBF measurement is easy to perform and can be repeated rapidly at the bedside in patients with severe SAH. Our preliminary observations suggest that serial measurements of CBF, $CMRO_2$, avDL and jugular bulb oximetry in addition to the established bedside monitoring may help to guide therapy in patients with CVS. The sensitivity of the new method to detect symptomatic CVS may be limited by the technique measuring global CBF values.

References

1. Clyde BL, Resnick DK, Yonas H, Smith HA, Kaufmann AM (1996) The relationship of blood velocity as measured by transcranial Doppler ultrasonography to cerebral blood flow determined by stable xenon computed tomographic studies after aneurysmal subarachnoid hemorrhage. Neurosurgery 38: 896–904
2. Fandino J, Kaku J, Schuknecht B, Valavanis A, Yonekawa Y (1998) Improvement of cerebral oxygenation patterns and metabolic validation of superselective intraarterial infusion of papaverine for the treatment of cerebral vasospasm. J Neurosurg 89: 93–100
3. Fandino J, Stocker R, Prokop S, Imhof HG (1999) Correlation between jugular bulb oxygen saturation and partial pressure of brain tissue oxygen during CO_2 and O_2 reactivity tests in severely head-injured patients. Acta Neurochir (Wien) 141: 825–834
4. Gopinath SP, Robertson CS, Contant CF, Hayes C, Feldman Z, Narayan RK, Grossman RG (1994) Jugular venous desaturation and outcome after head injury. J Neurol Neurosurg Psychiatry 57: 717–723
5. Keller E, Wietasch G, Ringleb P, Scholz M, Schwarz S, Stingele R, Schwab S, Hanley D, Hacke W (2000) Bedside monitoring of cerebral blood flow (CBF) in patients with acute hemispheric stroke. Crit Care Med 28: 511–516
6. Kety SS, Schmidt CF (1945) The determination of cerebral blood flow in man by the use of nitrous oxide in low concentrations. Am J Physiol 143: 53
7. Lennihan L, Mayer SA, Fink ME, Beckford A, Myunghee CP, Zhang H, Wu Y, Klebanoff LM, Raps EC, Solomon RA (2000). Effect of hypervolemic therapy on cerebral blood flow after subarachnoid hemorrhage. Stroke 31: 383–391
8. Mickey B, Vorstrup S, Voldby B, Lindewald H, Harmsen A, Lassen NA (1984) Serial measurements of regional cerebral blood flow in patients with SAH unsing ^{133}Xe inhalation and emission computerized tomography. J Neurosurg 60: 916–922
9. Obrist WD, Thompson HK, Wang HS, Wilkinson WE (1975) Regional cerebral blood flow estimated by ^{133}Xe inhalation. Stroke 6: 245–256
10. Robertson CS, Narayan RK, Ziya LG, Pahwa R, Grossman RG, Caram P, Allen E (1989) Cerebral arteriovenous oxygen difference as an estimate of cerebral blood flow in comatose patients. J Neurosurg 70: 222–230

Correspondence: Emanuela Keller, M.D., Department of Neurosurgery, University Hospital, Frauenklinikstrasse 10, 8091 Zürich, Switzerland.

Acta Neurochir (2001) [Suppl] 77: 135–138

Changes in Neuronal Metabolites in Brain Following Subarachnoid Haemorrhage Evaluated by Proton MR Spectroscopy

Y. Handa, H. Kimura, H. Arishima, M. Ishida, H. Ishii, and **T. Kubota**

Department of Neurosurgery and Radiology, Fukui Medical University, Fukui, Japan

Introduction

Recently, several advances in operative techniques and management of chronic cerebral vasospasm for patients with aneurysmal subarachnoid haemorrhage (SAH) have improved morbidity and mortality rates. However, even when the surviving SAH patients show no grossly evident neurological deficits, they frequently have subtle neurobehavioral problems [5, 9]. These problems have been suggested to result from widespread damage of neuronal cells from SAH [8], whereas ischaemic lesions observed by imaging study are not involved in such problems [9]. Though the details of the pathogenesis of this pathological condition is not obvious, possible causative mechanisms have been considered to explain: impairment of cerebral microcirculation at the onset of SAH and/or during chronic cerebral vasospasm [3], and secondary neuronal cell damage elicited by subarachnoid clot [6].

In vivo proton magnetic resonance spectroscopy (MRS) has been recognized as a valuable method for observation of the longitudinal changes in the biochemical status of the injured brain under various pathological conditions [1, 2, 4, 7] in which MRS could demonstrate remarkable changes in N-acetylaspartate (NAA) and/or choline compounds (Cho) concentrations [4, 7]. NAA, neuron specific amino acid, exists largely within the neurons and its decrease is an indication of neuronal cell loss. The changes in Cho concentration has been proposed to result from the destruction of the neuronal cell membrane or active membrane metabolism. When widespread neuronal cell damage presumably exists in the brain following SAH, it may be able to detect the changes in these neuronal metabolites by means of proton MRS. For confirmation of this hypothesis, we observed changes in the neuronal metabolites in the cerebral hemisphere by means of in vivo proton MRS to evaluate whether or how neuronal cells are affected by SAH and/or cerebral vasospasm.

Keywords: Cerebral aneurysm; proton magnetic resonance spectroscopy; subarachnoid hemorrhage.

Materials and Methods

For the present study, the objective cases were selected from the patients who underwent direct aneurysm surgery within three days after the onset of SAH, revealed no definitive focal neurological deficits at the chronic stage, and no apparent ischemic lesion on MRI, respectively. There were 14 men and 17 women whose age at operation ranged from 47 to 74 years (mean $\pm$ standard deviation, 57.4 ± 10.8 years). The grade of SAH was classified by the Hunt and Kosnik grading scale. The patients were subdivided into two groups: one group (6 cases) whose members showed a transient focal neurological deficit, presumably symptomatic vasospasm, at the acute stage of SAH and one group (25 cases) whose members showed no focal neurological deficit during their entire illness. In all cases, MRI and proton MRS were evaluated at the acute stage (7 to 10 days after SAH) and/or chronic stage (6 to 8 weeks after SAH).

MRS study was performed by using a 1.5-tesla MR imager on a prototype system (Signa Horizon, GEYMS). Before MRS measurements, routine multi-slice axial T1-weighted, T2-weighted images were obtained. The voxel of interest (VOI) ($20 \times 20 \times 20$ mm) for MRS was routinely prescribed from the axial image in the bilateral fronto-parietal subcortical white matter (centrum semiovale) (Fig. 1). The location of VOI was carefully determined to ensure the same location for each patient. Proton spectra were obtained in 96 scans by using a multiple-echo spectroscopy acquisition sequence with long echo (TR, 2000 ms; TE, 136 ms) and water-suppressed technique. Proton spectra from each case showed three peaks: NAA, Cho and sum of creatine and phosphocreatine (Cr). (Fig. 1) On the contrary, the peak of lactate could not be distinguished from other signals in the spectra in any patient at any stage of SAH. The peak areas of NAA, Cho and Cr were analyzed by planimetry from the area under each peak. The NAA/Cr and Cho/Cr ratios were calculated in each spectrum, and the average value of the bilateral hemisphere at each MRS measurement was evaluated.

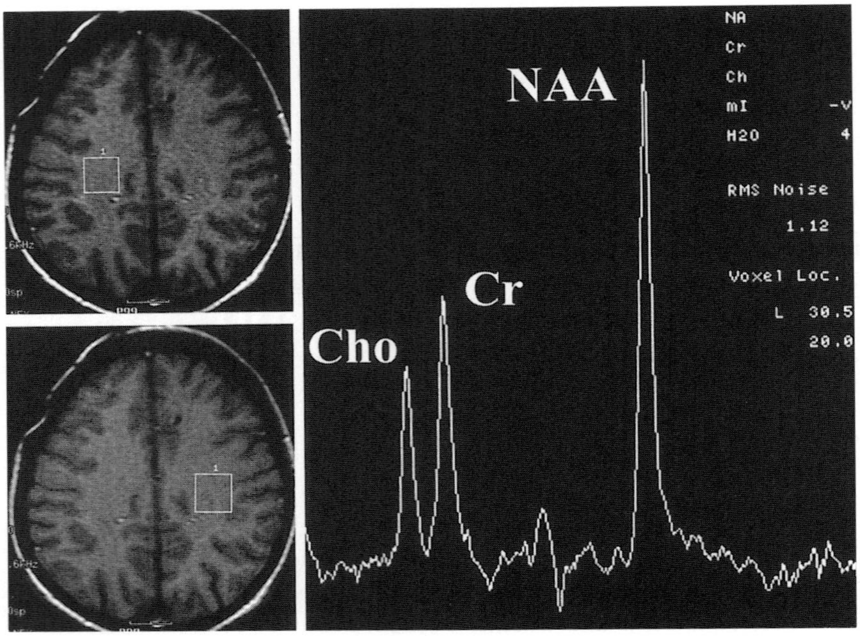

Fig. 1. Left: Axial MR images showing VOI in the bilateral centrum semiovale for proton MR spectrum. Right: peaks in the spectrum assigned to NAA, the sum of creatine and phosphocreatine (*Cr*), and choline compounds (*Cho*)

Table 1. *Ratios of Neuronal Metabolites in Normal Volunteers and SAH Patients*

	No	Cho/Cr		NAA/Cr	
Normal volunteers	11	1.15 ± 0.11		2.16 ± 0.26	
SAH patients		Acute	Chronic	Acute	Chronic
No symptomatic vs	25	1.25 ± 0.17	1.08 ± 0.13	2.16 ± 0.17	1.92 ± 0.23*
Symptomatic vs	6	1.52 ± 0.17*	1.07 ± 0.09	2.26 ± 0.21	1.85 ± 0.11*

Values are mean ± standard deviation. * $p < 0.05$, compared to control value in the normal volunteers. *Cho* Choline compounds; *Cr* sum of creatine and phosphocreatine, *NAA* N-acetyl-aspartate.

We studied 11 normal volunteers, who showed no apparent lesion in the cerebral hemisphere on MRI, as an age-matched control group. The mean age of the normal volunteers (57.1 ± 11.4 years) showed no significant difference compared to that in the SAH cases. The proton MRS study and evaluation were carried out the same way as in the SAH cases.

ANOVA test was used for statistical evaluation. A p value of <0.05 was regarded as significant in the analysis of the all data.

Results

Ratio of Neuronal Metabolite in Normal Volunteers

The mean Cho/Cr ratio calculated from the spectra in the age-matched normal volunteers was 1.15 ± 0.11 (mean ± standard deviation), and the NAA/Cr ratio was 2.16 ± 0.26. These ratios were used as normal control values in the present study (Table 1).

Changes in Ratio of Neuronal Metabolites in SAHe Patients

At the acute stage, the mean Cho/Cr ratio obtained from the patients without symptomatic vasospasm was higher but not significant compared to the control value, while the mean Cho/Cr ratios obtained from the patients with symptomatic vasosapsm were significantly ($p < 0.05$) higher than the control value. The value of this metabolite ratio in both SAH groups was reduced to the control level at the chronic stage of SAH. (Table 1, Fig. 2) The mean NAA/Cr ratio both

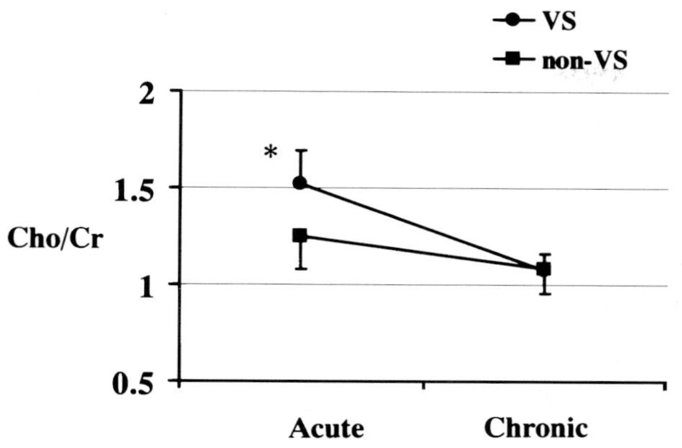

Fig. 2. Changes in Cho/Cr ratio at the acute and chronic stages of SAH. *VS* Patient group with symptomatic vasospasm, *non-VS* patient group with no focal neurological signs

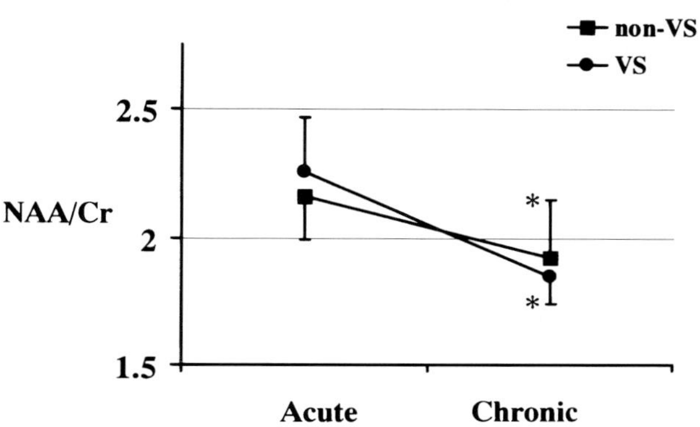

Fig. 3. Changes in NAA/Cr ratio at the acute and chronic stages of SAH. *VS* Patient group with symptomatic vasospasm, *non-VS* patient group with no focal neurological signs

in the patients with symptomatic vasospasm and no symptoms showed no significant difference compared to the normal control value at the acute stage. On the other hand, at the chronic stage, the mean NAA/Cr ratios in both of the two groups showed significant ($p < 0.05$) decreases compared to the control normal value. (Table 1, Fig. 3)

Correlation Between Severity of SAH and Neuronal Metabolites

To determine how the severity of SAH affects the changes in ratios of neuronal metabolites, the correlation between severity of SAH grade and changes in Cho/Cr ratio at the acute stage and changes in NAA/Cr ratio at the chronic stage were evaluated in all SAH patients. The mean value of Cho/Cr ratio from the patients with Grade 4 showed a significant ($p < 0.05$)

Table 2. *Changes in Ratios of Neuronal Metabolites and Grade of Subarachnoid Hemorrhage (SAH)*

H & K SAH Grade	Cho/Cr acute stage (No.)	NAA/Cr chronic stage (No.)
Grade 2	1.18 ± 0.16 (7)	2.03 ± 0.19 (6)
Grade 3	1.31 ± 0.16 (9)	1.96 ± 0.12 (15)
Grade 4	1.43 ± 0.30 (6)*	1.73 ± 0.27 (8)**

H & K Hunt and Kosnik. Values are mean ± standard deviation. * $p < 0.05$, compared to the value in the patients with Grade 2. ** $p < 0.05$, compared to the values in the patients with Grade 2 and 3.

increase compared to that from the patients with Grade 2. The severity of SAH grade correlated with a decrease in NAA/Cr ratio at the chronic stage of SAH, and the mean value showed a significant ($p < 0.05$) decrease in the patients with Grade 4 compared to those with Grade 2 and 3 (Table 2).

Discussion

We evaluated the changes in ratios of neuronal metabolites rather than their absolute concentrations in the brain following SAH. While evaluation of absolute metabolite quantification was tried to evaluate by means of the internal water standard method, this technique seems unsuitable for measurement in SAH patients because of the changes in the blood components or its lysates in the cerebrospinal fluid during time course. The tissue content of creatine plus phosphocreatine expressed as a single peak as total creatine concentration (Cr in the present study) and is recognized to remain relatively stable even during development of pathological condition. (1.2) Hence, we evaluated changes in NAA or Cho to Cr ratio as the changes in the neuronal metabolites in the present study. We selected the voxel for proton spectrum located only in the white matter, because it is suspected that blood components or secondary inflammated cells following SAH in the subarachnoid space over the cortex may possibly affect the proton spectrum.

Proton spectroscopy presents a decrease in NAA concentration even when MRI study shows no remarkable lesions in patients with AIDS encephalopathy [7] or Alzheimer disease [4]. Those patients show some degree of neuropsychological symptoms, as diffuse metabolic abnormalities in the neurons. A decrease in NAA concentration is also observed after an elevation of lactate concentration during development of cerebral infarction [2]. On the other hand, in the present study, we were able to observe a decrease in NAA without a definitive increase in lactate concentration in any stage of SAH or even in patients with symptomatic vasospasm. These results indicate that the present pathological condition in the brain after SAH, described by NAA depletion, somewhat differs from that in the development of cerebral infarction. The transient increase in Cho at the acute stage, which was correlated with the severity of SAH and affected by development of cerebral vasospasm, indicates the damage of cell membranes in a subpopulation of neurons or axons. Severity of SAH also correlated with a decrease in NAA at the chronic stage, while it is not obvious that these affected neurons in the acute stage result in neuronal cell loss at the chronic stage. These results confirm that SAH causes widespread neuronal injury, characterized by a non-ischaemic mechanism as seen in the development of an infarction, in the brain hemisphere during the time course of SAH. This pathological feature is suspected to be caused by some possible mechanisms such as impairment of microcirculation at the onset of SAH, impairment of cerebral circulation by development of chronic cerebral vasospasm [3] and neuronal injury caused secondarily by subarachnoid clot [6].

Ljunggren *et al.* [5] emphasized the fact that patients with a good recovery after SAH demonstrate a diffuse SAH-induced encephalopathy with impairment covering the whole spectrum of intellectual dysfunction from minor memory disturbance to numerous indications of higher intellectual processes. Postmortem histopathological study in SAH patients demonstrated the widespread multiple small lesions in the cerebral cortex presumably caused by impaired microcirculation following SAH, and this feature may be implicated in the etiology of psychological problems in SAH patients [8]. Some of the patients in the present study with a definitive decrease in NAA concentration revealed impairment of some aspects of intelligence by WAIS-R test (unpublished data). These results indicate that the widespread neuronal cell loss detected by NAA depletion is thought to be the main pathophysiological feature causing neurobehavioral dysfunction following SAH. Location of ruptured aneurysm is considered to also influence the development of neurobehavioral problems. However, in the present study, severity of SAH showed a relatively close correlation against the depletion of NAA concentration rather than the location of an aneurysm. It is important to study how spatially the brain tissues are affected, by means of mapping technique for metabolite changes in proton spectrum, in each ruptured aneurysm. We are planning to study the correlation among topographical changes in the neuronal metabolites and aspects of neurobehavioral dysfunction, which may present useful information implicated in this pathological feature following SAH.

References

1. Frahm J, Bruhn H, Gyngell ML, Mehrboldt KD, Hanicke W, Sauter R (1989) Localized proton NMR spectroscopy in different regions of the human brain in vivo: relaxation times and concentrations of cerebral metabolites. Magn Reson Med 11: 47–63
2. Graham GD, Blamire AM, Howseman AM, Rothman DL, Fayad PB, Brass LM, Petroff OA, Shulman RG Prichard JW (1992) Proton magnetic resonance spectroscopy of cerebral lactate and other metabolites in stroke patients. Stroke 22: 33–340
3. Handa Y, Kaneko M, Matuda T, Kobayashi H, Kubota T (1997) In vivo proton magnetic resonance spectroscopy for metabolic changes in brain during chronic cerebral vasospasm in primates. Neurosurgery 40: 773–781
4. Lazeyras F, Charles HC, Tupler LA, Erickson R, Boyko OB, Krichnan KR (1998) Metabolic brain mapping in Alzheimer disease using proton magnetic resonance spectroscopy. Psychiatry Res 82: 95–106
5. Ljunggren B, Sonesson B, Saveland H, Brandt L (1985) Cognitive impairment and adjustment in patients without neurological deficits after aneurysmal SAH and early operation. J Neurosurg 62: 673–679
6. Matz P, Massa SM, Weinstein PR, Turner C, Panter SS, Sharp FR (1996) Focal hyper expression of hemoxygenase-1 protein and messenger RNA in rat brain caused by cellular stress following subarachnoid injections of lysed blood. J Neurosurg 85: 892–900
7. Menon DK, Baudouin CJ, Tomlinson D, Hoyle C (1990) Proton MR spectroscopy and imaging of the brain in AIDS: Evidence of neuronal loss in regions that appear normal with imaging. J Comp Assist Tomogr 14: 882–885
8. Neil-Dwyer G, Lang DA, Doshi B, Gerber CJ, Smith PW (1994) Delayed cerebral ischemia: The pathological substrate. Acta Neurochir (Wien) 131: 137–145
9. Romner B, Sonesson B, Ljunggren B, Brandt L, Saveland H, Holtas S (1989) Late magnetic resonance imaging related to neurobehavioral functioning after subarachnoid hemorrhage. Neurosurgery 25: 390–397

Correspondence: Yuji Handa, M.D., Department of Neurosurgery, Fukui Medical University, Matsuoka, Yoshida-gun, Fukui 910-1193, Japan.

Microdialysis and Metabolic Monitoring

Acta Neurochir (2001) [Suppl] 77: 141–144

On-Line Microdialysis Following Aneurysmal Subarachnoid Hemorrhage

O. W. Sakowitz[1], **A. S. Sarrafzadeh**[1], **G. Benndorf**[2], **W. R. Lanksch**[1], and **A. W. Unterberg**[1]

[1] Department of Neurosurgery, Charité-Humboldt University Berlin, Berlin, Germany
[2] Department of Radiology, Charité-Humboldt University Berlin, Berlin, Germany

Introduction

Cerebral vasospasm (VSP) is one of the feared sequelae of subarachnoid hemorrhage (SAH). Symptomatic VSP, i.e. VSP leading to delayed ischemic neurological deficits (DIND), is still observed in approximately 30% of SAH patients and contributes considerably to the overall mortality and morbidity [11, 12].

Transcranial doppler sonography (TCD) is a noninvasive, inexpensive and easy-to-use method to monitor for cerebral vasospasm. However, in a number of studies it was found both insufficiently sensitive and specific to prognosticate or confirm the advent of cerebral VSP [4, 7, 13, 18].

Since the beginning of the 90s, microdialysis (MD) has been transferred from the laboratory into the ICU. A possible role of MD in neuro-intensive care monitoring has been repeatedly emphasized [10, 15]. Up to now in-vivo MD has been applied to a range of cerebrovascular diseases including aneurysmal SAH [5, 8, 9, 14].

Automated bedside devices allow continuous surveillance of brain metabolism by using enzymekinetic assays instead of analyzing samples off-line by time-consuming high pressure liquid chromatography (HPLC) [14, 16].

In this study bedside MD and serial TCD measurements were correlated with the development of DIND in patients following aneurysmal SAH. The following report summarizes these findings and experiences from routine neurometabolic monitoring in the setting of a neurosurgical intensive care unit.

Keywords: Cerebral vasospasm; doppler sonography; ischemia; microdialysis; subarachnoid hemorrhage.

Materials and Methods

Patients

A total of 78 patients with aneurysmal SAH were enrolled in a prospective study on cerebral metabolism monitored by bedside MD. SAH was confirmed by computerized tomography (CT) scanning. Distribution and pattern of hemorrhage was graded (Fisher). Clinical presentation was graded according to the WFNS-Scale. The presence of an aneurysm, its size and location were assessed using four-vessel digital subtraction angiography.

Blood flow velocities were obtained at least once daily by TCD (TC2-64, EME, Tubingen, Germany). Cerebral angiography was performed routinely in all patients upon admittance. According to the time course of VSP, control angiography was performed on day 7–8 after bleeding or earlier in case of neurologic deterioration. Only patients presenting with DIND, i.e. the insidious onset of confusion, appearance of a focal neurological deficit or both, were treated with "triple-H" (hypertension, hypervolemia and hemodilution) therapy.

Ethics

Intensive-care monitoring of SAH patients using the microdialysis-technique was approved by the local medical ethics committee. Written informed consent was obtained from the patient or the closest relative.

Neurochemical Monitoring

Following aneurysm clipping MD catheters (CMA70, CMA, Sweden; 10 mm membrane) were placed 25–35 mm into the brain parenchyma of the vascular territory most likely to be affected by VSP, e.g. the temporal lobe in patients with a middle cerebral (MCA) or an internal carotid artery (ICA) aneurysm or into the frontal lobe in patients with anterior communicating artery (Acom) aneurysms. Catheters were perfused (CMA 106 microdialysis pump, CMA, Sweden) with sterile Ringer's solution at a fixed flow rate of 0.3 $\mu l\ min^{-1}$.

Perfusates were collected in microvials, exchanged hourly and analyzed immediately for concentrations of glucose, lactate, pyruvate and glutamate. All analyses were carried out at bedside using the CMA600 enzyme-kinetic analyzer (CMA, Sweden).

Table 1. *Patient Characteristics*

Age	52 ± 12 yrs				
Gender	55F/23M				
WFNS Grade [†]	[1]	[2]	[3]	[4]	[5]
n =	26 (33%)	11 (14%)	9 (12%)	18 (23%)	14 (18%)
Fisher Grade [‡]	[1]	[2]	[3]	[4]	
n =	3 (4%)	22 (28%)	16 (21%)	37 (47%)	
Time to surgery [*]	39 ± 71 hrs				
Time to MD	46 ± 69 hrs				
Total time of MD [**]	155 ± 73 hrs				

Demographical data of 78 patients monitored post-operatively. [†]: initial WFNS grade on scene or after resuscitation; [‡]: initial CT scan; [*]: early operation (<72 hrs post SAH) in 69 cases (88%); [**]: total MD duration exceeded 96 hrs in 61 cases (78%)

Table 2.

	Asymptomatic	AIND	DIND
Glucose (mM)	3.1 ± 1.0	1.8 ± 1.2 (*)	2.8 ± 1.5
Lactate (mM)	2.7 ± 1.8	8.6 ± 4.7 (*)	4.3 ± 3.4
Pyruvate (μM)	115.0 ± 55.6	151.3 ± 109.2	155.4 ± 83.8
LPR	25 ± 10	89 ± 117 (*)	28 ± 14
Glutamate (μM)	3.5 ± 2.3	83.5 ± 151.7 (*)	14.0 ± 21.0

Baseline values of ECF glucose, lactate and glutamate according to clinical courses. Individually determined as median values of the first 72 hours. Group means and standard deviation. *AIND* Acute ischemic neurological deficit, *DIND* delayed ischemic neurological deficit. [*] $p < 0.05$ compared with asymptomatic patients

Criteria for Sensitivity and Specificity

For the analysis of sensitivity and specificity in the verification of DIND only patients with control angiography were regarded. Angiographic VSP was defined as moderate to severe vessel narrowing that reduced vessel calibers by more than 30% compared to baseline values obtained on admission.

In serial TCD studies flow velocities greater 120 cm/s were regarded pathologic [1]. To determine sensitivity and specificity of MD in detecting secondary neurological deterioration lactate concentrations above 4 mM and glutamate concentrations above 3 μM were considered pathologic [16]. These had to persist for at least 6 consecutive hours.

Data Analysis

All statistics were done using SPSS 8.0 (SPSS) Inc., Chicago, IL, USA). Post-hoc data reduction of MD-values was achieved by calculation of intraindividual medians. Data averaged among groups are reported as means and standard deviation. Contingency tables were evaluated using Chi-square-statistics. Nonparametric testing was used for comparison of MD values between (Mann-Whitney-U) and within groups (Wilcoxon). A p-value less than 0.05 was considered significant.

Results

Patient Characteristics

The clinical courses of 78 SAH patients were prospectively evaluated. Demographical data of this group are summarized in Table 1. There were no complications (hemorrhagic, infectious) related to MD. Overall in-hospital mortality was 13%.

Acute ischemic neurological deficits (AIND, i.e. ischemia secondary to extensive intracerebral hemorrhage, thromboembolic events, clip stenosis or generalized brain swelling) were encountered in 19 (24%) patients. MD became pathologic in 17 (89%) of these cases. DIND was encountered in 15 (19%) patients.

Estimates of sensitivity, specificity and likelihood-ratios are based on those cases in whom control angiography was performed within the time of monitoring ($n = 30$).

Cerebral Metabolism Following SAH

Considering baseline values, distinct patterns of cerebral metabolism were associated with clinical courses following SAH (Table 2).

In patients with AIND glucose concentrations were significantly lower when compared with asymptomatic patients ($p < 0.05$). Lactate and glutamate were significantly elevated (both $p < 0.05$).

In contrast, patients with DIND did not differ from asymptomatic patients in baseline concentrations of glucose, lactate and glutamate initially. Glutamate

Table 3.

	DSA		TCD		MD	
	(+)	(−)	(+)	(−)	(+)	(−)
DIND (+)	11	0	7	4	9	2
DIND (−)	9	10	7	12	2	17
Sensitivity	1.00 (1.00 − 1.00)		0.64 (0.46 − 0.81)		0.82 (0.68 − 0.96)	
Specificity	0.53 (0.35 − 0.70)		0.63 (0.46 − 0.80)		0.89 (0.78 − 1.00)	
LHR	2.1		1.7		7.8	

Two-by-two tables of detecting (+) or missing (−) delayed ischemic neurological deficits (DIND +) or their absence (DIND −). Comparison of methods regarding sensitivity, specificity and likelihood-ratios of three tests to confirm symptomatic VSP. Likelihood-ratios (*LHR*) calculated as *sensitivity*/(1 − *specificity*). *DSA* Digital subtraction angiography, *TCD* transcranial doppler ultrasonography, *MD* microdialysis

concentrations, however, were of considerable inter-individual variance.

Sensitivity and Specificity

Serial TCD studies and continuous MD were compared regarding their ability to verify DIND. Threshold conditions were defined to mark the occurrence of ischemia. Sensitivity, specificity and likelihood-ratios to verify DIND were calculated for all patients with control angiography within the monitoring period (asymptomatic n = 19; DIND n = 11).

As shown in Table 3 sensitivity of DSA was superior to MD and TCD. DSA, however, had the lowest specificity followed by TCD. MD proved to be the most specific method to confirm DIND. Consecutively, the likelihood ratio of a positive test related with delayed ischemia was highest for MD, being considerably lower for DSA and TCD.

Discussion

Different clinical courses of patients after SAH are associated with early alterations in MD parameters. Moreover, on-line MD reveals characteristic metabolic changes during vasospasm and is capable of confirming its diagnosis with a high specificity.

In general, alterations in MD parameters correlate well with the clinical condition of patients suffering from cerebral ischemia [8, 14]. In this study AIND was often reflected in pathological MD values in the initial post-operative phase. In view of this, MD could become a valuable tool to detect early deterioration and react to acute ischemic events more timely.

"Normal" values of extracellular lactate and glutamate have been reported [16]. However these were assessed intraoperatively, i.e. relatively short after probe placement, and may thus overestimate physiological conditions. This may explain why by using even lower threshold values (e.g. 3 μM for glutamate in this study) an excellent specificity to verify DIND was obtained.

In regard to DIND prognostication, this study investigated the sensitivities and specificities of 3 methods to *verify* DIND. It still has to be clarified which metabolic patterns in MD enable to predict this condition.

In previous studies sensitivity of TCD ranged from 59% to 88%, while specificity ranged from 72% to 100% [6, 17]. These values, however, were calculated with the predefined condition being *angiographic* VSP. Our study reflects that angiography itself has a low specificity; approximately 60–70% of SAH patients display angiographic VSP to a certain degree whereas only 30% develop DIND [6, 12].

Reasons for false negative and false positive TCD results have been discussed in the literature. In correlative studies of regional CBF-measurements and TCD considerable rates of false positive test results were related to mistaking hyperemia for ischemia [3]. The known inter-observer variability may be another source of error [2].

Conclusion

"On-line" MD is an invasive but safe monitoring technique to assess regional cerebral metabolism. As the current study demonstrates, it can be carried out routinely in the ICU-setting to detect and monitor patterns of metabolic impairment. Compared to TCD it has a remarkable specificity making it a well-suited method to monitor for DIND following aneurysmal hemorrhage.

Acknowledgments

This study was supported by the Deutsche Forschungsgemeinschaft (DFG), grant Un56/7-3.

References

1. Aaslid R, Huber P, Nornes H (1984) Evaluation of cerebrovascular spasm with transcranial doppler ultrasound. J Neurosurg 60: 37–41
2. Ceravolo M, Minciotti P, Orlandini M, Provinciali L (1992) Intra- and inter-observer variability of basal flow velocity and vascular reactivity measurements using transcranial doppler sonography. Neurol Res 14: 122–124
3. Clyde B, Resnick D, Yonas H, Smith H, Kaufmann A (1996) The relationship of blood velocity as measured by transcranial doppler ultrasonography to cerebral blood flow as determined by stable xenon computed tomographic studies after aneurysmal subarachnoid hemorrhage. Neurosurgery 38: 896–904
4. Creissard P, Proust F, Langlois O (1995) Vasospasm diagnosis: theoretical and real transcranial doppler sensitivity. Acta Neurochir (Wien) 136: 181–185
5. Enblad P, Valtysson J, Andersson J, Lilja A, Valind S, Antoni G, Langstrom B, Hillered L, Persson L (1996) Simultaneous intracerebral microdialysis and positron emission tomography in the detection of ischemia in patients with subarachnoid hemorrhage. J Cereb Blood Flow Metab 16: 637–644
6. Grolimund P, Seiler R, Aaslid R, Huber P, Zurbruegg H (1987) Evaluation of cerebrovascular disease by combined extracranial and transcranial doppler sonography. Experience in 1,039 patients. Stroke 18: 1018–1024
7. Grosset D, Straiton J, McDonald I, Cockburn M, Bullock R (1993) Use of transcranial doppler sonography to predict development of a delayed ischemic deficit after subarachnoid hemorrhage. J Neurosurg 78: 183–187
8. Hamberger A, Runnerstam M, Nystrom B, Starmark J, von Essen C (1995) The neuronal environment after subarachnoid haemorrhage – correlation of amino acid and nucleoside levels with post-operative recovery. Neurol Res 17: 97–105
9. Kanthan R, Goplen G, Griebel R, Miyashita H, Burbridge B, Kalra I, Shuaib A (1995) Clinical evaluation of vasospasm in subarachnoid haemorrhage by in vivo microdialysis. J Neurol Neurosurg Psychiatry 59: 646–647
10. Landolt H, Langemann H (1996) Cerebral microdialysis as a diagnostic tool in acute brain injury. Eur J Anaesthesiol 13: 269–278
11. Lanzino G, Kassell N (1999) Double-blind, randomized, vehicle-controlled study of high-dose tirilazad mesylate in women with aneurysmal subarachnoid hemorrhage. Part ii. A cooperative study in North America. J Neurosurg 90: 1018–1024
12. Lanzino G, Kassell N, Dorsch N, Pasqualin A, Brandt L, Schmiedek P, Truskowski L, Alves W (1999) Double-blind, randomized, vehicle-controlled study of high-dose tirilazad mesylate in women with aneurysmal subarachnoid hemorrhage. Part i. A cooperative study in Europe, Australia, New Zealand, and South Africa. J Neurosurg 90: 1011–1017
13. Laumer R, Steinmeier R, Gonner F, Vogtmann T, Priem R, Fahlbusch R (1993) Cerebral hemodynamics in subarachnoid hemorrhage evaluated by transcranial doppler sonography. Part 1. Reliability of flow velocities in clinical management. Neurosurgery 33: 1–8
14. Nilsson O, Brandt L, Ungerstedt U, Saveland H (1999) Bedside detection of brain ischemia using intracerebral microdialysis: subarachnoid hemorrhage and delayed ischemic deterioration. Neurosurgery 45: 1176–1184
15. Persson L, Hillered L (1992) Chemical monitoring of neurosurgical intensive care patients using intracerebral microdialysis. J Neurosurg 76: 72–80
16. Reinstrup P, Stahl N, Mellergard P, Uski T, Ungerstedt U, Nordstrom C (2000) Intracerebral microdialysis in clinical practice: baseline values for chemical markers during wakefulness, anesthesia, and neurosurgery. Neurosurgery 47: 701–709
17. Sloan M, Haley E, Kassell N, Henry M, Stewart S, Beskin R, Sevilla E, Torner J (1989) Sensitivity and specificity of transcranial doppler ultrasonography in the diagnosis of vasospasm following subarachnoid hemorrhage. Neurology 39: 1514–1518
18. Vora Y, Suarez-Almazor M, Steinke D, Martin M, Findlay J (1999) Role of transcranial doppler monitoring in the diagnosis of cerebral vasospasm after subarachnoid hemorrhage. Neurosurgery 44: 1237–1247

Correspondence: Dr. Oliver W. Sakowitz, Department of Neurosurgery, Charité-Campus Virchow-Klinikum, Augustenburger Platz 1, D-13353 Berlin, Germany.

Acta Neurochir (2001) [Suppl] 77: 145–147

Time Course of Various Interstitial Metabolites Following Subarachnoid Hemorrhage Studied by on-Line Microdialysis*

A. S. Sarrafzadeh, O. W. Sakowitz, W. R. Lanksch, and **A. W. Unterberg**

Department of Neurosurgery, Charité Campus Virchow Medical Clinic, Humboldt University of Berlin, Germany

Introduction

Subarachnoid hemorrhage (SAH) is one of the most devastating of all cerebrovascular disorders [10]. One of the most serious complications of SAH remains vasospasm [2, 9]. Bedside cerebral microdialysis is a recently available method to sample and directly analyze extracellular concentration of cerebral metabolites next to the patient [7]. It monitors the energy metabolites glucose, pyruvate and lactate, the excitatory amino acid glutamate and glycerol, a marker of cell membrane damage. The usefulness of the microdialysis technique in a clinical setting of a neurointensive care unit has been reported previously [4, 5, 6]. Since changes of brain extracellular metabolites were shown to correlate with the neurological condition, the microdialysis techniques may be powerful in monitoring the progression of ischemia in SAH patients [6].

In a prospective clinical trial we studied the time course of various interstitial metabolites in patients with clinical symptoms of acute and delayed ischemic neurological deficits by bedside microdialysis.

Keywords: Cerebral metabolism; microdialysis; subarachnoid hemorrhage; vasospasm.

Materials and Methods

This study was in accordance with the local medical ethics policies in the study of human subjects and written informed consent was obtained from the patient or nearest family relative.

Patient Characteristics and Management

72 patients (WFNS Grade 0–5) with diagnosis of aneurysmal SAH were enrolled in a prospective, non randomized study on cerebral metabolism monitored by bedside microdialysis. Following preoperative resuscitation, patients were treated with early surgery (within 72 hrs after hemorrhage) unless the patient already exhibited symptoms of clinical vasospasm. At surgery, it was uniform policy to insert an external ventricular drainage and to clear all accessible subarachnoid clot in addition to clipping or wrapping the aneurysm. The diagnosis of vasospasm was clinically based, using classic symptoms of symptomatic vasospasm (onset occurring from day 2–14 post-SAH; worsening of headache, stiff neck; insidious onset of confusion, disorientation, and/or drowsiness; and focal deficits, which often were fluctuating) and no other identifiable cause of neurological deterioration such as electrolyte disturbance or seizure present.

Bedside Microdialysis

A microdialysis catheter (CMA 70, CMA, Sweden) was inserted immediately after clipping of the aneurysm into brain parenchyma of the respective vascular territory most likely to be affected by vasospasm, e.g. the temporal lobe in patients with a middle (MCA) cerebral artery aneurysm. The catheters (membrane length 10 mm, diameter 0.6 mm, molecular weight limit 10.000) were tunneled through a burr hole of the bone flaps underneath the scalp and fixed to the skin with sutures. Immediately after surgery, a microdialysis syringe placed in a microinfusion pump (CMA 106, Sweden) was connected to the inlet tubing. Catheters were perfused with sterile Ringer's at a flow rate of 0.3 µl/minute. On the outlet tube perfusates were collected in microvials, exchanged hourly and immediately analyzed bedside in a mobile photometric, enzyme-kinetic analyzer (CMA 600, Sweden) for concentrations of glucose, pyruvate, lactate, glutamate and frozen for later analyzes of glycerol.

Data Analysis

All data were collected during days 1–14 after admission due to SAH and are presented as mean ± SEM if not otherwise indicated. To calculate group specific differences the 72-hrs median for days 0 to 2, 3 to 5 and 6 to 8 post hemorrhage were calculated. Differences

* Supported by Deutsche Forschungsgemeinschaft Un-56/7

Table 1. *Demographic Characteristics of Patients with SAH*

	Asymptomatic (n = 42)	AIND (n = 18)	DIND (n = 12)
Age (yr)	51.5 ± 1.8	53.1 ± 2.6	47.1 ± 2.5
Admission WFNS grade	2.5 ± 0.2	3.1 ± 0.4	3.0 ± 0.3
Fisher score	2.8 ± 0.1	3.6 ± 0.3	3.3 ± 0.2
Location of aneurysm			
ACI	9	5	2
ACM	8	7	4
ACoA	21	5	5
ACoP	4	1	1
Duration microdialysis (hrs)	139 ± 10 hrs	146 ± 13 hrs	178 ± 13 hrs

were considered statistically significant at $p < 0.05$. All statistics were done using SPSS 8.0 (SPSS Inc., Chicago, IL, USA).

Results

Patient Characteristics

Demographic data are listed in Table 1. There were no complications related to the MD-catheter insertion (hemorrhagic, infectious). Patients were classified according to the post-operative clinical course as asymptomatic or presenting symptoms of acute (AIND) or delayed ischemic neurological deficits (DIND) (Table 1). Patient groups were comparable for age ($p = 0.2$) and WFNS score ($p = 0.1$).

Cerebral Metabolic Changes After SAH

For data analysis the first 6 hours after insertion were excluded. There were significant group differences in the extracellular lactate, glutamate and the lactate-pyruvate ratio for all time points after SAH (72, 144, 216 hrs after SAH), for the 72 hrs-glucose and the 72-, and 144-hrs glycerol, $p < 0.01$). In asymptomatic patients (n = 42), extracellular glucose and glycerol concentrations were stable during monitoring time (glucose: 2.7 ± 0.5 mM; glycerol: 70.8 ± 8.1 mM). There was a moderate increase in extracellular lactate over time (Fig. 1). Glutamate levels decreased after insertion and were generally low compared to symptomatic patients (Fig. 1). Patients with AIND (n = 18) developed immediate microdialysis alterations if the probe was close to the malperfused region. These patients had low glucose concentrations (in average 1.4 ± 0.6 mM), and significantly higher lactate, glutamate and glycerol (in average 313.7 ± 237.5 μM) concentrations compared to asymptomatic and DIND patients, indicative of anaerob metabolism, ischemia and membrane degradation (Fig. 1, $p < 0.01$). In DIND patients (n = 12), glutamate was

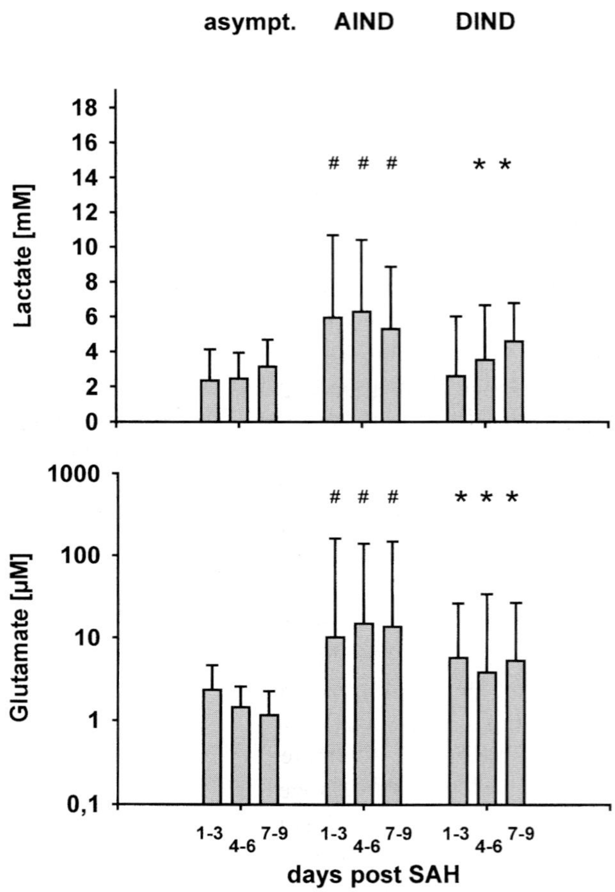

Fig. 1. Temporal course of extracellular lactate and glutamate concentrations in three different patient groups: asymptomatic patients, patients with acute ischemic neurological deficits (*AIND*) and patients with delayed ischemic neurological deficits (*DIND*). Data are given as 72-hours median ± SD. # indicates $p < 0.05$ asymptomatic versus AIND patients. * Indicates $p < 0.05$ asymptomatic versus DIND patients. *SAH* Subarachnoid hemorrhage

generally high and lactate secondarily increased over time (Fig. 1).

Discussion

Morbidity and mortality after aneurysmal SAH often result from ischemia secondary to vasospasm. Since the onset of clincal vasospasm is within a wide range between day 3 and day 10 after initial bleeding, continuous monitoring is desirable for early detection of ischemia. Only recently, microdialysis – a well established neurochemistry technique – is available for bedside detection of cerebral biochemical changes in patients [7]. So far, no adverse effect has been observed in patients and because of its small size, the dialysis catheter is expected to cause only minimal damage [4, 5]. Several investigators have studied the metabolic changes of the extracellular milieu by microdialysis in aneurysmatic subarachnoid hemorrhage patients. Säveland and colleagues [6] measured the levels of glutamate and aspartate using microdialysis in 7 SAH-patients in different vascular territories of the brain. They observed highly variable levels of excitatory amino acids in correlation with the clinical course and the vascular territory where the vasospasm occurred. Asymptomatic patients ($n = 2$) had low glutamate (0.6 mM) and aspartate (0.03 mM) levels, while patients with acute ischemic neurological deficits ($n = 2$) had relatively high glutamate (12 μM) and aspartate (4.3 mM) levels. These observations were confirmed by our study which showed that patients had significantly higher extracellular lactate and glutamate concentrations in the presence of neurological symptoms compared to asymptomatic patients. As extracellular levels of glutamate were found to increase in severe ischemia [1], changes in extracellular glutamate have been proposed as useful indicators to predict the outcome from these conditions [3, 8]. Additional interpretation of the energy metabolism may help to differentiate between a glutamate increase due to ischemia versus high glutamate levels due to cellular leakage, such as seen as transient effect directly after insertion of a microdialysis probe.

Conclusion

On-line MD has become a valuable tool in neurointensive care monitoring of SAH patients. Distinct patterns of alterations in MD parameters can be monitored in good accordance with clinical presentation. In patients presenting clinical symptoms of acute and delayed ischemic neurological deficits, the extracellular concentrations of lactate and glutamate are significantly higher compared to asymptomatic patients. In our view, bedside microdialysis is a valuable technique for early detection of cerebral ischemia in SAH patients.

References

1. Benveniste H, Drejer J, Schousboe A, Diemer NH (1984) Elevation of the extracellular concentrations of glutamate and aspartate in rat hippocampus during transient cerebral ischemia monitored by intracerebral microdialysis. J Neurochem 43: 1369–1374
2. Kassell NF, Haley EC Jr, Apperson-Hansen C, Alves WM (1996) Randomized, double-blind, vehicle-controlled trial of tirilazad mesylate in patients with aneurysmal subarachnoid hemorrhage: a cooperative study in Europe, Australia, and New Zealand. J Neurosurg 84(2): 221–228
3. Mendelowitsch A, Sekhar LN, Wright DC, Nadel A, Miyashita H, Richardson R, Kent M, Shuaib A (1998) An increase in extracellular glutamate is a sensitive method of detecting ischaemic neuronal damage during cranial base and cerebrovascular surgery. An in vivo microdialysis study. Acta Neurochir (Wien) 140(4): 349–355
4. Nilsson OG, Brandt L, Ungerstedt U, Saveland H (1999) Bedside detection of brain ischemia using intracerebral microdialysis: subarachnoid hemorrhage and delayed ischemic deterioration. Neurosurgery 45(5): 1176–1184
5. Persson L, Valtysson J, Enblad P, Warme PE, Cesarini K, Lewen A, Hillered L (1996) Neurochemical monitoring using intra-cerebral microdialysis in patients with subarachnoid hemorrhage. J Neurosury 84: 606–616
6. Saeveland H, Nilsson OG, Boris-Moeller F, Wieloch T, Brandt L (1996) Intracerebral microdialysis of glutamate and aspartate in two vascular territories after aneurysmal subarachnoid hemorrhage. Neurosurgery 38: 12–20
7. Ungerstedt U (1991) Microdialysis: Principles and applications for studies in animals and man. J Intern Med 230: 365–373
8. Vespa P, Prins M, Ronne-Engstrom E, Caron M, Shalmon E, Hovda DA, Martin NA, Becker DP (1998) Increase in extracellular glutamate caused by reduced cerebral perfusion pressure and seizures after human traumatic brain injury: a microdialysis study. J Neurosurg 89(6): 971–982
9. Weaver JP, Fisher M (1994) Subarachnoid hemorrhage: an update of pathogenesis, diagnosis and management. J Neurol 125(2): 119–131
10. Yanagihara T, Piepgras DG, Atkinson JLD (1998) Subarachnoid hemorrhage: An overview. In: Yanagihara T, Piepgras DG, Atkinson JLD (eds) Subarachnoid hemorrhage. Medical and surgical management. Marcel Dekker, Inc, New York

Correspondence: Asita S. Sarrafzadeh, Charité Campus Virchow Medical Clinic, Humboldt University of Berlin, Augustenburger Platz 1, 13353 Berlin, Germany.

Acta Neurochir (2001) [Suppl] 77: 149–153

Monitoring Subtle Neurometabolic Changes in Subarachnoid Hemorrhage Patients Using Microdialysis: A Study on 16 Cases

E. De Micheli[1], **G. Pinna**[2], **E. Piovan**[2], **R. Prisco**[3], **L. Hillered**[4], **L. Persson**[4], **L. Monolo**[1], and **A. Bricolo**[2]

[1] Department of Neurosurgery, Lecco City Hospital, Italy
[2] Department of Neurosurgery, Verona University Hospital, Italy
[3] Department of Finance, Industry and Technological Studies, School of Business, University of Verona, Italy
[4] Department of Neurosurgery, Uppsala University Hospital, Sweden

Introduction

Microdialysis (MD) is a new technique which allows the continuous acquisition of samples from a limited area of the brain with good temporal resolution. This method enables the retrieval of critical biochemical substances from the extracellular fluid (ECF) of the brain, thus representing a valid tool for studying the mechanisms of cerebral secondary ischemia in humans [10, 11, 12]. One of the most common causes of unfavorable outcome following subarachnoid aneurysmal hemorrhage (SAH) is cerebral vasospasm-induced delayed ischemia, often leading to reversible or permanent neurological deficits as a consequence of neuronal damage or death [6, 10]. Vasospasm is generally a focal rather than diffuse phenomenon and development is not always detected early by TCD evaluation nor by routine neuroradiological exams; therefore, a technique such as MD may be important for direct neurochemical monitoring.

The objectives of this study were to test the sensitivity of MD in detecting vasospasm-induced neurometabolic abnormalities in patients with non-severe SAH and to identify neurochemical pathological patterns which may be used to predict the development of cerebral ischemia. The authors investigated if a correlation exists between ECF levels of important endogenous substances retrieved by MD and neurological course, brain imaging (CT), cerebral blood flow velocity measured by TCD and regional cerebral blood flow (rCBF) measured using Xenon-CT (Xe-CT).

Keywords: Microdialysis; aneurysmal subarachnoid hemorrhage; brain metabolism; cerebral ischemia.

Materials and Methods

Patient Criteria

Inclusion criteria for this study was based on the following: 1) patient age (>18 years); 2) admission in good neurological condition (Hunt & Hess Grades I–III and World Federation of Neurological Surgeons Scale Grades 1–3); 3) SAH diagnosis by clinical history and confirmed by Computerized Tomography (CT); 4) angiography demonstrating a saccular aneurysm; 5) early surgical intervention (<72 hours after SAH).

Methods

During hospitalization, patients underwent repeated CT and TCD exams; flow velocity was calculated based on the middle cerebral artery (MCA) mean value, ipsilateral to the MD catheter. MCA flow velocity values above 80 cm/sec were considered pathologic [13]. In selected cases, Xe-CT was performed to measure rCBF between Days 3–4 and 6–10 after SAH. The rCBF was calculated using the arithmetic mean of 10 overlapping ROI (each 20 mm in diameter) of the frontal or temporal cortex of each hemisphere in relation to the MD catheter location. The absolute rCBF values (ml/100 g/min) in the area of the MD catheter were compared with values of the contralateral homologous area as well as the normal values obtained from an age-matched control group; rCBF changes were expressed as a percentage difference.

Patient outcome was evaluated based on neurological examination according to the Glasgow Outcome Scale (GOS) and CT scans performed 6 and 12 months after SAH.

During surgery, a 10 mm flexible microdialysis catheter with an external diameter of 0.6 mm (CMA/70 custom catheter, CMA/Microdialysis, Solna, Sweden) was inserted in the subfrontal (patients with AcoA and ACA aneurysm) or temporal (ICA and MCA) cortex, and perfused with artificial CSF at a rate of 0.3 μl/min using a microinjection pump (CMA 106, CMA/Microdialysis, Solna, Sweden). An equilibration period of 60 minutes without sampling was allowed after catheter implantation. Dialysate was collected every 6 hours. Microdialysis samples were divided into aliquots and analyzed enzymatically on two different High Performance Liquid Cromatography (HPLC) systems. Glucose, lactate, pyruvate and glycerol were analyzed using an enzymatic technique (CMA 600

Table 1. *Clinical Characteristics of 16 Patients with Non-Severe SAH who Underwent Post-Operative Intracerebral Microdialysis*

Case	Admission grade (H & H)	Aneurysm location	Surgery day	Catheter location	MD[1] days	TCD vasospasm	Clinical vasospasm	Ischemia on CT	Outcome (GOS [12])
1	III	ACoA	1	L F	9	yes[2]	yes	no	GR
2	II	R ICA	3	R T	11	yes[2]	yes	yes	Md
3	III	L ICA	2	L T	9	yes	yes	no	GR
4	II	L MCA	2	L T	11	yes[2]	no	no	GR
5	II	L ACA	2	L F	2	no	no	no	GR
6	II	ACoA	3	L T	6	no	yes	no	GR
7	II	ACoA	2	R F	9	yes	no	no	GR
8	II	ACoA	3	L F	9	yes	no	no	GR
9	II	R MCA	2	R T	11	yes[2]	yes	yes	GR
10	II	ACoA	3	R F	8	yes	yes	yes	GR
11	II	R ICA	2	R T	9	no	no	no	GR
12	II	R MCA	3	R T	6	yes	no	no	GR
13	II	R ICA	2	R T	6	yes[2]	no	no	GR
14	II	ACoA	1	R F	5	yes[2]	yes	no	GR
15	III	ACoA	3	R F	12	no	yes	yes	GR
16	II	ACoA	2	R F	5	yes	yes	no	GR

ACA Anterior cerebral artery; *ACoA* anterior communicating artery; *CT* computerized tomography; *F* Frontal; *GOS*[12] Glasgow Outcome Scale; *GR* good recovery; *H & H* Hunt & Hess; *ICA* internal carotid artery; *L* left; *MCA* middle cerebral artery; *Md* moderate disability; *R* right; *T* Temporal; *TCD* transcranial doppler; *Xe-CT* Xenon-computerized tomography.

[1] MD Days refers to duration of microdialysis measurement.

[2] Blood flow velocity values > 120 cm/sec.

Analyser, CMA/Microdialysis, Solna, Sweden). Adenosine was detected at 254 nm, according to the method of Fredholm and Sollevi (1981) [2]. Amino acids were fluorimetrically detected following precolumn derivatization with o-phtaldialdehyde. The study was approved by the Hospital Ethics Committee and patients gave informed consent.

Statistics

The results were analyzed by simple regression analysis using commercially available software (Stat View 5.0, Abacus Concepts Inc., Berkeley, CA.; SPSS 8.0; SPSS Inc., Chicago, IL.). Differences with a probability value of less than 0.05 were considered statistically significant.

Results

Sixteen patients were included in this study. Clinical characteristics of the patients are illustrated in Table 1. Nine patients presented vasospasm-related clinical disturbances during the microdialysis period (Cases 1–3, 6, 9, 10, 14–16); transient in 8 patients, and persistent in 1 (Case 2). In these cases, MD data showed a progressive increase of lactate and decrease of glucose. This trend was also seen in patients with increased blood flow velocity but with an uneventful clinical course. Increased TCD velocities were found in 12 patients (Cases 1–4, 7–10, 12–14, 16) at some point during the study, exceeding 120 cm/sec in 6 (Cases 1, 2, 4, 9, 13, 14). Increasing TCD values correlated with decreasing glucose/lactate (G/L) ratios and increasing adenosine levels in 8 patients (Cases 1–3, 6, 10, 11, 15, 16). In 9 patients (Cases 8–16), ECF pyruvate levels were also measured; Lactate/Pyruvate (L/P) ratios were found to be above the reported "normal" threshold of 25 [11] in 8 cases, while no correlation between L/P ratio and clinical status was found.

In all patients, CT scans were obtained before, during and after the microdialysis study, and at the 3-month follow-up. In 4 cases (Cases 2, 9, 10, 15), sequential CT showed a delayed development of a persistent hypodense lesion (cerebral infarction). In 2 patients (Cases 9 and 10), in which the cerebral infarct was adjacent to the catheter site, MD revealed increasing glutamate levels eventually reaching the highest values found in this study. Glutamate levels (mean 4.4 μmol/l) are comparable to those previously found in SAH patients with favorable outcome [11]. In addition, glutamate was also found to positively correlate with lactate (Fig. 1), but not with G/L ratio or L/P ratio, as in severe SAH [11].

In selected patients (Cases 3–8, 10, 15, 16), repeated rCBF measurements were obtained with Xe-CT in the cortical area where the MD catheter was located. Absolute rCBF values were compared to normal values obtained from an aged-matched control group. In 5 patients (Cases 3, 4, 6, 7, 15), rCBF values were sig-

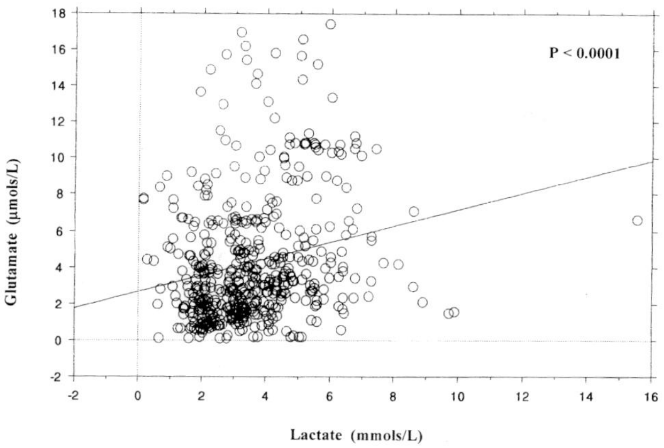

Fig. 1. Scatter plot showing correlation between glutamate and lactate in patient dialysate samples ($p < 0.0001$)

nificantly different from the controls, lower in 4 cases (% difference from normal value: Case 3, 27.8%; Case 4, 34.8%; Case 6, 25.8%; Case 15, 18.6% and 41%), and higher in 1 (% difference from normal value: Case 7, 27.1%). In patients with rCBF significantly lower than the control values, the G/L ratio was found <1 (Case 3: 0.38; Case 4: 0.28; Case 6: 0.77; Case 15: 0.36 and 0.4), whereas >1 when rCBF was higher than the control value (Case 7: 1.14). In 4 patients, significant changes between interhemispheric rCBF asymmetries on repeated Xe-CT exams correlated with G/L and lactate (Cases: 3, 6, 7, 15), and glutamate and adenosine (Cases: 3, 7, 15) fluctuations (Fig. 2).

Clinical outcome according to the Glasgow Outcome Scale (GOS) was assessed at 6 and 12 months after SAH. Fifteen patients made a good recovery, and one was evaluated as moderately disabled (Case 2).

Discussion

Aneurysmal subarachnoid hemorrhage is a cerebrovascular event with high morbidity and mortality [7, 8]. The major causes related to poor outcome are the effects of initial bleeding, surgical complications, and delayed ischemic deterioration due to cerebral vasospasm; the latter is the leading cause of disability and death in these patients, and accounts for nearly 30% of unfavorable outcomes [7, 8, 12]. Since arterial vasospasm is more often a focal rather than diffuse phenomenon, cerebral blood flow velocities, which are measured with TCD from the large cerebral arteries, may not always reflect microcirculatory alterations. Intracerebral microdialysis is a more sophisticated technique to monitor metabolic changes in cerebral areas which are considered at risk for secondary ischemia development [11, 12]. Since it is generally accepted that vasospasm rarely occurs immediately after SAH, monitoring the fluctuations in the ECF levels of neurochemical markers may be useful in predicting impending cerebral hypoxic and/or ischemic phenomena.

The physiopathology of vasospasm-induced ischemic damage is still poorly understood; yet two mechanisms, progressive cellular energy failure and massive extracellular release of excitotoxic amino acids, have been suggested to play a crucial role [9]. Glucose, lactate and adenosine have demonstrated to be reliable biochemical markers of disturbed neuronal energy metabolism, thus reflecting the bioenergetic status of the cell [4, 9]. ECF glucose levels indicate the availability of the major substrate for brain energy metabolism, the supply being directly dependent on blood flow. Interstitial lactate level is a marker of cellular oxygen deficiency which indicates cellular anaerobic energy production. In response to mild to moderate hypoxia, when the oxidative phosphorylation is preserved, glycolysis increases with a higher production of both lactate and pyruvate, and with a less marked increase of the L/P ratio. In this condition, lactate has proven to be a more sensitive marker of cellular energy imbalance than the L/P ratio [10], as confirmed also in this study, where a significant positive correlation between glutamate and lactate was found. During hypoxia, adenosine is formed rapidly within the nervous cell from 5′ AMP and then released into the extracellular space where levels reflect cellular bioenergetic state [1]. It has been proposed that adenosine exerts neuroprotection from a concerted cooperation of different actions: it inhibits Ca^{2+} fluxes in neuronal tissue; reduces formation of free radicals; and inhibits an excessive release of the excitatory transmitter glutamate [3]. Excitatory amino acids are of particular importance for ischemic neuronal damage, and their massive release into the extracellular space may exert excitotoxic effects eventually leading to cell death. Our study suggests that sustained high levels of glutamate (>6 µmol/l), when associated with increasing lactate production, may predict the development of irreversible ischemic processes. Following cellular energy metabolic failure, Ca^{2+} influx activates intracellular phospholipases leading to the split of cellular and subcellular membrane phospholipids into free fatty-acids and glycerol. Thus glycerol harvested by microdialysis

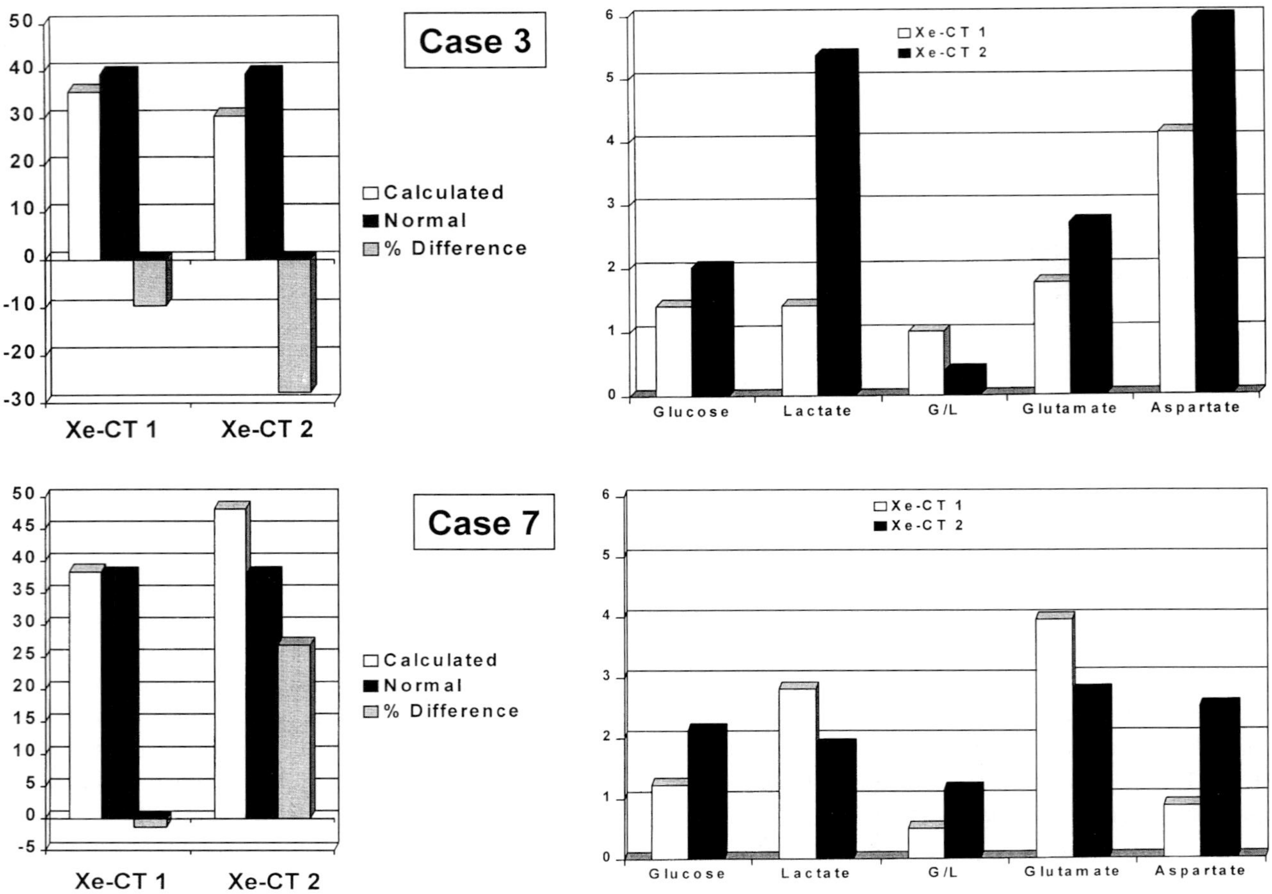

Fig. 2. Cases 3 and 7. rCBF in the cortical areas where the MD catheter was located: calculated and normal control values are expressed in ml/100 g/min; % differences are from normal control values. Absolute glucose (mmol/l), lactate (mmol/l), glutamate (μmol/l), aspartate (μmol/l) values, and glucose/lactate ratios at first and second Xenon-CT exam

has been proposed as a marker of phospholipid membrane breakdown [5].

Conclusions

The results of this study suggest the following: cerebral metabolic perturbation occurs to a certain degree also in non-severe SAH patients with uneventful clinical course and good outcome; in mild-to-moderate hypoxia, lactate is a more sensitive marker of the cellular energy metabolism state than the L/P ratio; in hypoxic conditions, a positive correlation between glutamate and lactate exists; adenosine is an early and sensitive marker of energetic metabolic imbalance, and elevated adenosine levels may exert neuroprotection by inhibiting a massive release of glutamate; sustained release of glutamate but not aspartate, when associated with increased lactate production, may represent a pattern predicting an impending condition of cellular ischemia; and lastly, ECF glycerol may be a reliable marker of the degree of cellular structural degeneration [5]. This study demonstrates the sensitivity of intracerebral microdialysis in revealing subtle metabolic abnormalities in patients with non-severe SAH. Consequently, MD may prove to be a useful neurochemical monitoring tool for early detection of impending spasm-induced cerebral ischemia in routine clinical practice.

References

1. De Micheli E, Pinna G., Ravenna G *et al* (1998) Intracerebral microdialysis of adenosine and glutamate in non-severe aneurysmal subarachnoid hemorrhage. In: von Wild KRH (ed) Pathophysiological principles and controversies in neurointensive care. Zuckschwerdt Verlag, München, pp 91–95

2. Fredholm BB, Sollevi A (1981) The release of adenosine and inosine from canine subcutaneous adipose tissue by nerve stimulation and noradrenaline. J Physiol 313: 351–367
3. Hagberg H, Sandberg M (1998) Nonglutamatergic neurotransmission in brain ischemia. In: Ginsberg MD, Bogousslavsky J (eds) Cerebrovascular disease, vol 1. Blackwell Science, Malden, MA, USA, pp 403–422
4. Hillered L, Persson L (1991) Microdialysis for metabolic monitoring in cerebral ischemia and trauma: experimental and clinical studies. In: Robinson TE, Justice JB Jr (eds) Microdialysis in the neurosciences VII: techniques in the behavioural and neural sciences. Elsevier, Amsterdam, pp 389–405
5. Hillered L, Valtysson J, Enblad P *et al* (1985) Interstitial glycerol as a marker for membrane phospholipid degradation in the acutely injured human brain. J Neurol Neurosurg Psychiatry 64: 486–491
6. Kassell NF, Sasaki T, Colohan ART, Nazar G (1985) Cerebral vasospasm following aneurysmal subarachnoid hemorrhage. Stroke 16: 562–572
7. Kassel NF, Torner JC, Haley EC Jr, Jane JA, Adams HP, Kongable GL (1990) The international cooperative study on the timing of aneurysm surgery, part 1: overall management results. J Neurosurg 73: 18–36
8. Kassel NF, Torner JC, Jane JA, Haley Jr EC, Adams HP (1990) The international cooperative study on the timing of aneurysm surgery, part 2: surgical results. J Neurosurg 73: 37–47
9. Lipton SA, Rosenberg PA (1994) Excitatory amino acids as a final common pathway for neurologic disorders. N Engl J Med 330: 613–622
10. Persson L, Hillered L (1992) Chemical monitoring of neurosurgical intensive care patients using intracerebral microdialysis. J Neurosurg 76: 72–80
11. Persson L, Valtysson J, Enblad P, Watme PE, Cesarini K, Lewen A, Hillered L (1996) Neurochemical monitoring using intracerebral microdialysis in patients with subarachnoid hemorrhage. J Neurosurg 84: 606–616
12. Saveland H, Nilsson O, Boris-Moller F, Wieloch T, Brandt L (1996) Intracerebral microdialysis of glutamate and aspartate in two vascular territories after aneurysmal subarachnoid hemorrhage. Neurosurgery 38: 12–20
13. Seiler RW, Grolimund P, Aaslid R, Huber P, Nornes H (1986) Cerebral vasospasm evaluated by transcranial ultrasound correlated with clinical grade and CT-visualized subarachnoid hemorrhage. J Neurosurg 64: 594–600

Correspondence: E. De Micheli, M.D., Department of Neurosurgery, Lecco City Hospital, Via Ghislanzoni 22, 23900 Lecco, Italy.

Acta Neurochir (2001) [Suppl] 77: 155–157

Microdialysis Nitric Oxide Levels and Brain Tissue Oxygen Tension in Patients with Subarachnoid Hemorrhage

M. Reinert[1,2], A. Zauner[1], A. Khaldi[1], R. Seiler[2], and R. Bullock[1]

[1] Division of Neurosurgery, Medical College of Virginia, VCU, Richmond, VA, USA
[2] Department of Neurosurgery, University of Bern, Inselspital Bern, Switzerland

Introduction

Nitric oxide (NO) is a highly reactive molecule that is believed to be involved in many physiological events. In the brain, nitric oxide has been implicated in a number of biological responses such as neurotransmitter modulation, retrograde neurotransmitter and synaptic plasticity. Nitric oxide diffuses across membranes and has guanylate cyclase in the smooth muscle as its primary target, by which nitric oxide leads to vasodilation thus regulating cerebral blood flow [3].

There are three isoforms of nitric oxide synthase (NOS), and all are expressed in the brain. The two constitutive, endothelial and neuronal (eNOS and nNOS), are believed to be primarily responsible for cerebral perfusion. On the other hand, microglial cells express inducible NOS (iNOS) in response to different stimuli such as lipopolysaccharids and cytokines. The role of the these different isoforms in brain injury is not yet well understood. NO is formed from the conversion of L-Arginin to L-Citruline. However the stoichiometric role of molecular diluted O_2 in brain tissue in this reaction has not been clearly established [1].

In animal and clinical studies, different groups have shown that vasospasm from SAH can be reversed by infusing nitric oxide donor [5]. Further it has been shown that brain tissue oyygen ($p_{ti}O_2$) is closely correlated with cerebral blood flow (CBF) [2]. In this study, we monitored local nitric oxide metabolites using intracerebral microdialysis in SAH patients along with a multi-parameter probe measuring $p_{ti}O_2$ and brain tissue carbon dioxide ($p_{ti}CO_2$). Global nitric oxide production in the CSF was also correlated with these local changes in brain tissue.

Keywords: Brain tissue oxygen; carbon dioxide; nitrate; nitric oxide; nitrate; subarachnoid hemorrhage.

Patients and Methods

12 patients suffering subarachnoid hemorrhage (SAH) with a Hunt and Hess grade of 3 or greater, were studied. A triple lumen transcranial bolt was threaded and tapped into the frontal skull as described by Zauner *et al.* The bolt was used to grip and immobilize the ventricular catheter, the microdialysis probe and the multiparameter sensor.

A multiparameter, Neurotrend 7 (Codman, Johnson and Johnson, USA) was used for continuous measurements of $p_{ti}O_2$, $p_{ti}CO_2$. A custom built sterile 10 mm flexible microdialysis probe (CMA Microdialysis, Acton, MA) with an external diameter of 0.5 mm and a molecular weight cut-off of 20,000 Dalton. The microdialysis probe was perfused at two microliter per minutes using sterile 0.9% saline. Sixty microliter dialysates were collected every half-hour. For total NO production (nitrite and nitrate) measurement, a fraction of the microdialysis sample (25 µl) was incubated with 5 µl of nitrite reductase (10 units/ml), 1 µl NADPH (4 mM), 5 µl 10X PBS and 14 µl 0.9% saline for 1 hour at room temperature. After which, 15 µl of sulfanilamide (1 mg/ml with 60 µl of phosphoric acid) and 15 µl of N-naphthylenediamine (10 mg/ml) was added for 10 minutes. The total volume (80 µl) was measured for absorbance at 545 nm. Every 4 to 6 hours a total NO (nitrate and nitrite) measurement was performed from the dialysate. The automatically recorded data, $p_{ti}O_2$, $p_{ti}CO_2$ were downloaded every 5 minutes. In order to compare the patients, the percent change of $p_{ti}O_2$ or $p_{ti}CO_2$ and total NO over the whole study were calculated.

Results

Of the 12 patients, 3 made a good recovery, 3 became moderately disabled, 1 stayed in vegetative state and 5 died.

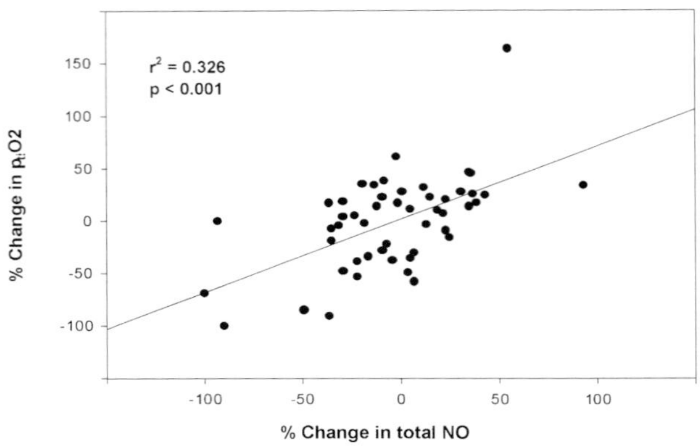

Fig. 1. The percent change of brain tissue oxygen ($p_{ti}O_2$) from the mean was correlated with the precent change of NO (Nitrate and Nitrite) from the mean. (N = 6 patients; $r^2 = 0.326$; $p < 0.001$)

Dialysate NO Metabolites and $p_{ti}O_2$

Dialysate NO production in microdialysis significantly changed over time. There was a close correlation between percentual change in NO metabolites and percentual change in $p_{ti}O_2$. A decrease in NO is associated with decreased $p_{ti}O_2$ levels while an increase in NO positively correlates with $p_{ti}O_2$ ($r^2 = 0.326$; $p < 0.001$) (Figs. 1 and 2a,b)

Nitrite/Nitrate in CSF

The levels of NO in CSF were calculated and the overall values were stable. The values of CSF NO metabolites were similar to previous studies, however showed little or no change in CSF NO production. Moreover, the relative changes in CSF NO metabolites did not significantly correlate with $p_{ti}O_2$ ($r^2 = 0.018$; $p = 0.734$). (Figs. not shown)

Dialysate NO Metabolites and Brain Tissue Energy Determinants

There was no significant correlation between NO and brain metabolites (glucose; $p = 0.098$, lactate; $p = 0.006$, $p_{ti}CO_2$ $p = 0.832$) within each patient or between patients. (Figs. not shown)

Discussion

The significance of increased NO production in pathological conditions is not well understood. In animal models, it has been shown that there is an increase in NO production after ischemia. The role of NO in pathogenesis ranges from neurotoxic to neuroprotective to neutral in nature. However NO is a known vasodilator [4] and its primary target in the brain is the guanylate cyclase in the smooth muscle. This is consistent with previous data that showed that cerebral perfusion is influenced by NO levels [3]. Moreover, the addition of nitric oxide donors reverses vasospasm in SAH animal models [5].

Measuring NO metabolites, nitrite and nitrate, in cerebral microdialysis samples indicates localized changes in NO production. These local changes are however not accompanied by a global change in NO

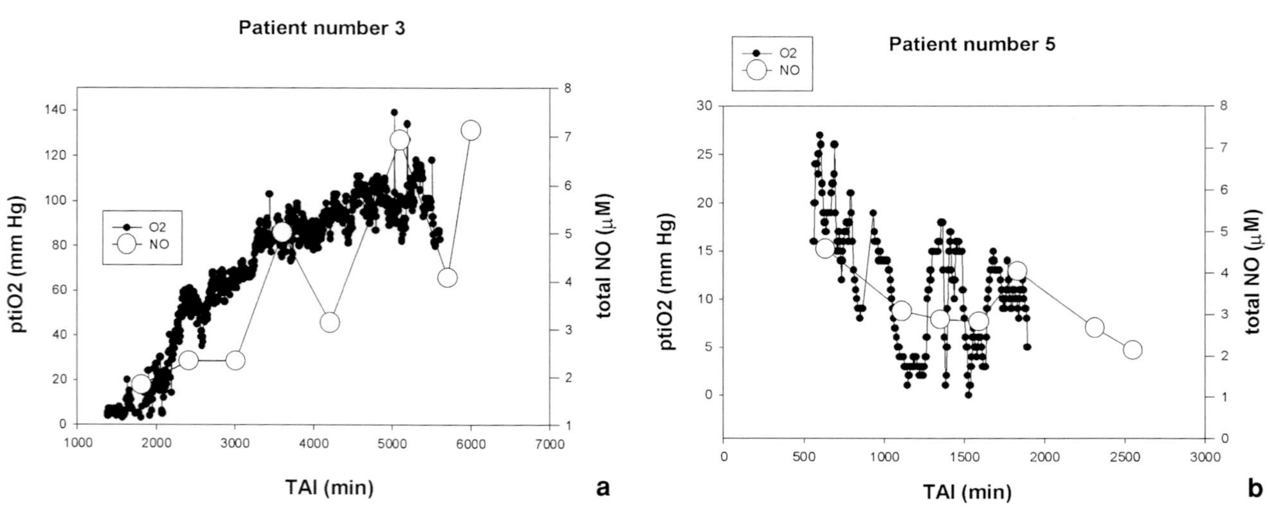

Fig. 2 (a,b) Two patients with SAH showing NO and $p_{ti}O_2$ values over monitoring time. The progress over time is different, but the correlation remains positive in both examples. Patient 3 had a good outcome and patient 5 died

production as seen from the CSF levels. The increase in dialysate NO production significantly correlated with local changes in brain tissue oxygen, whereas global CSF NO did not. These changes are however not accompanied with changes in metabolic parameters such as carbon dioxide, glucose and lactate levels in brain tissue. It has been shown that CBF positively influences brain tissue oxygen and that NO is involved in the regulation of CBF. However, under certain circumstances NO has been shown to influence metabolism as well, and thus may be indirectly responsible for changes in brain tissue oxygen. Nevertheless this mechanism seems less probable, as the metabolic parameters such as glucose, lactate and $p_{ti}CO_2$ were not influenced by changes in NO metabolites in this study. As encouraging as these results appear, the stoichiometric importance of molecular O_2 in the formation of NO needs to be taken into consideration, and further efforts need to be pursued in this direction such as an oxygen challenge and NO measurements in the animal model, in order to confirm our positive correlation between $p_{ti}O_2$ and NO.

Conclusion

In this study, a decline in NO production was accompanied by a decrease in brain tissue oxygen, while an increase in NO production was simultaneously accompanied by an increase in oxygen delivery ($p < 0.001$). These results further encourage the ongoing trials of NO substitution [6] after subarachnoid hemorrhage.

References

This study was supported N1H grant No. 9012587. Michael Reinest was supported by the Swiss National Foundation and by the Novartis Foundation.

1. Beal M (1997) Therapeutic effects of nitric oxide synthetase inhibition in neuronal injury. In: Bär P, Beal M (eds) Neuroprotection in CNS diseases. Marc Decker, New York Basel Hong Kong, pp 131–146
2. Doppenberg E, Zauner A, Bullock R, Ward JD, Fatouros PP, Young HF (1998) Correlations between brain tissue oxygen tension, carbon dioxide, pH and cerebral blood flow – a better way of monitoring the severely injured brain? Surg Neurol 49: 650–654
3. Faraci F, Brian J (1994) NO and cerebral circulation. Stroke 25: 692–703
4. Furchgott R, Zawadzki J (1980) The obligatory role of endothelial cells in the relaxation of arterial smooth muscle by acetylcholine. Nature 288
5. Pluta R, Oldfield E, Boock R (1997) Reversal and prevention of cerebral vasospasm by intracarotid infusion of nitric oxide donors in a primate model of subarachnoid hemorrhage. J Neurosurg 87: 746–751
6. Thomas J, Rosenwasser R (1999) Reversal of severe cerebral vasospasm in three patients after aneurysmal subarachnoidal hemorrhage: initial observations regarding the use of intraventricular sodium nitroprusside in humans. Neurosurgery 44: 48–57

Correspondence: Michael Reinert, Department of Neurosurgery, Inselspital Bern, University of Bern, 3010 Bern, Switzerland.

Prevention of Vasospasm by Clot Lysis

Acta Neurochir (2001) [Suppl] 77: 161–165

Cisternal Washing Therapy for the Prevention of Cerebral Vasospasm Following Aneurysmal Subarachnoid Hemorrhage

T. Nakagomi, K. Takagi, K. Narita, H. Nagashima, and **A. Tamura**

Department of Neurosurgery, Teikyo University School of Medicine, Tokyo, Japan

Introduction

Cerebral vasospasm is still one of the major causes of mortality and morbidity (M & M) in patients with subarachnoid hemorrhage (SAH) [1]. In spite of intense and extensive investigation over the past four decades, the optimal treatment of cerebral vasospasm has not yet been established. Clinical studies have clearly demonstrated the relationship between the location and volume of the subarachnoid clots and the incidence, distribution, and severity of vasospasm [3, 4, 11]. In 1988, Kodama *et al.* reported that cisternal irrigation therapy with urokinase and ascorbic acid was effective in preventing cerebral vasospasm [5]. In 1990, Suzuki *et al.* demonstrated that head-shaking method enhanced the fibrinolysis in cisternal irrigation [10]. In January 1994, we combined these two methods in order to achieve better outcome in Fisher CT group 3 patients and started cisternal irrigation therapy with urokinase combined with head-shaking, i.e., cisternal washing therapy. In this paper, we retrospectively analyzed 250 consecutive cases with SAH, who had clipping surgery within 3 days following SAH, and investigated the effect of this fibrinolytic therapy in preventing symptomatic vasospasm.

Keywords: Vasospasm; head-shaking; fibrinolysis; urokinase.

Materials and Methods

This study consists of 250 consecutive patients with aneurysmal SAH who had been admitted to the Teikyo University Hospital from January 1988 to January 2000. All patients underwent clipping surgery within 3 days from the onset of SAH. The SAH degree of the patients was assessed by preoperative CT scan and classified into 3 groups according to Fisher's criteria. Preoperative condition of the patient was estimated with WFNS score. The patients were divided into two groups; 100 cases from January 1988 to December 1993 (group A) and 150 cases from January 1994 to January 2000 (group B). In group B, 82 patients with Fisher CT group 3 (group C) had cisternal washing therapy. In patients with supratentorial aneurysms, cerebrospinal fluid was aspirated to let the brain relax through a ventricular tube which was placed just after the craniotomy. After aneurysm clipping, an irrigation tube was placed in the carotid cistern or in the chiasmatic cistern. The prepontine clot was removed when possible after opening the Liliequist's membrane. However, extensive removal of the clot distant from the ruptured aneurysm was not performed to avoid further damage to the brain. In patients with infratentorial aneurysms an infusion tube was inserted into the lateral ventricle through the burr hole in the occipital region, and a drainage tube was placed in the subarachnoid space near the ruptured aneurysm. In order to prevent postoperative hemorrhagic complications, meticulous hemostasis was performed during the surgery.

All patients had CT scans just after the surgery. Patients who had a hemorrhagic complication or massive intracranial air on postoperative CT scan were not rendered to the cisternal washing therapy. After the patients returned to the recovery room, fibrinolytic therapy was started by irrigating the subarachnoid space. Lactated Ringer's solution containing urokinase (60,000 IU/500 ml) was infused from the ventricular tube at a rate of 60–120 ml/hour. The pressure for cisternal irrigation was not set over a height of 25 cm H2O from the external auditory meatus. The intracranial pressure control system was usually set at a height of 5–10 cm H2O from the external auditory meatus. Then the head of the patients were rested on the head-shaking device (Neuroshaker), and were shaken periodically at the rate of 1–1.5 c/s. Almost all patients in group C could tolerate head-shaking up to 48 hours.

Cisternal washing therapy was terminated when total amount of urokinase reached 420,000 IU or high density areas in the Sylvian fissure disappeared on CT scan. Mean intervals for head-shaking and ventriculo-cisternal irrigation were 2.6 and 3.4 days, respectively. If the patients showed one of the initial symptoms due to vasospasm after termination of this therapy, additional treatments were given immediately to the patients, which included intrathecal injection of nicardipine and/or intraarterial injection of papaverine.

In these three groups, incidence of transient symptomatic vasospasm (transiently symptomatic without infarction) and cerebral infarction on CT were analyzed. Outcome of the patient at 6 months following SAH was assessed according to the Glasgow Outcome Scale. Overall mortality and morbidity (below moderately disabled) (M & M) at 6 months following SAH, and M & M due to vasospasm at 6 months following SAH were analyzed. Statistical analysis was done using Student's t-test or chi-square test. The values were considered to be significantly different when $p < 0.05$.

Results

The age, sex, timing of surgery, preoperative WFNS grade, preoperative Fisher CT grade, and site of the aneurysm are shown in Table 1. In group B, the patients were significantly ($p < 0.05$) older than those in group A. In group B, the numbers of vertebro-basilar artery aneurysms were more than those in group A. There were, however, no significant differences in sex distribution, interval from the onset of SAH to the surgery, preoperative WFNS grade, preoperative Fisher CT grade, and the site of the ruptured aneurysms.

By the cisternal washing therapy, thick subarachnoid clot in the prepontine, quadrigeminal, carotid,

Table 1. *Summary of Cases*

	1988–1993		1994–2000	
Age				
Range	19–77		26–87	
Mean ± SD	52.0 ± 10.5		57.8 ± 12.5	
Sex				
M	34	34%	49	32.7%
F	66	66%	101	67.3%
Total	100		150	
WFNS grade				
I	44	44%	72	48.0%
II	30	30%	44	29.3%
III	12	12%	7	4.7%
IV	9	9%	21	14.0%
V	5	5%	6	4.0%
mean ± SD	2.0 ± 1.18		1.97 ± 1.20	
CT grade (Fisher)				
2	40	40%	36	24.0%
3	56	56%	113	75.3%
4	4	4%	4	2.7%
mean ± SD	2.6 ± 0.58		2.78 ± 0.47	
Timing of surgery				
0	8	8%	35	23.3%
1	58	58%	80	53.3%
2	19	19%	23	15.3%
3	15	15%	12	8.0%
mean ± SD	1.4 ± 0.84		1.08 ± 0.84	
Site of aneurysm				
AC	45	45%	55	36.7%
IC	31	31%	46	30.7%
MC	22	22%	39	26.0%
V-B	2	2%	10	6.7%

AC Anterior cerebral artery, *IC* internal carotid artery, *MC* middle cerebral artery, *V-B* vertebrobasilar artery.

and chiasmatic cisterns disappeared almost completely within 24 hours. Thick subarachnoid clot in the distal Sylvian fissure, however, could not be removed completely in some patients. Seven patients showed one of the initial symptoms due to vasospasm after termination of this therapy. Additional treatments were given immediately to these patients. Despite all these efforts, 2 patients developed cerebral infarction on the follow-up CT scan. Cerebral infarction in the MCA territory was noted in another patient, who did not show any of the symptoms of cerebral vasospasm.

In group A patients, incidence of transient symptomatic vasospasm and cerebral infarction on CT were 5% and 23% (Table 2). On the other hand, in group B, they were 4.4% and 7.3%, respectively. There was no significant difference in the incidence of the transient symptomatic vasospasm between the groups. Incidence of cerebral infarction, however, decreased significantly after induction of cisternal washing therapy. In 82 cases in group C, incidence of transient symptomatic vasospasm and cerebral infarction on CT were 6.1% and 3.6%. In Fisher CT group 3 patients in group A ($N = 56$), incidence of transient symptomatic vasospasm and cerebral infarction on CT were 7.1% and 35.7%. On the other hand, in Fisher CT group 3 patients in group B ($N = 110$) were 5.4% and 9.1%, respectively. Incidence of cerebral infarction on CT in group C was approximately one tenth of that in Fisher CT group 3 patients in group A. Overall M & M and M & M due to vasospasm at 6 months after SAH in group A were 38% and 16% (Table 2). On the other hand, in group B patients, they were 19.3% and 3.3%, respectively. In 82 cases in group C, overall M & M and M & M due to vasospasm at 6 months following SAH were 19.5% and 3.6%. After 1994, there was no mortality due to cerebral vasospasm. Overall M & M and M & M due to vasospasm decreased approximately by 50% and by 80% after induction of cisternal washing therapy, respectively. Incidence of M & M due to vasospasm was significantly ($P < 0.01$) decreased after the induction of cisternal washing therapy.

Certain complications occurred in 4 patients during the cisternal washing therapy. Three patients developed hemorrhagic complications. One patient had a new bleeding in the hematoma cavity. Two patients had enlargement of intracerebral hematoma and subdural hematoma, respectively. None of them, however, needed a further craniotomy. These hemorrhagic complications did not affect the outcome of the pa-

Table 2. *Incidence of Symptomatic Cerebral Vasospasm and Clinical Outcome*

	1988–1993		1994–2000			
			total		cisternal washing	
Case	100		150		82	
Vasospasm						
symp only	5	5%	7	4.7%	5	6.1%
infarction	23	23%	11	7.3%	3	3.6%
total	28	28%	18	12.0%	8	9.7%
GOS						
GR(1)	62	62%	122	81.3%	67	81.7%
MD(2)	14	14%	15	10.0%	7	8.5%
SD(3)	8	8%	5	3.3%	4	4.9%
V(4)	7	7%	1	0.7%	0	0.0%
D(5)	9	9%	7	4.7%	3	3.6%
mean ± SD	1.87 ± 1.35		1.37 ± 0.95		1.32 ± 0.89	
M&M						
PBD	11	11%	6	4.0%	2	2.4%
Med C	4	4%	10	6.7%	6	7.3%
Surg C	7	7%	8	5.3%	5	6.1%
vasospasm	16	16%	5	3.3%	3	3.6%
total	38	38%	29	19.3%	16	19.5%

GOS Glagow Outcome Scale, *M&M* Mortality and Morbidity, *GR* Good recovery, *MD* moderately disabld, *SD* severely disabled, *V* vegetative, *D* dead, *PBD* primary brain damage, *Med C* medical complication, *Surg C* surgical complication.

tients, who were discharged from the hospital without any neurological deficits. One patient had tinnitus after head-shaking, but it was only transient. No meningitis was observed.

Discussion

According to a literature review of more than 30,000 cases by Dorsch and King, symptomatic vasospasm or delayed ischemic neurological deficits (DIND) occurred in 32.5% of the cases [1]. Thirty percent of the patients with DIND died, and permanent neurological deficits occurred in 34% of the patients. In the present study, of the 100 patients from 1988 to 1993, 23 patients (23%) developed cerebral infarction on CT and 5 patients (5%) showed transient symptomatic vasospasm. Incidence of total symptomatic vasospasm (transient symptomatic vasospasm without infarction and cerebral infarction) in the patients from 1988 to 1993 in the present study was almost the same as the incidence of symptomatic vasospasm reported by Dorsch and King. On the other hand, after induction of cisternal washing therapy (1994–2000), only 11 patients (7.3%) developed cerebral infarction on CT and 7 patients (4.7%) showed transient symptomatic vasospasm of the 150 patients. There was no significant difference in the incidence of transient symptomatic vasospasm between the two groups. Incidence of total symptomatic vasospasm, however, decreased significantly ($p < 0.01$) after induction of cisternal washing therapy. In 82 patients from 1994 to 2000 (cisternal washing group), incidence of cerebral infarction on CT was 3.6%. In Fisher CT group 3 patients from 1988 to 1993 ($N = 56$), however, incidence of cerebral infarction on CT were 35.7%. Decrease in cerebral infarction in the Fisher CT group 3, therefore, can be attributed to cisternal washing therapy. The incidence of total symptomatic vasospasm was much less than that in the review by Dorsch and King. Kodama *et al.* recently reported that, of the 217 patients who had cisternal irrigation therapy with urokinase and ascorbic acid, 5 patients (2.3%) developed cerebral infarction on CT [6]. Our result can be compared to that by Kodama *et al.*

The present study demonstrates that overall M & M and M & M due to vasospasm decreased approximately by 50% and by 80% after induction of cisternal washing therapy, respectively. Outcome of the patients having suffered from SAH was much better than that in the review by Dorsch and King. In the present study, thick subarachnoid clot in the basal cisterns was completely removed by cisternal washing therapy within 24 hours. Thick subarachnoid clot in the distal Sylvian fissure, however, could not be removed completely by this method. Seven patients showed one of the initial symptoms due to vasospasm after termination of this therapy. Three patients developed cerebral infarction in the territory of the branch of middle cerebral artery (MCA) on the follow-up CT scan. To decrease the symptomatic vasospasm in cisternal washing therapy, therefore, it is necessary to remove the clot surrounding the MCA, particularly, in the region below the M2 portion of the MCA. Insertion of the tip of another irrigation tube deeply into the distal portion of the Sylvian fissure, or bolus injection of urokinase into the distal Sylvian fissure during the surgery will be needed.

Cisternal washing therapy always carries the risk of hemorrhage, because urokinase is a fibrinolytic agent. In the present study, complications occurred in 4 patients (5%) during the cisternal washing. Three patients (4%) developed hemorrhagic complications. One patient had a new bleeding in the hematoma cavity. Two patients had enlargement of previously existing intracerebral hematoma or subdural hematoma, respectively. However, follow-up study disclosed that these patients had no neurological deficits. Kodama *et al.* reported that complications occurred in 8 patients (4%) during irrigation therapy with urokinase and ascorbic acid; two patients developed meningitis, two patients experienced seizures, and four patients had an intracranial hemorrhage [6]. Two patients who had intracranial hematoma required hematoma evacuation. All of these patients recovered without neurological deficits. Recent studies have demonstrated the efficacy of tissue-type plasminogen activator (tPA) in preventing symptomatic vasospasm [2, 7, 8, 9, 12, 13]. However, many hemorrhagic complications have been reported in tPA studies, with the incidence between 0 70%. Compared to the fibrinolytic therapy using tPA, cisternal washing therapy could minimize the risk of bleeding through the use of relatively low dose of urokinase and continuous irrigation. In the present study, one patient had tinnitus after head-shaking, but it was only transient. The patient could well tolerate this complication.

In the present study, mean intervals for head-shaking and ventriculo-cisternal irrigation were 2.6 and 3.4 days, respectively. Almost all patients in the cisternal washing group could well tolerate head-shaking up to 48 hours. On the other hand, the duration of cisternal irrigation therapy reported by Kodama *et al.* is rather long (mean 9.9 days) and patients are forced to be bedridden during this period [6]. Moreover, great energy and care were demanded of the medical staff during the cisternal irrigation. There seems to be no significant difference in the incidence of cerebral infarction on CT between our study and that by Kodama *et al.* Therefore, cisternal washing therapy is recommended as a fibrinolytic therapy for the prevention of symptomatic vasospasm.

References

1. Dorsch NWC, King MT (1994) A review of cerebral vasospasm in aneurysmal subarachnoid hemorrhage. J Clin Neurosci 1: 19–26
2. Findlay JM, Kassell NF, Weir BKA, Haley EC Jr, Kongabel G, Germanson T, Truskowski L, Alves WM, Holnesso RO, Knuckey NW, Yonas H, Steinberg GK, West M, Winn HR, Ferguson G (1995) A randomized trial of intraoperative, intracisternal tissue plasminogen activator for the prevention of vasospasm. Neurosurgery 37: 168–178
3. Fisher CM, Kistler JP, Davis JM (1980) Relation of cerebral vasospasm to subarachnoid hemorrhage visualized by computerized tomographic scannning. Neurosurgery 6: 1–9
4. Fraser J, Johnson S, Ray M, Robertson JT (1980) Prediction of cerebral vasospasm with subarachnoid hemorrhage due to ruptured intracranial aneurysm by computerized tomography. Neurosurgery 6: 686–687
5. Kodama N, Sasaki T, Yamanobe K, Sato M, Kawakami M (1988) Prevention of vasospasm: cisternal irrigation therapy with urokinase and ascorbic acid. In: Wilkins (ed) Cerebral vaasospasm. Raven Press, New York, pp 415–418
6. Kodama N, Sasaki T, Kawakami M, Sato M, Asari J (2000) Cisternal irrigation therapy with urokinase and ascorbic acid for prevention of vasospasm after aneurysmal subarachnoid hemorrhage. Surg Neurol 53: 110–118
7. Mizoi K, Yoshimoto T, Takahashi A, Fujiwara S, Koshu K, Sugawara T (1993) Prospective study on the prevention of cerebral vasospasm by intrathecal fibrinolytic therapy with tissue-type plasminogen activator. J Neurosurg 78: 430–437
8. Ohman J, Servo A, Heiskanen O (1991) Effect of intrathecal fibrinolytic therapy on clot lysis and vasospasm in patients with aneurysmal subarachnoid hemorrhage. J Neurosurg 75: 1970–201
9. Sasaki T, Ohta T, Kikuchi H, Takakura K, Usui M, Ohnishi H, Kondo A, Tanabe H, Nakamura J, Yamada K, Kobayashi N, Ohnishi Y (1994) A phase II clinical trial of recombinant human tissue-type plasminogen activator against cerebral vasospasm after aneurysmal subarachnoid hemorrhage. Neurosurgery 35: 597–605
10. Suzuki I, Shimizu H, Takahashi H, Ishijima B (1990) Effect of head-shaking method on clot removal in cisternal irrigation. In: Sano K (ed) Cerebral vasospasm. University of Tokyo Press, Tokyo, pp 314–316
11. Suzuki J, Komatsu S, Sato T, Sakurai Y (1980) Correlation between CT findings and subsequent development of cerebral infarction due to vasospasm in subarachnoid hemorrhage. Acta Neurochir (Wien) 55: 63–70
12. Usui M, Saito N, Hoya K, Todo T (1994) Vasospasm prevention with postoperative intrathecal thrombolytic therapy. A retrospective comparison of urokinase, tissue plasminogen activator, and cisternal drainage alone. Neurosurgery 34: 235–245
13. Zabramski JM, Spetzler RF, Lee HKS, Papadopoulos SM, Bovill E, Zimmerman RS, Bederson JB (1991) Phase I trial of

tissue plasminogen activator for the prevention of vasospasm in patients with aneurysmal subarachnoid hemorrhage. J Neurosurg 75: 189–196

Correspondence: Tadayoshi Nakagomi, M.D., Department of Neurosurgery, Teikyo University School of Medicine 2-11-1, Kaga, Itabashi-ku, Tokyo 173-8605, Japan.

Acta Neurochir (2001) [Suppl] 77: 167–169

Sequential Changes of Oxyhemoglobin in Drained Fluid of Cisternal Irrigation Therapy – Reference to the Effect of Ascorbic Acid

Y. Konno, T. Sato, K. Suzuki, M. Matsumoto, T. Sasaki, and **N. Kodama**

Department of Neurosurgery, Fukushima Medical School, Fukushima, Japan

Introduction

We have been using cisternal irrigation therapy with urokinase (UK) and ascorbic acid (AsA) for prevention of symptomatic vasospasm after aneurysmal subarachnoid hemorrhage (SAH), and excellent results were obtained [3]. In this therapy, UK is used to dissolve the residual clot and AsA is added to degenerate oxyhemoglobin (Oxy-Hb), one of the strongest spasmogenic substances [4]. Previous experimental studies [1, 5] revealed the effect of AsA in degenerating Oxy-Hb. The present study intends to evaluate the effect of AsA in clinical cases by measuring Oxy-Hb concentration of drained fluid sequentially.

Keywords: Ascorbic acid; cisternal irrigation; oxyhemoglobin; subarachnoid hemorrhage; urokinase.

Materials and Methods

Since April 1984, cisternal irrigation therapy has been applied in 222 patients with aneurysmal SAH. This series consisted of 60 recent patients treated with cisternal irrigation therapy with UK and AsA (irrigation group) and 21 patients with cisternal drainage during the same period (drainage group). In the irrigation group, 29 patients were male and 31 were female, ranging in age from 31 to 83 years (average 56 years). In the drainage group, seven patients were male and 14 were female, ranging in age from 43 to 85 years (average 62 years). Cisternal irrigation therapy was chosen when the preoperative computed tomography (CT) scan demonstrated SAH degree classified as Fisher CT group 3 and the highest CT number (Hounsfield number) of the clot exceeded 60, indicating a significant risk for symptomatic vasospasm. In contrast, cisternal drainage was applied, when the CT scan showed SAH of Fisher CT group 2 or 3 and the highest CT number of the clot was less than 60.

All patients underwent acute surgery within 72 hours from the onset of SAH. At surgery, a drainage tube was placed in the prepontine or chiasmal cistern. In the irrigation group, an infusion tube was inserted deeply into the Sylvian fissure. After surgery, lactated Ringer's solution without UK and AsA was infused for 12 hours to prevent postoperative hemorrhage. Then 120 IU/ml UK and 4 mg/mL AsA were added. The irrigation fluid was adjusted to the same pH (7.2–7.6) and osmotic pressure (280–300 mOsm/kg) as those of normal cerebrospinal fluid. Infusion was performed at a rate of 30 ml/hour. The mean duration of the therapy was about 10 days in this series.

To examine the effect of AsA, Oxy-Hb concentration was measured using the spectrometric method. The absorption spectrum of the drained fluid was measured daily and the sequential changes of the Oxy-Hb specific 576 nm peak [5] in both groups were compared.

Results

In the irrigation group, the Oxy-Hb specific peak at 576 nm decreased day by day and the peak became undetectable by Day 4. This finding was observed in 56 out of 60 patients. The other 4 cases showed atypical pattern of continuous high level of Oxy-Hb peak. In these cases, preoperative CT scans showed massive intracerebral hematoma and postoperative CT scans revealed residual hematoma (Fig. 1).

On the other hand, in the drainage group, the Oxy-Hb peak decreased in the early stage, but the values increased again and remained high in most cases (Fig. 2).

Sequential changes of mean values of the spectrometric peak of Oxy-Hb were compared in both groups. The peak of Oxy-Hb in the cisternal irrigation group decreased by Day 5 and the values remained low. In contrast, the peak of Oxy-Hb of the drainage group increased from Day 3, with the highest value on Day 8. The values remained higher than those of the irrigation group until Day 12 (Fig. 3).

Symptomatic vasospasm did not appear in any patients of either group.

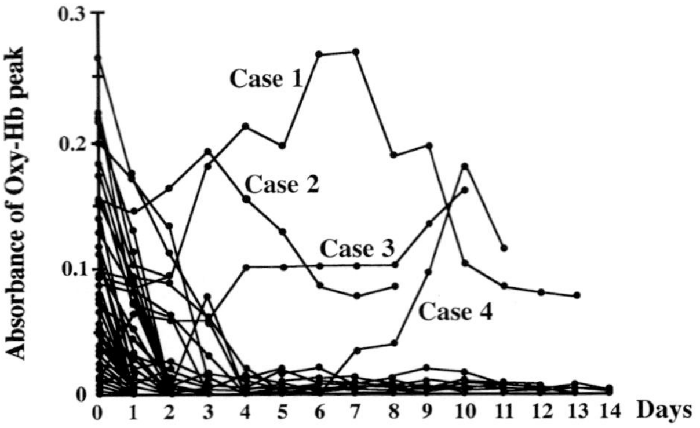

Fig. 1. Sequential changes of the absorption spectrum in 60 cases treated with cisternal irrigation. In 56 cases, the peak of Oxy-Hb at 576 nm disappeared within 4 days. In cases 1 to 4, pre- and postoperative CT scan showed intracerebral hematoma and high values of Oxy-Hb peak continued during cisternal irrigation

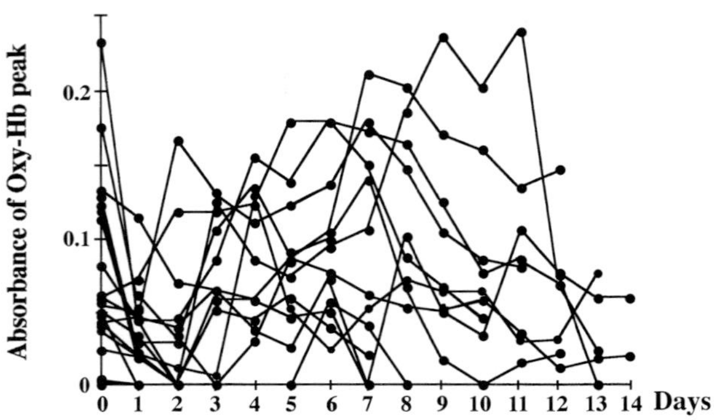

Fig. 2. Sequential changes of the absorption spectrum in 21 cases treated with cisternal drainage. In most cases, the peak of Oxy-Hb at 576 nm remained high during cisternal drainage

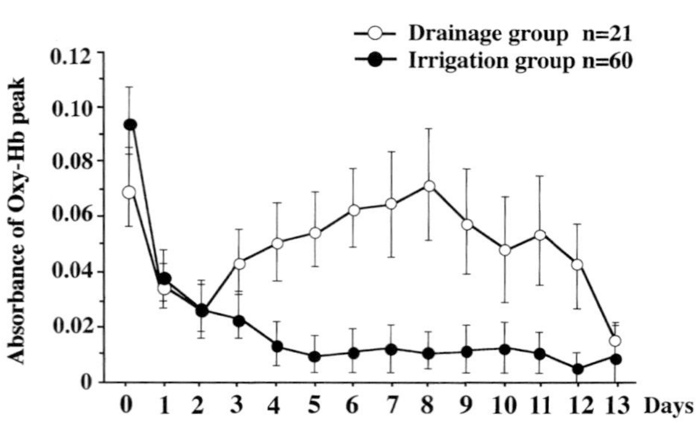

Fig. 3. Sequential changes in mean values of the spectrometric peak of Oxy-Hb (mean ± SE). The peak of Oxy-Hb at 576 nm decreased by Day 5 and the values remained low in the irrigation group (n = 60). In contrast, the peak of Oxy-Hb in the drainage group (n = 21) without irrigation increased from Day 3, with the highest value on Day 8. It remained higher than that in the irrigation group until Day 12

Discussion

In previous experimental studies, it was confirmed that AsA did degenerate Oxy-Hb into reduced Hb and finally into verdoheme-like products, which were non-spasmogenic [1, 5]. The present study demonstrated the effect of AsA in clinical cases. Cisternal irrigation therapy with AsA could decrease the Oxy-Hb level in drained fluid, however, cisternal drainage could not. It suggests that Oxy-Hb was degenerated by AsA. In four cases with residual intracerebral hematoma on postoperative CT scan, the Oxy-Hb peak remained in high values during the cisternal irrigation. It is presumed that Oxy-Hb is oozing from intracerebral or intraventricular hematoma.

In the drainage group, high values of Oxy-Hb peak in the early stage was caused by mechanical damage of erythrocytes at surgery. The Oxy-Hb peak was decreased temporarily by drainage. Due to spontaneous erythrolysis, the Oxy-Hb concentration increased again from Day 3. The maximum level of increase was observed on Day 8. Then the Oxy-Hb peak gradually decreased, finally to the same level as that of the cisternal irrigation group at Day 14. This sequential change in the drainage group corresponds with the life span of extravascular erythrocytes and the period of vasospasm [2].

No patients experienced symptomatic vasospasm in this series. Therefore, the correlation with Oxy-Hb peak and incidence of symptomatic vasospasm was unclear. We, however, considered that AsA was effective for the prevention of symptomatic vasospasm because very low Oxy-Hb concentrations were observed and symptomatic vasospasm did not occur in the cisternal irrigation group even with massive SAH on preoperative CT scan, which suggested a significant risk for symptomatic vasospasm.

Conclusion

To evaluate the effect of AsA in the cisternal irrigation therapy with UK and AsA, Oxy-Hb concentration in drained fluid was sequentially measured using the spectrophotometric method. Oxy-Hb concentrations of the cisternal irrigation group with UK and AsA were lower than those of the cisternal drainage group without UK and AsA. Symptomatic vasospasm was not observed in the irrigation group even with massive SAH on preoperative CT scan. These results suggest that AsA is effective in degenerating Oxy-Hb into non-spasmogenic substances and in preventing symptomatic vasospasm after aneurysmal SAH.

References

1. Kawakami M, Kodama N, Toda N (1991) Suppression of the cerebral vasospastic actions of oxyhemoglobin by ascorbic acid. Neurosurgery 28: 33–40
2. Kodama N, Mizoi K, Sakurai Y, Suzuki J (1980) Incidence and onset of vasospasm. In: Wilkins RH (ed) Cerebral arterial vasospasm. Williams and Wilkins, Baltimore, p 361–365
3. Kodama N, Sasaki T, Kawakami M, Sato M, Asari J (2000) Cisternal irrigation therapy with urokinase and ascorbic acid for prevention of vasospasm after aneurysmal subarachnoid hemorrhage: outcome in 217 patients. Surg Neurol 53: 110–118
4. Osaka K (1977) Prolonged vasospasm by the breakdown products of erythrocytes. J Neurosurg 47: 403–411
5. Sato M (1987) Prevention of cerebral vasospasm: experimental studies on the degradation of oxyhemoglobin by ascorbic acid. Fukushima J Med Sci 33: 55–70

Correspondence: Y. Konno, M.D., Department of Neurosurgery, Fukushima Medical School, 1 Hikarigaoka, Fukushima 960-1295, Japan.

Acta Neurochir (2001) [Suppl] 77: 171–174

Cisternal Irrigation Therapy with Urokinase and Ascorbic Acid for Prevention of Vasospasm

N. Kodama, M. Matsumoto, T. Sasaki, Y. Konno, and **T. Sato**

Department of Neurosurgery, Fukushima Medical School, Fukushima, Japan

Introduction

Although cerebral vasospasm is one of the most serious complications of aneurysmal subarachnoid hemorrhage (SAH), the optimal treatment of cerebral vasospasm has not yet been established. It has been reported previously that subarachnoid clots are related to the vasospasm and that vasospasm can be induced by spasmogenic substances released from the clot. Although removal of this thick clot is performed in acute stage surgery for ruptured aneurysms to prevent the occurrence of vasospasm, it is still very difficult to completely remove all of the clot.

Over the last 14 years, we have developed a novel method for preventing the occurrence of cerebral vasospasm following acute stage surgery. Cisternal irrigation therapy with urokinase and ascorbic acid was introduced to prevent symptomatic vasospasm following aneurysmal SAH. To dissolve and wash out the subarachnoid clot, cisternal irrigation with urokinase has been used. Ascorbic acid is added to degenerate oxy-hemoglobin, one of the strongest spasmogenic substances, into verdoheme-like products which are non-spasmogenic. The efficacy and safety of this therapy were evaluated.

Keywords: Subarachnoid hemorrhage; cerebral vasospasm; cisternal irrigation; urokinase.

Materials and Methods

This therapy was performed consecutively in 222 patients (Table 1). The degree of SAH of the patients was classified as Fisher CT group 3, and the highest CT number (Hounsfield number) exceeded 60 in the SAH, which suggested a significant risk for symptomatic vasospasm (Fig. 1). All patients underwent surgery within 72 hours from the onset of SAH. After clipping the aneurysm, irrigation tubes were placed in the Sylvian fissure (inlet) unilaterally or bilaterally and in the prepontine or chiasmal cistern (outlet) (Fig. 2).

Table 1. *Summary of Cases of Irrigation Therapy with Urokinase and Ascorbic Acid*

No. of cases	222
Age (yrs.)	
Range	27–87
Mean	59.2
Sex (male/female)	93/129
Site of aneurysm	
Acom A	89
ICA	63
MCA	55
VBA	11
ACA	4
Preoperative grade (Hunt & Kosnik)	
I	6
II	107
III	73
IV	35
V	1

Acom A anterior communicating artery; *ICA* internal carotid artery; *MCA* middle cerebral artery; *VBA* vertebrobasilar artery.

In order to prevent postoperative hemorrhage, only lactated-Ringer's solution without UK was infused for 12 hours, followed by UK and ascorbic acid irrigation. Lactated-Ringer's solution with UK (120 IU/ml) [10] and ascorbic acid (4 mg/ml) [7] was infused at a rate of 30 ml/hour/side. The solution for irrigation was adjusted to the same pH (7.2–7.6) and osmotic pressure (280–300 mOsm/Kg) as that of the normal cerebrospinal fluid. A microdrop system was used to control the flow rate, and a milliporefilter was also connected to the infusion tube to prevent infection. The total volume of infused and drainaged fluid was measured every hour to avoid excessive infusion. The intracranial pressure control system was set usually at a height of 10 cm H_2O (Fig. 3).

Termination of irrigation was determined on the basis of the number of days from the onset of SAH, the absence on CT of a high density area near the Sylvian fissures, and data from drainage fluid in which the levels of RBC and FDP were below 10,000 /mm^3 and

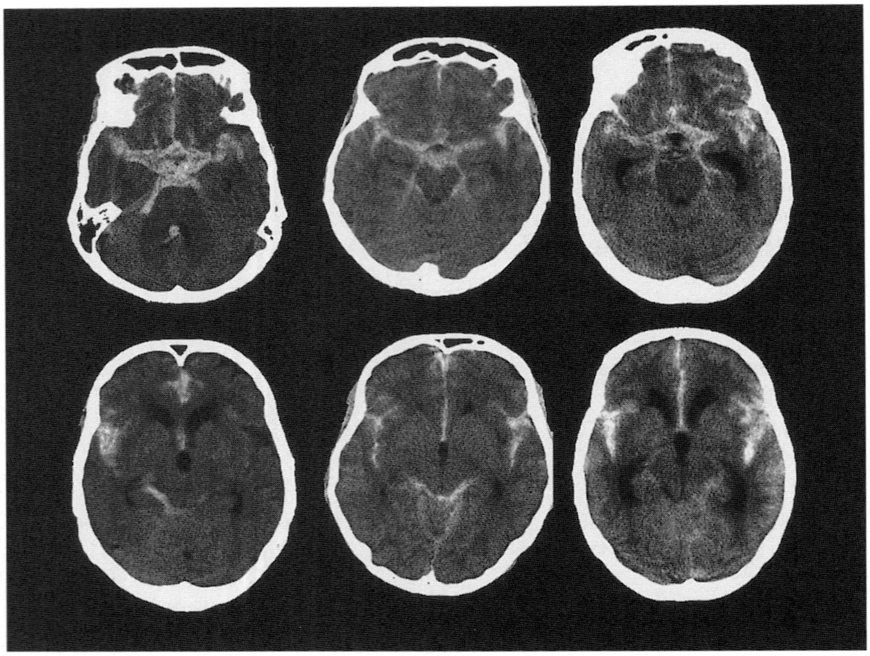

Fig. 1. Preoperative computed tomography (CT) scans of 3 representative cases. Inclusion criteria included a Fisher CT group 3 classification and a CT number (Hounsfield number) greater than 60 in the highest area of subarachnoid hemorrhage

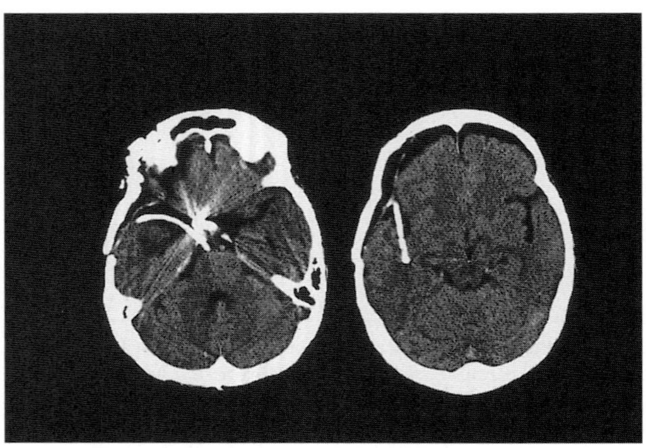

Fig. 2. Position of irrigation tubes on a representative CT scan. An outlet tube was placed in the prepontine cistern and an inlet tube in the Sylvian fissure

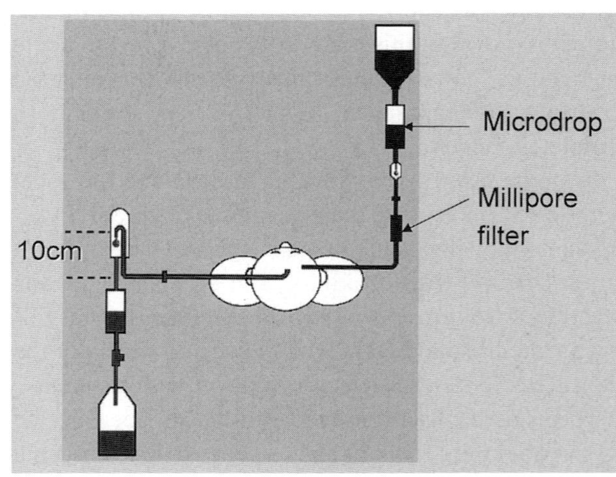

Fig. 3. Schematic drawing of cisternal irrigation. A microdrop was used to control the flow rate, and a milliporefilter was connected to the tube to prevent infection. The intracranial pressure control system was set usually at a height of 10 cm H_2O

10 μg/ml, respectively. The duration of cisternal irrigation therapy ranged from 2 to 18 days (mean duration, 9.9 days).

Results

Among 222 patients, all of whom had a high risk of vasospasm based on the CT findings mentioned above, symptomatic vasospasm was observed in 6 cases (2.7%). Four patients developed transient symptoms. Three of these patients developed transient hemiparesis on the day following removal of the irrigation tube. One patient developed permanent hemiparesis. In that case, because the irrigation tube was not inserted deeply enough into the Sylvian fissure, the subarachnoid clot could not be washed out sufficiently. CT scan revealed a new low density area, and the outcome was fair at the time of discharge. Another patient experienced consciousness disturbance without any localizing sign, and the outcome was fair.

The outcome assessed at discharge from the hospital was excellent in 122 cases, good in 58, fair in 24, poor in 12, and 6 patients died. The morbidity and mortality rates were 16.2% and 2.7%, respectively. The morbidity due to cerebral vasospasm was 0.9%, and the mortality was 0%. Six patients who died had no symptoms of vasospasm. Hydrocephalus occurred in 79 patients (35.6%). All of them underwent ventriculo-peritoneal shunting.

Certain complications occurred in 8 patients during irrigation therapy; 2 patients experienced seizures, 2 developed meningitis, and 4 had an intracranial hemorrhage. However, all of these patients recovered without neurological deficits.

Discussion

Fisher, *et al.* [2], reported that vasospasm was found in almost all cases of SAH associated with a thick and widespread subarachnoid clot on CT scan (group 3 according to their classification). The location of the cerebral vasospasm was clinically well correlated with the site of SAH and the volume of the clot. It is now generally accepted that the factors in the subarachnoid clot induce the arterial constriction, although the precise mechanism is still not understood. Suzuki, *et al.* [9], reported that the CT density of a clot is a useful index of the quantity of the SAH and the risk of vasospasm. The best means to prevent vasospasm, therefore, is to remove as much of the clot as possible and as early as possible during acute surgery. However, complete evacuation of the clot during surgery is technically impossible. In the present study, our hypothesis is that the chemical lysis of the clot and neutralization of one of the spasmogenic factors following surgery would prevent vasospasm and improve the ultimate outcome [4, 6]. Attention was paid to oxy-Hb [5], which is a strong vasoconstrictor.

We previously reported that UK at a concentration of either 60 or 120 IU/ml was most effective for optimal clot dissolution in vitro [10]. In initial cases, both kinds of concentration of UK were used. Considering the absorption into the bottle and tube, and the dilution of UK by cerebro-spinal fluid, the concentration of 120 IU/ml is currently used. We have also reported that Oxy-Hb was converted to verdohemelike products by ascorbic acid in vitro and that ascorbic acid suppressed the ability of Oxy-Hb to constrict the cerebral arteries in vivo and in vitro [3, 7]. At present, considering the reaction time for the conversion of Oxy-Hb, the concentration of 4 mg/ml is used.

Based on the results of these prior studies, we have performed cisternal irrigation therapy with UK and ascorbic acid following acute stage surgery for aneurysmal SAH since 1984 [4, 6]. According to a literature review of more than 30,000 cases by Dorsch and King [1], symptomatic vasospasm or delayed ischemic deficit (DID) occurred in 32.5% of the cases. Thirty percent of the patients with DID died, and permanent neurological deficit occurred in 34% of the patients. As mentioned above, in the irrigation group, morbidity due to cerebral vasospasm was 0.9% and mortality was 0%. These results demonstrate that cisternal irrigation therapy with UK and ascorbic acid is effective in preventing symptomatic vasospasm following aneurysmal SAH.

Recently, many studies on intrathecal fibrinolytic therapy have demonstrated the efficacy of tissue-type plasminogen activator (tPA) in preventing vasospasm [8]. All of those studies found tPA to be of significant benefit; however, the number of patients in these studies was relatively small (less than 30). It was found that there was no difference between the incidence of symptomatic vasospasm in the placebo patients (37.7%) and that in the tPA-treated patients (39.6%). TPA would be good for clotlysis but single injection method could not flow out the bloody CSF continuously. We believe continuous flow out is an important factor to reduce the incidence of symptomatic vasospasm.

In our present study, we performed irrigation therapy on all patients in whom there was a strong possibility of the occurrence of vasospasm. It is impossible to predict which patients may develop symptomatic vasospasm, therefore, it was necessary to perform irrigation therapy on all patients. Furthermore, future studies must determine the subset of patients most likely to develop symptomatic vasospasm.

There are still some problems that we must resolve before this therapy can be widely used. The most adequate length of this treatment still remains unclear. The duration of this therapy is rather long (mean: 9.9 days) and patients are forced to be bedridden during this period. Moreover, greatest energy and care were demanded of the medical staff during the irrigation. However, since only two patients (0.9%) developed symptomatic vasospasm that caused permanent sequela, the benefit from cisternal irrigation therapy appears to far exceed its disadvantages.

Conclusion

These results suggest that cisternal irrigation therapy with urokinase and ascorbic acid is effective in preventing symptomatic vasospasm following aneurysmal SAH.

References

1. Dorsch NWC, King MT (1994) A review of cerebral vasospasm in aneurysmal subarachnoid hemorrhage. J Clin Neuroscience 1: 19–26
2. Fisher CM, Kistler JR, Davis JM (1980) Relation of cerebral vasospasm to subarachnoid hemorrhage visualized by computerized tomographic scanning. Neurosurgery 6: 1–9
3. Kawakami M, Kodama N, Toda N (1991) Suppression of the cerebral vasospastic actions of oxyhemoglobin by ascorbic acid. Neurosurgery 28: 33–40
4. Kodama N, Sasaki T, Kawakami M, Sato M, Asari J (2000) Cisternal irrigation therapy with urokinase and ascorbic acid for prevention of vasospasm after aneurysmal subarachnoid hemorrhage. Outcome in 217 patients. Surg Neurol 53: 110–118
5. Osaka K (1977) Prolonged vasospasm produced by the breakdown products of erythrocytes. J Neurosurg 47: 403–411
6. Sasaki T, Kodama N, Kawakami M, Sato M, Asari J, Sakurai Y, Watanabe K, Onuma T, Matsuda T (2000) Urokinase cisternal irrigation therapy for prevention of symptomatic vasospasm after aneurysmal subarachnoid hemorrhage – a study of urokinase concentration and fibrinolytic system. Stroke 31: 1256–1262
7. Sato M (1987) Prevention of cerebral vasospasm: experimental studies on the degradation of oxyhemoglobin by ascorbic acid. Fukushima J Med Sci 33: 55–70
8. Steinberg GK, Vanefsky MC, Marks MP, Adler JR Jr, Koenig GH (1994) Failure of intracisternal tissue plasminogen activator to prevent vasospasm in certain patients with aneurysmal subarachnoid hemorrhage. Neurosurgery 34: 809–814
9. Suzuki J, Komatsu S, Sato T, Sakurai Y (1980) Correlation between CT findings and subsequent development of cerebral infarction due to vasospasm in subarachnoid hemorrhage. Acta Neurochir (Wien) 55: 63–70
10. Yamanobe K (1987) Prevention of vasospasm: experimental studies on lysis of urokinase. Fukushima Med J (Jap) 37: 27–39

Correspondence: Namio Kodama, M.D., Department of Neurosurgery, Fukushima Medical School, 1, Hikarigaoka, Fukushima, 960-1295, Japan.

Endovascular Treatment of Cerebral Vasospasm

Acta Neurochir (2001) [Suppl] 77: 177–180

Endovascular Treatment of Cerebral Vasospasm Following S.A.H.

X. Barreau, M. Pastore, M. Piotin, C. Spelle, and **J. Moret**

Introduction

Cerebral vasospasm (CV) remains one of the most feared complication of subarachnoid hemorrhage associated with severe morbidity and mortality. After HHH therapy and intravenous nimodipine infusion, some patients still show evidence of neurological deficit due to CV. Many studies have demonstrated the benefits of papaverin infusion but this drug appeared to have a transient and moderate efficiency on the patient outcome and may be reserved for diffuse CV. Percutaneous angioplasty associated with vasodilating drugs has been shown to offer greater chance of long-lasting re-opening of the narrowed vessels. This articles reviews different techniques for endovascular management of CV and several studies relating to efficacies of PTA and or papaverine/nimodipine intra-arterial infusion.

Keywords: Cerebral vasospasm; intracranial angioplasty.

Epidemiology

Cerebral vasospasm (CV) is defined as a significant narrowing of the cerebral arteries occurring after subarachnoid hemorrhage (SAH). The frequency of this feared complication of SAH has been widely studied. Angiographic vasospasm occurs in approximately 70% of aneurysmal SAH [4]. The incidence of CV is influenced by the time between the SAH and the angiographic study, and is more frequent between the sixth and eighth day after SAH. Clinical manifestations are encountered in 30 to 50% of CV [8, 9, 27], demonstrating that the non-symptomatic CV is more frequent than the symptomatic one.

The international cooperative study on the timing of aneurysm surgery [27] stated that 13,5% of the patients die or are disabled secondary to vasospasm.

Mechanisms of CV

General Considerations

The initial trigger for CV is blood effusion into the subarachnoid space. Following SAH, the vascular response is divided into two phases. The first phase consists of an acute vasoconstriction occurring 1 to 3 days after hemorrhage. This phase is responsible for high mortality related to intracranial pressure elevation [13], cerebral blood flow [1] and cerebral perfusion diminution [24]. The second phase is a delayed phase responsible for severe neurological deficits and is believed to be more refractory to treatment than the first phase.

Biomolecular Mechanisms of Cerebral Vasospasm

In a recent paper Dietrich [3] reported the fundamental mechanism of CV. In his review CV is demonstrated to be related to different cellular responses specially directed at endothelial and vascular smooth muscle cells regulation.

Briefly, oxyhemoglobin and bilirubin initiate the vascular response. These substances are released in the subarachnoid space after clot lysis and disturb the equilibrium between vasoconstrictor and vasodilator systems.

Endothelium-dependent relaxation is impaired by nitric oxyde (NO) scavenging and oxygen radical release. As hemoglobin can bind NO, this reaction may result in a decrease of guanylate cyclase activity triggering vasoconstriction. Moreover, the production of a vasodilatating prostacyclin (PGI 2) decreases after SAH while vasoconstrictive prostaglandin is increased (PGF 2 α, Thromboxane A2 ...). The decrease of PGI 2 may be caused by eicosanoids and free radical release stimulated by oxyhemoglobin [20].

Smooth muscle cell response seems to be related to many different factors, but calcium channels, potassium channels, and increased protein kinase activity may be the major keys to vasospasm. The activation of these ion-channels can be triggered by cell depolarization or ligation with ATP (for example). Protein kinase C is activated by hemolysate and causes prolonged vasoconstriction via the contractile proteins phosphorylation. Another major pathway of smooth muscle cell regulation is myosin light chain phosphorylation by a Ca-calmodulin dependent protein kinase (MLCK). The action of an antivasospastic agent inhibiting MLCK demonstrated a slight reduction of cerebral vasospasm in dogs [12].

Pathologic Study of Spastic Vessels

10 to 12 days after SAH several modifications can be observed within the arterial wall. The intima and internal elastic layer become creased. Platelets aggregate on the wall foldings, but thrombosis or distal embolization is rarely observed. Endothelial and smooth muscle cells become vacuolized and a new type of «myo-intimal» cell proliferates. The production of the extra-cellular matrix (Type V collagen) and the inflammatory cells adventitial infiltration leads to a fibrous cap surrounding the artery and stabilizing the spasm. Cerebral ischemia is related to the reduced contractility and compliance associated with an impairment of autoregulatory vasodilatation [26].

Endovascular Therapy of CV

Many different therapeutic options have been used to treat CV. Surgical washing of the cisternal clots, nimodipine, intraventricular thrombolysis, 21-aminosteroid tirilazad, hypertensive-hypervolemic therapy ... All these techniques will not be further discussed and only endovascular treatment of CV will be described. Chemical vasodilators and percutaneous transluminal angioplasty (PTA) are the two techniques available for the emergency treatment of CV.

Intra Arterial Infusion of Vasodilator Agents

Papaverine is the most common agent used for chemical angioplasty. This alkaloid has the ability to relax smooth muscle cells and to increase cerebral blood flow (CBF). This relaxant action which appears as a dynamic effect is believed to be more efficient if performed in the first phase of CV. Papaverine is injected through a micro-catheter proximal to the spastic vessel. Three hundred milligrams mixed in 100 ml of saline are slowly delivered manually or using an injector.

The vasodilatation seems to be as effective on the circle of Willis vessels as on the distal circulation.

Most of the time the immediate angiographic results of papaverine administration are good. After prolonged infusion (20 to 60 min.) CBF, mean transit time [16] and the vessel diameter are increased in only 25 to 50% of the cases [14, 23]. But the main problem of papaverine administration (especially if used alone) remains its transient effect. Up to 100% of the patients [16] demonstrate a quick recurrence of vasospasm 1 hour to 1 day after the infusion. This transient effect is probably due to the short half-life of papaverine (45 to 60 min.) in the circulation. Some authors tried to vary the dose or to repeat the infusion with various results but only a few cases have been studied [19]. Some adverse effects must be emphasized, i.e. the risk of visual impairment in the case of injection in the ophthalmic artery, seizures, severe hypotension or cardiac arrhythmia.

As the efficacy of papaverine remains uncertain, other drugs are used in some centers in order to improve the neurological outcome or to facilitate PTA.

In our center we are using the intra-arterial injection of nimodipine. This drug is available in France for intra-arterial use which has not been well documented yet. Only a few reports have been published from Japan and the use of arterial nimodipine is still not allowed in the US. We usually mix 2 mg of nimodipine with 10 ml. of serum followed by a slow manual injection (10 min.) through the microcatheter proximal to the spasm. Although our experience is limited, it appears to us that the vasodilating effect remains stable over days after treatment. The effects of nimodipine have not been compared with papaverine in a controlled trial and it must be said that we always use it with PTA. Whatever the effectiveness of chemical angioplasty, it clearly appears that chemical angioplasty must be combined with balloon angioplasty. PTA warrants a long lasting re-opening of the lumen and chemical vasodilators must be used to facilitate PTA, to open a severe spasm and to allow balloon to cross the stenosis.

Intracranial Balloon Angioplasty of Vasospasm

Multiple studies have demonstrated that angioplasty of cerebral vasospasm is able to reverse the arterial constriction occurring after SAH. Histological changes in the arterial wall can be reversed after PTA [11]. Zubkov [28] was the first to publish a study about PTA in 33 patients in 1984 with promising results. With improvements in balloon technology, more studies have been successively published. Some studies have confirmed that PTA improves cerebral perfusion distally to the dilated vasospasm. These results have been observed using transcranial doppler [5], SPECT [15] or perfusion CT [7]. Many authors reported on short-term outcome. Clinical improvement and results are between 31 to 100% [10]. Bejjani [2] reported that PTA dramatically improves clinical outcome in 23 out of 31 patients treated within the first day after vasospasm and refractory to HHH therapy. Eskridge [6] reported that 61% of 50 patients showed sustained improvement in neurological function within 72 hours after treatment, if PTA was performed within 12 hours of the onset of symptoms. For Polin [21], PTA successfully reversed angiographic vasospasm but no significant difference has been found concerning immediate or 3-month-outcome in 38 patients when compared to a control group. The timing of angioplasty remains unclear but according to some studies it seems to be evident that the sooner PTA is performed, the better it is. Newell [18] recommends early PTA before 12 hours and Rosenwasser [22] found 70% rate of clinical improvement if PTA is performed within 2 hours. Even if the time window is not clearly defined yet, it is reasonable to think that early re-opening of CV limits cerebral infarction and warrants a long lasting dilatation of the vessel while narrowing is still spastic and no fibrous narrowing occurred. Some authors recently proposed prophylactic PTA for patients with high risk of CV [17].

Balloons and Techniques

The two main balloons currently used for PTA are the Endeavor Balloon and the Solstice balloon. In our unit we are used to the Solstice balloon which is also often used for the remodeling technique for the aneurysm embolizations. This silicon balloon (10 mmx 3,5 mm) can be inflated after occlusion of its distal part by the micro-guidewire. The use of such a system is quite easy and allows us to perform PTA on all circle of Willis and most of the time to treat the distal spasm as in M2, P1 or A2.

We perform several inflations of 0.1 ml using a syringe, pushing the device through the stenosis after each dilatation. Generally each inflation is maintained 30 seconds. Occasionally we use intra-arterial nimodipine infusion to complete the dilatation or to allow the balloon to cross a severe spasm.

Complications

PTA complications are rare with this technique and the most feared complication is balloon rupture [6, 25]. Branch occlusion, clip displacement, inguinal or retroperitoneal hematoma have been reported [2, 21]. The recurrence of CV after PTA appears to be very rare, which is one of the main advantages of PTA.

Conclusion

PTA of CV appears a very promising technique to treat cerebral ischemia following sub-arachnoid hemorrhage. Mainly due to technical improvements of balloons and better comprehension of pathogenesis of CV, PTA now allows neuro-interventionists to improve the neurological outcome of patients. It appears reasonable to associate PTA and vasodilator agents infusion in order to facilitate balloon placement and to re-open distal vessels in case of distal vasospasm. In our institution, CV occurs in approximately 15 to 20% of the patients already treated with intravenous nimodipine and according to many authors, PTA is still advocated in case where CV is refractory to medical treatment. The time window for PTA seems to be very short and must definitely be performed promptly within 0–8 hours after the onset of symptoms.

References

1. Asano T, Sano K (1977) Pathogenetic role of no-reflow phenomenon in experimental subarachnoid hemorrhage in dogs. J Neurosurg 46: 454–466
2. Bejjano GK, Bank WO, Olan WJ, Sekhar LN (1998) The efficacy and safety of angioplasty for cerebral vasospasm after subarachnoid hemorrhage. Neurosurg 42(5): 979–986
3. Dietrich HH, Ralph GD (2000) Molecular keys to the problems of cerebral vasospasm. Neurosurgery 46: 517–530
4. Dorsch NWC (1990) Incidence, effects and treatment of ischemia following aneurysm rupture. In: Sano K, Takakura K, Kassell NF, Saaki T (eds) Cerebral vasospasm. University of Tokyo Press, Tokyo, pp 495–498
5. Elliot JP, Newell DW, Lam DJ (1998) Comparison of balloon

angioplasty and papaverine infusion for the treatment of vasospasm following aneurysmal subarachnoid hemorrhage. J Neurosurg 88: 277–284

6. Eskridge JM, McAuliffe W, Song JK (1998) Balloon angioplasty for the treatment of vasospasm: results of the 50 first cases. Neurosurgery 42: 510–517
7. Firlik AD, Kaufmann AM, Jungreis CA, Yonas H (1997) Effect of transluminal angioplasty on cerebral blood flow in the management of symptomatic vasospasm following subarachnoid hemorrhage. J Neurosurg 86: 830–839
8. Fisher CM (1975) Clinical syndromes in cerebral thrombosis, hypertensive hemorrhage and ruptured saccular aneurysm. Clin Neurosurg 22: 117–147
9. Fisher CM, Roberson GH, Ojemann RG (1977) Cerebral vasospasm with ruptured saccular aneurysm. The clinical manifestations. Neurosurg 1: 245–248
10. Hiroshi Katoh, Katsuji Shima, Akira Shimizu, Katoh H, Shima K, Shimizu A, Takiguchi H, Miyazawa T, Umezawa H, Nawashiro H, Ishihara S, Kaji T, Makita K, Tsuchiya K (1999) Clinical evaluation of percutaneous transluminal angioplasty and intra arterial papaverine infusion for the treatment of vasospasm following aneurysmal subarachnoid hemorrhage. Neurol Res 21: 195–203
11. Honma Y, Fujiwara T, Irie K, Ohkawa M, Nagao S (1995) Morphological changes in human cerebral arteries after PTA for vasospasm caused by subarachnoid hemorrhage. Neurosurgery 36: 1073–1081
12. Inkyeom K, Leinweber B, Morgalla M, Butler WE, Minoru S, Yasuharu S, Peterson J, Morgan K (2000) Thin and thick filament regulation of contractility in experimental cerebral vasospasm. Neurosurgery 46: 440–447
13. Kassel NF, Torner JC, Haley EC, Jane JE, Adams HP, Kongable GL (1990) The International cooperative study on the timing of aneurysm surgery: part 1- overall management results. J Neurosurg 73: 18–30
14. Kassel NF, Helm G, Simmons N, Phillips CD, Cail W (1992) Treatment of cerebral vasospasm with intra-arterial papaverine. J Neurosurg 77: 842–847
15. Lewis DH, Eskridge JM, Newell DW, Grady MS, Cohen WA, Dalley RW, Loyd D, Grothaus-King A, Young P, Winn HR (1992) Brain SPECT and the effect of cerebral angioplasty in delayed ischemia due to vasospasm. J Nucl Med 10(33): 1789–1796
16. Milburn JM, Moran CJ, Cross TD, Diringer MN, Pilgram TK, Dacey RG Jr (1998) Increase in diameters of vasospastic intracranial arteries by intra-arterial papaverine administration. J Neurosurg 88: 38–42
17. Muizelaar JP, Zwienenberg M, Rudisill NA, Hecht ST (1999) The prophylactic use of transluminal angioplasty in patients with Fisher Grade 3 subarachnoid hemorrhage: a pilot study. J Neurosurg 91: 51–58
18. Newell DW, Eskridge JM, Mayberg JM, Grady MS, Lewis D, Winn HR (1992) Endovascular treatment of intracranial aneurysm and cerebral vasospasm. Clin Neurosurg 39: 348–360
19. Numaguchi Y, Zoarsky GH, Clouston JE, Zagardo MT, Simard JM, Aldrich EF, Sloan MA, Maurer PK, Okawara SH (1997) Repeat intra-arterial papaverine for recurrent cerebral vasospasm after SAH. Neuroradiology 39: 751–759
20. Pasqualin A (1998) Epidemiology and physiopathology of cerebral vasospasm following subarachnoid hemorrhage. J Neurosurg Sci 42: 15–21
21. Polin RS, Coenen VA, Hansen CA, Shin P, Baskaya MK, Nanda A, Kassell NF (2000) Efficacy of transluminal angioplasty for the management of symptomatic cerebral vasospasm following subarachnoid vasospasm hemorrhage. J Neurosurg 92: 284–290
22. Rosenwasser RH, Armonda RA, Thomas GE, Benitez RP, Gannon PM, Harrop J (1999) Therapeutic modalities for the management of cerebral vasospasm: timing of endovascular options. Neurosurgery 44: 975–980
23. Sawada M, Hashimoto N, Tsukahara T, Nishi S, Kaku Y, Yoshimura S (1997) Effectiveness of intra-arterially infused papaverine solutions at various concentrations for the treatment of delayed cerebral vasospasm. Acta Neurochir (Wien) 139(8): 706–711
24. Tranquart F, Ades PE, Groussin P, Rieant JF, Jan M, Baulieu JL (1993) Postoperative assessment of cerebral blood flow in subarachnoid hemorrhage by means of TC 99m-HMPAO tomography. Eur J Nucl Med 20: 53–58
25. Volk EE, Prayson RA, Perl J II (1997) Autopsy findings of fatal complications of posterior cerebral artery angioplasty. Arch Pathol Lab Med 121: 738–740
26. Yundt KD, Grubb RL, Diringer HM, Povers WJ (1998) Autoregulatory vasodilatation of parenchymal vessels is impaired during cerebral vasospasm. J Cereb Blood Flow Metab 18: 419–424
27. Zabramsky JM, Hamilton MG (1997) Cerebral vasospasm. In: Carter LP, Spetzler RF (eds) Neurovascular surgery. Mc Graw-Hill, New York, pp 583–602
28. Zubkov YN, Nikiforov BM, Shustin UA (1984) Balloon catheter technique for dilatation of constricted cerebral arteries after aneurysmal SAH. Acta Neurochir (Wien) 70: 65–69

Correspondence: Prof. J. Moret, Interventional Neuroradiology Service, Rothschild Foundation, 25-29 Rue Manin, 75940 Paris, France.

Acta Neurochir (2001) [Suppl] 77: 181–183

Current Indications and Results of Cerebral Angioplasty

D. W. Newell[1], **J. M. Eskridge**[2], and **R. Aaslid**[3]

[1] Department of Neurological Surgery, University of Washington, Seattle, Washington
[2] Department of Neurological Surgery and Radiology, University of Washington, Seattle, Washington
[3] University of Washington, Seattle, Washington

Introduction

Historical Background

Balloon angioplasty was first made possible by advances in micro-catheter technology and neuro-interventional imaging. Zubkov *et al.* reported the first use of balloon angioplasty for cerebral vasospasm in humans in 1984 [8]. Subsequent reports by others confirmed the results that vasospasm of the cerebral arteries induced by subarachnoid hemorrhage could be successfully treated by cerebral angioplasty with micro-balloon catheters [3, 6]. These initial case series reported immediate reversal of angiographic vasospasm as well as sustained improvement in vessel caliber as measured by transcranial Doppler and improvements in cerebral blood flow. Improvements in neurological deficits caused by vasospasm were also reported. Initial reports emphasized the need for careful selection of patients and also reported several associated complications including vessel occlusion, rupture of unsecured aneurysms as well as re-perfusion hemorrhage.

Technique of Angioplasty

Angioplasty is accomplished using transfemoral catheterization with super selective catheterization of major intracranial arteries. A road mapping technique is essential to facilitate the procedure. The procedure is done with the aid of heparinization. Patients are normally given 5000–7000 IU of heparin to attempt to achieve an activated clotting time of >300, prior to placing the catheters in the intracranial vessels. It is important to also immobilize the head and utilize general anesthesia if necessary to prevent movement which may increase complications such as vessel rupture.

Normally the treatment is limited to the basal intracranial vessels including the supraclinoid internal carotid arteries, middle cerebral arteries bilaterally, to the proximal M-2 branches and more recently, anterior cerebral artery [7]. The posterior circulation including the intracranial vertebral arteries, basal arteries, and P1 segments also can be treated by angioplasty.

Initial Indications for Angioplasty

Following the initial experience with the technique and observation of complications, initial indications for treatment became established. These included treatment of symptomatic patients refractory to other treatments such as calcium channel blockers and hypertensive hypervolemic and hemodilution (triple-H) therapy. It was recommended that angioplasty be avoided in patients with unprotected aneurysms due to previous experience with aneurysm ruptures. It was also initially recommended that angioplasty initially not be done if low density lesions appear on CT due to concern for re-perfusion hemorrhage. At many centers, angioplasty also was limited to symptomatic vessels only, however further experience led to the observation that initially asymptomatic vessels with a milder degree of vasospasm would often progress to severe vasospasm if left untreated. This led to the approach in our Institution to treat all vessels affected by vasospasm at the initial treatment session. It was also noted by our group and others that some low density areas on CT, which appear destined for infarction can undergo resolution to a normal appearance when vessels supplying these areas are treated by cerebral angioplasty.

Intra-Arterial Papaverine

The use of intra-arterial papaverine for the treatment of vasospasm was reported by Kassell *et al.* in 1992 [4]. An initial report appeared describing the use in 12 patients who were candidates for balloon angioplasty and were treated with a micro-catheter infusion of intra-arterial papaverine. Eight patients had reversal of angiographic vasospasm and 4 patients showed reversal of delayed ischemic neurological deficits (DINDS). Two patients had recurrent DINDS five days following treatment. Both of these patients had recurrent severe vasospasm when examined angiographically. Other groups also reported early angiographic resolution of vasospasm treated with intra-arterial papaverine and also observed transient effects of the treatment in some patients.

Our group also utilized intra-arterial papaverine either alone or in combination with a balloon angioplasty. We conducted a review of patients either treated only with papaverine or only with angioplasty and compared the results of both treatments [1]. The results of this comparison showed that angioplasty was superior to papaverine treatment alone in basal intracranial arteries for permanent reversal of vasospasm and improvement in blood flow and improvement in DINDS. Transcranial Doppler measurement of velocities in the intracranial vessels showed that the effect of balloon angioplasty was largely permanent, whereas papaverine treatment only resulted in temporary reduction in velocities indicating temporary reversal of vasospasm. The cerebral blood flow measurements also revealed that transluminal angioplasty had a more permanent effect on reversal of cerebral blood flow changes.

Clinical results revealed a similar phenomenon with more patients treated with papaverine requiring repeat treatment and crossover to balloon angioplasty compared to those patients treated with balloon angioplasty alone initially. Following the evaluation of these procedures in patients, advantages and disadvantages of each treatment were observed. Table 1 lists features of angioplasty and papaverine for treatment of cerebral vasospasm. It has subsequently become apparent that the indications for angioplasty could be expanded, and patients with progressive severe sonographic spasm by Doppler, and reductions in cerebral blood flow, who are in poor neurological condition, were also candidates for treatment since these patients were at risk for infarctions before clinical deficits become manifest.

Table 1. *Angioplasty vs Papaverine*

Angioplasty	*Papaverine*
Experienced Interventional neuroradiologist required	less skill required to perform
Lasting effect on cerebral vessels	less permanent effect on cerebral vessels
Improvement in CBF	improvement of CBF
Reversal / prevention of DIND	– distal effects
Success dependent of timing of treatment	may require multiple treatments
Potential complications	adjunct to angioplasty
– Vessel rupture	allows treatment of distal vessels
– Hemorrhage	potential complications
– Dissection	– increased ICP, respiratory depression
	– thrombocytopenia
	– hemorrhage
	– blindness
	– midriasis

Current Indications for Angioplasty

Current indications for angioplasty include symptomatic patients, poor grade patients with sonographic spasm and decreased perfusion. Early low density changes are now not an absolute contra-indication for treatment and currently all accessible vessels which are observed to be in spasm are usually treated with balloon angioplasty.

With expanded indications our success rate for reversal of symptomatic neurological deficits defined by an improvement in Glasgow Coma Score or improvement in motor score by two points within 72 hours have been recorded. The percentage of patients with improvement on a neurologic score is slightly less than previously reported [2], however, many other patients have stabilized and not progressed to infarction. Table 2 lists current results for our series of angioplasty regarding clinical response. One reason for decreased improvement includes early treatment of patients

Table 2. *Results of Balloon Angioplasty in 109 Patients with Symptomatic Vasospasm at The University of Washington*

Improved within 72 hours	47/109 (44%)
Remained unchanged	31/109 (28%)
Deteriorated	31/109 (28%)

without clinically manifest deficits and also more aggressive treatment of poor grade patients with evidence of early infarction.

Trends in Treatment and Future Directions

Recent data from animals and also observations in humans have indicated that prophylactic treatment of vessels exposed to perivascular blood or subarachnoid blood is often effective in preventing vessels from undergoing severe contraction [5]. This observation has led to a prophylactic trial in humans with severe subarachnoid hemorrhage in which patients are randomized to either balloon treatment versus standard management before the onset of vasospasm.

Conclusions and Unanswered Questions Remain Regarding the Effectiveness of Angioplasty

Comparison of the results of treated patients to the natural history of the condition or comparison to standard therapy including hypertensive, hypervolemic, hemodilution, and calcium channel blocker treatment are needed. Questions also remain regarding treatment of symptomatic patients only, versus treatment of severe spasm in asymptomatic patients and pre-emptive angioplasty in high risk patients. Data regarding long term follow-up is also needed.

Agreed upon criteria for evaluation of treatment are also needed including assessment of effectiveness. Criteria for improvement should be established as well as criteria for stabilization. Effect of treatment on outcome will also be needed to be established in clinical trials which include the assessment of treatment intensity of other modalities.

References

1. Elliott JP, Newell DW, Lam DJ, Eskridge JH, Douville CM, LeRout PD, Lewis DH, Mayberg MR, Grady MS, Winn HR (1998) Comparison of balloon angioplasty and papaverine infusion for the treatment of vasospasm following aneurysmal subarachnoid hemorrhage. J Neurosurg 88: 277–284
2. Eskridge JM, McAuliffe W, Song JK, Deliganis AV, Newell DW, Lewis DH, Mayberg MR, Winn HR (1998) Balloon angioplasty for the treatment of vasospasm: results of first 50 cases. Neurosurgery 42: 510–516, discussion 516–517
3. Higashida RT, Halbach VV, Cahan LD, Brant-Zawadzki M, Barnwell S, Dowd C, Hieshima GB (1989) Transluminal angioplasty for treatment of intracranial arterial vasospasm. J Neurosurg 71: 648–653
4. Kassell NF, Helm G, Simmons N, Phillips CD, Cail WS (1992) Treatment of cerebral vasospasm with intra-arterial papaverine. J Neurosurg 77: 848–852
5. Muizelaar JP, Zwienenberg M, Rudisill NA, Hecht ST (1999) The prophylactic use of transluminal balloon angioplasty in patients with Fisher Grade 3 subarachnoid hemorrhage: a pilot study. J Neurosurg 91: 51–58
6. Newell DW, Eskridge JM, Mayberg MR, Grady MS, Winn HR (1989) Angioplasty for the treatment of symptomatic vasospasm following subarachnoid hemorrhage. J Neurosurg 71: 654–660
7. Newell DW, Elliott JP, Eskridge JM, Winn HR (1999) Endovascular therapy for aneurysmal vasospasm. Crit Care Clin 15: 685–699, v
8. Zubkov YN, Nikiforov BM, Shustin VA (1984) Balloon catheter technique for dilatation of constricted cerebral arteries after aneurysmal subarachnoid hemorrhage. Acta Neurochir (Wien) 70: 65

Correspondence: David W. Newell, M.D., Department of Neurological Surgery, University of Washington School of Medicine, Harborview Medical Center, 325 Ninth Avenue, Seattle, Washington 98104.

Acta Neurochir (2001) [Suppl] 77: 185–190

Balloon Prophylaxis of Aneurysmal Vasospasm

J. P. Muizelaar and **L. K. Madden**

Department of Neurological Surgery, University of California, Davis

Introduction

Mechanical treatment with transluminal balloon angioplasty (TBA) is now a well established treatment for vasospasm refractory to medical treatment [1, 3, 4, 6, 8, 9, 12, 13, 15, 18, 21, 25, 29, 30, 34]. The time-window for performing effective TBA in symptomatic vasospasm is short, and is successful in reversal of delayed ischemic neurological deficit (DIND) in only 31 to 77% of the cases, leaving substantial numbers of patients with neurological deficits from vasospasm [2, 3, 6, 12].

Experiments using a dog model of vasospasm have shown that transluminal balloon prophylaxis (TBP) on day zero totally prevents the development of angiographic narrowing on day seven, which has been ascribed to the blood vessels becoming unresponsive to a large number of constrictive (as well as to dilatory) agents [23]. Because the effect of TBP was better than any previously described pharmacological treatment in experimental vasospasm, and because TBP in patients can be performed at a time that secondary insults are usually not important as yet, we have advocated for an investigation of TBP in patients with aneurysmal SAH [24]. TBP is an invasive procedure. Therefore, we felt that a pilot study of TBP should include only patients at greatest risk to develop vasospasm (i.e. Fisher grade III SAH [7]).

Keywords: Subarachnoid hemorrhage; cerebral vasospasm; transluminal balloon prophylaxis; aneurysm.

Materials and Methods

The Human Subjects Review Committee (HSRC) approved this study. The experimental nature of the treatment was explained to the patients and/or their families and informed consent was obtained before performing TBP.

Enrollment Criteria

All patients considered for TBP had SAH from a ruptured aneurysm, and Fisher Grade III [7] on a CT scan obtained within the first two days after SAH. Patients were only included after surgical or neurointerventional treatment of the ruptured aneurysm and any coincidental unruptured aneurysm, and when TBP could be performed within three days from the bleed. Patients included in our sample did not have angiographic evidence of vasospasm prior to the TBP treatment. There were no age limits for inclusion. Pregnancy was not a reason for exclusion. To be included in the prophylactic treatment group, TBP had to be performed in at least two of the three parts of the intracranial circulation (right and/or left carotid system and/or vertebrobasilar system), including the arteries directly leading to the treated ruptured aneurysm.

Surgical and Medical Management

Within two days of rupture, all patients underwent GDC embolization by a neurointerventionalist or clipping of their aneurysms via the classic transsylvian approach as described by Yasargil and Fox [33]. Perivascular blood was cleaned only from cisterns, which were easily accessible. No cisternal drains were left in place. All patients received oral Nimodipine and magnesium supplementation to obtain plasma levels of around 2.2 mg/l [32]. The patient's hematocrit was kept between 30–35, and ample fluids, including 500 ml/24 hours of albumin were infused for prophylactic hyperdynamic therapy. No other plasma expanders were used [31].

Transluminal Balloon Prophylaxis

After surgery, the first nine patients were allowed to wake up to check for any new neurological deficits, and the last nine patients remained intubated for TBP immediately following surgery or coiling. Arterial access was gained via a 6 FR sheath (Pinnacle, Meditech, Watertown, MA) percutaneously placed in the femoral artery. A 100 cm, 5.8 FR thin wall guide catheter (P5.8-NT-100-M-NS-0, Cook, Inc., Bloomington, IN) was advanced into the internal carotid and vertebral arteries. After diagnostic angiography to check for vasospasm, a 4 mm × 10 mm 0.1 cc occlusion balloon type angioplasty balloon catheter (NDSB 8501/20002, Interventional Therapeutics Corp., Fremont, CA) was coaxially advanced through a 6 French guide catheter. Angioplasty target goals for the carotid circulation were the A1 segment of the anterior cerebral artery (ACA), the M1 segment of the middle cerebral artery (MCA) and the supraclinoid internal carotid artery (ICA). Vertebral artery target goals were the P1 segment of the posterior cerebral arteries (PCA)

Table 1. *Grading of Cerebral Vasospasm Using TCD*

Mean blood flow velocity (cm/sec)	Severity of vasospasm
150–200	mild
201–250	moderate
>250	severe

bilaterally, the basilar artery (BA) and the ipsilateral distal vertebral artery (VA). All balloon manipulations were performed with systemic heparinization and roadmapping technique. A single 5000 u bolus of heparin was administered immediately prior to balloon introduction. Balloons were inflated to the vessel diameter with approximately 1 mm of balloon elongation. Inflation duration was five seconds [4, 5]. Arteries were not expanded beyond their native diameter during angioplasty. As the type of balloon used ruptures at approximately 6 atmosphere, and no balloon ruptures were encountered, all arteries treated experienced radial pressures of less than 6 atmosphere.

Diagnosis of Vasospasm and Delayed Neurological Deficit

For 10–14 days after onset of SAH, Transcranial Doppler (TCD) Ultrasonography was performed on all vessels comprising the circle of Willis. Cerebral vasospasm was graded by peak mean velocities, according to the scale shown in Table 1 [20].

DIND was thought to be due to vasospasm if it occurred between days three and fourteen after the SAH in a vascular distribution judged to be at risk (focal deficits for all vessels and/or a decline in the Glasgow Coma Scale score of two or more for midline vessels), and when there was no other discernable cause of deterioration such as post-operative hematoma, hydrocephalus, seizure or metabolic derangement [10, 11]. In cases with suspected DIND the protocol called for angiographic evaluation and if indicated, therapeutic TBA. Outcome was assessed at three months (plus or minus two weeks) using the Glasgow Outcome Scale by an experienced, blinded assessor [14]. Outcome rating was assessed by the operating surgeon only in cases of early unequivocal good outcome (i.e. returned to former work prior to 3-month window).

Results

Patient characteristics and results are outlined in Tables 2 and 3. Within a period of seventeen months (June, 1997 to May, 1998; April, 2000 to August, 2000), a total of eighteen patients were enrolled and underwent TBP as planned (study group, Table 2). During the same period nine patients presented with a Fisher Grade III SAH CT but were not included in our treatment group for various reasons (excluded group, Table 3).

The eighteen patients in the study group consisted of five males and thirteen females ranging in age from 29–75 years (mean age of 48 years). Patients presented with the following Hunt and Hess scores: Grade I (one patient) Grade II (four patients), Grade III (seven patients), Grade IV (five patients) and grade V (one patient). The ruptured aneurysms were located as follows: anterior communicating artery (ACoA) (eleven patients), MCA (one patient), posterior communicating artery (PCoA) (three patients), BA tip (three patients).

During the study period we found two patients who were unable to receive TBP because severe arthero-

Table 2. *Characteristics of 18 Patients with Fisher Grade III SAH Treated with Balloon Prophylaxis*

Sex/age	H&H Adm	H&H pre-op	Site	TCD MCA PVel	TCD ACA PVel	Angiogr Vasosp	GOS score
1. F/41	4	3	ACoA	196 (day 5)	132		GR
2. M/32	4	3	ACoA	176	90		GR
3. M/38[1]	3	3	ACoA	146	70		MD
4. F/44	3	3	ACoA	165	106		GR
5. F/29[1]	2	2	ACoA	172	102		GR
6. M/43	4	4	PCoA	*	*		GR
7. F/47	3	3	BA	90	122		MD
8. F/75[1]	4	5	ACoA	115	143		D
9. F/43[1]	2	2	PCoA	–	–	no	D
10. F/64[1]	5	4	ACoA	127	179		D
11. F/73	3	3	PCoA	83	85		GR
12. M/45[1]	3	3	ACoA	119	62		MD
13. F/48	2	2	MCA	112	223**	yes	GR
14. F/65[1]	4	4	BA	110	114		GR
15. M/39	3	3	ACoA	202 (day 13)	194 (day 13)		MD
16. F/43	3	3	BA	190 (day 14)	96		MD
17. F/45	2	2	ACoA	165	134		GR
18. F/41	1	1	ACoA	164	124		GR

D Dead; *GR* good recovery; *MD* moderate disability

[1] Patient with Fisher Grades III&IV. – Unable to obtain TCD velocities due to early death. * TCD machine broken. ** Untreated.

Table 3. *Characteristics of 9 Patients with Fisher Grade III SAH not Treated with Balloon Prophylaxis*

Sex/age	H&H Adm	H&H pre-op	Site	TCD MCA PVel	TCD ACA PVel	Angiospasm	Exclusion reason	GOS
a. M/78	3	3	PCoA	122	91	NA	severe athero	D
b. F/71	5	3	PCoA	215	198	NA	severe athero	D
c. F/74	5	4	ACoA	147	–	NA	only 2 vessels	D
d. F/62	2	2	BA	135	44	yes	early vasospasm	V
e. F/72	4	4	ACoA	158	126	NA	only 2 vessels	GR
f. M/69	5	5	ACoA	[1]	[1]	yes	delay hosp adm	D
g. M/40	2	2	BA	86	68	NA	refused treat	GR
h. F/37	3	3	ACoA	220	163	yes	control	GR
i. F/48	3	3	PCoA	209	137	yes	control	MD

[1] Unable to insonate.

sclerotic and tortuous arteries precluded angioplasty (#a, #b). These patients were 71 and 78 years old. Two other patients (#c, #e) received TBP in only one part of the intracranial circulation, mostly due to severe atherosclerotic changes and vascular abnormalities. These patients were respectively 74 and 72 years, suggesting that this treatment may not be feasible with some patients in the older age range. Three patients presented to our hospital several days after their SAH. One of the patients (#d) represented in Table 3 showed angiographic evidence of vasospasm just prior to angioplasty. This excluded her from the prophylactic treatment group. One patient (#g) refused to be included in the study. Two patients (#h, #i) have been enrolled in our multicenter study and randomized to the control group. The patient characteristics and results of these patients are outlined in Table 3.

Transcranial Doppler Ultrasonography Findings

In the study group TCD velocities were between 150 and 200 cm/s in four patients, graded as mild vasospasm and 202 cm/s in one patient, graded as moderate vasospasm. There were not any velocities in excess of 250 cm/s (severe vasospasm). In the exclusion group, one patient had mild vasospasm, and three patients had moderate vasospasm. Due to a temporarily broken probe a complete TCD exam could not be obtained in all patients.

Complications

One patient (#9) died of a rupture of the posterior inferior cerebellar artery (PICA) during TBP. No other complications were encountered.

Delayed Ischemic Neurological Deficit and Outcome

DIND did not develop in a single patient in the study group. In the exclusion group symptomatic vasospasm occurred in at least six cases.

Outcome assessment in the study group revealed twelve patients with good recovery and three patients with moderate disability, for a favorable outcome rate of 83%. Three patients died, one because of a vessel rupture during TBP. Two older patients, 75 and 64 years of age, were in very poor clinical condition preoperatively (Hunt & Hess grade IV–V). Both improved to following commands and spontaneous eye opening around day ten, suggesting no occurrence of clinical vasospasm or DIND, but later died from pulmonary complications.

In the exclusion group three patients had a good recovery, one patient remained vegetative and four patients died. One patient died in a nursing facility because of pulmonary complications (#a) and another patient (#c) with an extensive medical history of congestive heart failure and rhythm disturbances died of respiratory failure in the course of her hospital stay. Two patients died and one patient remained vegetative because of vasospasm (#b, #f, and #d, respectively).

Discussion

Transluminal balloon prophylaxis, within three days after SAH from a ruptured berry aneurysm, proved to be feasible in this pilot study with eighteen patients. In this series, no patient had TCD documented moderate-to-severe vasospasm nor developed DIND. Fifteen patients (83%) had a favorable outcome and three patients (17%) died, one because of a vessel rupture during TBP and two patients presum-

Table 4. *Presence of DIND Correlated with Outcome in TBA Treated Study and Exclusion Groups Compared with Reports in the Literature and Historical Controls*

Group & study	No. of patients	Fisher Grades included	% with DIND	% with favorable outcomes
BPAV group, this study	18	III, III & IV	0	83%
Exclusion group, this study	9	III, III & IV	67	44
Nicardipine, Haley, *et al.*, 1993	457	All	46	56
Cyclosporine, Manno, *et al.*, 1997	9	III	56	56
Matched controls, this study	12	III, III & IV	33	67

ably because of the combination of severe initial damage and older age.

Comparison of the data of the previously published studies and our own characteristics-matched patients (historical controls) with those from this pilot-study suggests a much lower incidence of vasospasm in the study-group (Table 4). From this small sample-size, however, it cannot be determined whether preventive TBP is more effective than therapeutic TBA for symptomatic vasospasm in leading to better outcome.

The time window and best technique (degree and duration of dilation) for preventive TBP to be effective cannot be established from our study. In the experimental study by Megeysi *et al.*, the vessels were dilated to a mean of 166% of baseline (range 148–200%) just before the placement of the blood clot, and on day seven the vessels were still at 164% of baseline [22]. In our study, TBP was performed much later. It should be noted that arteries prophylaxed in this study were not dilated beyond their normal anatomic confines, hence the term balloon prophylaxis rather than angioplasty. A force was definitely applied to the intima of the prophylaxed arteries, since there was 1–2 mm elongation of balloon length once the balloon diameter achieved the native artery diameter. Moreover, in the experimental study each segment was dilated twice for ten seconds, while we dilated only once for five seconds as we usually do for the treatment of clinical vasospasm [9]. Any of these technical differences, species differences, or the lesser severity of the experimental SAH compared to clinical aneurysmal SAH (none of the dogs with the untreated vessels with a diameter of 69% of baseline on day seven developed neurological deficits) could also account for the seemingly larger efficacy under experimental conditions.

We aimed at performing TBP in no less than ten vessels (one VA, the BA, both P1 segments of the PCA, bilateral ICA's and M1 segments of the MCA's and A1 segments of the ACA's), but this goal could not be reached in a single case. Short duration of cerebral angiographic procedures is associated with increased safety [19]. Given that there was no proved therapeutic utility of TBP while our study data were collected, shorter procedure duration at the expense of prophylaxis of fewer vessels was favored over longer procedure duration with more target vessels prophylaxed. No guidewires or over-the-wire balloon systems were used. If longer procedural duration had been accepted, and if a greater array of devices had been employed, then more target vessels could have been prophylaxed in each patient.

Another frequently encountered problem was severe atherosclerosis or vessel tortuosity in older patients precluding navigation of the balloon into more than none or one of the three parts of the intracranial circulation (as specified by our protocol). In view of the preliminary character of our study, it was not felt to be justified to become overly aggressive with our attempts to dilate the intracranial vessels. Considering the encouraging results of this study and the high incidence of poor outcome due to vasospasm in the elderly [16, 23], a more persistent attitude seems warranted.

The most severe and clinically relevant vasospasm seems to occur in the system with the ruptured aneurysm [28]. Thus, it might be sufficient to only dilate the right ICA and right M1 segment for a ruptured right sided MCA aneurysm, or the right ICA, A1 segment for an ACoA aneurysm with a dominant right A1, or only the VBA system for posterior circulation aneurysms, etc.

Because at the time of this study we did not measure the Lindegaard index or cerebral blood flow (CBF), it is not possible to tell whether these higher velocities in the treated vessels were due to narrowing of the conductance vessels or less spasm in the medium and small resistance vessels leading to a better run-off. This would be an important question to answer, though, because it could shed light onto the mechanism by which preventive TBP prevents DIND; with better run-off one might assume that preventive TBP prevents the release of some (endothelium-derived?) constricting factor into the downstream circulation, which in turn would make the internal manipulation of the blood vessels more important than dilation per se.

The single procedural death during TBP warrants particular attention. TBP carries risks both from the angiographic technique and from the actual dilatation. From a retrospective study of 597 post aneurysm surgery diagnostic angiograms, it was concluded that post-operative angiography is safe and should be routinely performed [17]. The highest quoted mortality from TBA associated with vessel rupture, derived from a large series of patients is 4% [5], all in non-intubated patients. Later series describe 0% mortality in intubated, paralyzed patients [2, 5, 26]. The initial protocol (employed in the first nine patients) called for treating the patients who had balloon prophylaxis exactly as they would have been had TBP not been performed. This decision was made to avoid confounding variables and theoretically to avoid excess morbidity related to prolonged or repeat intubation. In the first eight patients TBP was successfully performed without intubation and chemical paralysis. In the ninth patient roadmap misregistration due to patient movement resulted in unintended entry of the balloon into the PICA, with subsequent rupture of that vessel resulting in death. The protocol was immediately modified, such that patients remained intubated until TBP was performed, permitting chemical paralysis during angioplasty and assuring reliable roadmapping.

Schwartz and Lellouch have proposed a distinction between 'pragmatic' (does the therapy under investigation improve outcome?) and 'explanatory' (does the therapy under investigation do what it is supposed to do?) trials [27]. In this sense, ours is explanatory as we aimed to research whether preventive TBP could prevent DIND and lead to less vasospasm by TCD criteria. In this sense, TBP appears to work as anticipated. In two cases, we found substantially higher TCD velocities in the MCA of the treated side than in the non-treated side (the reverse was never found). Whether preventive TBP improves outcome and whether the costs of this treatment in all patients are offset by great savings in some patients, can only be determined in a much larger randomized study in patients with Fisher Grade III SAH. Such a study is presently underway.

References

1. Barnwell SL, Higashida RT, Halbach VV *et al* (1989) Transluminal angioplasty of intracerebral vessels for cerebral arterial spasm. Reversal of neurological deficits after delayed treatment. Neurosurg 25: 424–429
2. Bejjani GK, Bank WO, Olan WJ *et al* (1998) The efficacy and safety of angioplasty for cerebral vasospasm after subarachnoid hemorrhage. Neurosurgery 42: 979–987
3. Coyne TJ, Montanera WJ, MacDonald RL *et al* (1994) Percutaneous transluminal angioplasty for cerebral vasospasm after subarachnoid hemorrhage. Can J Surg 37: 391–396
4. Elliott JP, Newell DW, Lam DJ *et al* (1998) Comparison of balloon angioplasty and papaverine infusion for the treatment of vasospasm following aneurysmal subarachnoid hemorrhage. J Neurosurg 88: 277–284
5. Eskridge J, Song JK (1997) A practical approach to the treatment of vasospasm. Am J Neuroradiol 18: 1653–1660
6. Firlik AD, Kaufmann AM, Jungreis CA *et al* (1997) Effect of transluminal angioplasty on cerebral blood flow in the management of symptomatic vasospasm following aneurysmal subarachnoid hemorrhage. J Neurosurg 86: 830–839
7. Fisher CM, Kistler JP, Davis JM (1980) Relation of cerebral vasospasm to subarachnoid hemorrhage visualized by computerized tomographic scanning. Neurosurg 6: 1–9
8. Fujii Y, Takahashi A, Ezura M *et al* (1995) Balloon angioplasty, immediately after surgical clipping for symptomatic vasospasm on admission. Report of four cases. Neurosurg Rev 18: 79–84
9. Fujii Y, Takahashi A, Yoshimoto T (1995) Effect of balloon angioplasty on high grade symptomatic vasospasm after subarachnoid hemorrhage. Neurosurgical Rev 18: 7–13
10. Haley EC, Kassell NF, Torner JC (1993) A randomized trial of Nicardipine in subarachnoid hemorrhage; angiographic and transcranial doppler ultrasound results. J Neurosurg 78: 548–553
11. Haley Jr EC, Kassel NF, Torner JC (1993) A randomized controlled trial of high-dose intravenous Nicardipine in aneurysmal subarachnoid hemorrhage: A report of the Cooperative Aneurysm study. J Neurosurg 78: 537–545
12. Higashida RT, Halbach VV, Cahan LD *et al* (1989) Transluminal angioplasty for treatment of intracranial arterial vasospasm. J Neurosurg 71: 648–653
13. Higashida RT, Halbach VV, Dowd CF *et al* (1992) Intravascular balloon dilatation therapy for intracranial arterial vasospasm: Patient selection, technique and clinical results. Neurosurg Rev 15: 89–95
14. Jennet B, Bond M (1975) Assessment of outcome after severe brain damage. A practical scale. Lancet 1: 480–484
15. Konishi Y, Maemura E, Sato E *et al* (1990) A therapy against vasospasm after subarachnoidal hemorrhage: Clinical experience of balloon angioplasty. Neurol Research 12: 103–105
16. Lanzino G, Kassell NF, Germanson TP *et al* (1996) Age and outcome after aneurysmal subarachnoid hemorrhage: why do older patients fare worse. J Neurosurg 85: 410–418
17. Le Roux PD, Elliot JP, Eskridge JM *et al* Risks and benefits of diagnostic angiography following aneurysm surgery: a retrospective analysis of 597 studies (submitted)
18. Le Roux PD, Newell DW, Eskridge J *et al* (1994) Severe symptomatic vasospasm: The role of immediate postoperative angioplasty. J Neurosurg 80: 224–229
19. Mani RL ER (1978) Complications of catheter arteriography: analysis of 5,000 procedures. II. Assessment of arteries injected, contrast medium used, duration of the procedure, and age of patient. Am J Roentgenol 131: 871–874

20. Manno EM, Gress DR, Ogilvy CS *et al* (1997) The safety and efficacy of cyclosporine A in the prevention of vasospasm in patients with Fisher Grade 3 subarachnoid hemorrhage: a pilot study. Neurosurgery 40: 289–293
21. Mayberg M, Eskridge J, Newell DW *et al* (1990) Angioplasty for symptomatic vasospasm. In: Sano K, Takakura K, Kassel NF *et al* (eds) Cerebral vasospasm. University of Tokyo Press, Tokyo
22. Megyesi JF, Findlay JM, Vollrath B *et al* (1997) In vivo angioplasty prevents the development of vasospasm in canine carotid arteries. Pharmacological and morphological analysis. Stroke 28: 1216–1224
23. Muizelaar JP, Vermeulen M, Van Crevel H *et al* (1988) Outcome of aneurysmal subarachnoid hemorrhage in patients 66 years of age and older. Clin Neurol Neurosurg 90: 203–207
24. Muizelaar JP (1997) In vivo angioplasty prevents the development of vasospasm in canine carotid arteries: editorial comment. Stroke 28: 1224
25. Newell DW, Eskridge JM, Mayberg MR (1992) Endovascular treatment of intracranial aneurysms and cerebral vasospasm. Clin Neurosurg 39: 348–360
26. Rosenwasser RH, Armonda RA, Thomas JE *et al* (1999) Therapeutic modalities for the management of cerebral vasospasm: timing of endovascular options. Neurosurg 44: 975–979
27. Schwartz D LJ (1967) Explanatory and pragmatic attitudes in therapeutic trials. J Chronic Dis 20: 637–648
28. Seiler RW, Grolimund P, Aaslid R (1986) Cerebral vasospasm evaluated by transcranial ultrasound correlated with clinical grade and CT-visualized subarachnoid hemorrhage. J Neurosurg 64: 594–699
29. Terada T, Kinoshita Y, Yokote H *et al* (1997) The effect of endovascular therapy for cerebral arterial spasm, its limitation and pitfalls. Acta Neurochir (Wien) 139: 227–234
30. Terada T, Nakamura Y, Yoshida H *et al* (1993) Percutaneous transluminal angioplasty for the M2 portion vasospasm following SAH: Development of the new microballoon and report of cases. Surg Neurol 39: 13–17
31. Trumble ER, Muizelaar JP, Myseros JS *et al* (1995) Coagulopathy with the use of hetastarch in the treatment of aneurysmal vasospasm. J Neurosurg 82: 44–47
32. Warren BB, Muizelaar JP, Choi SC (1993) Magnesium's role in cerebral vasospasm and outcome in patients with aneurysmal subarachnoid hemorrhage. In: Findlay JM (ed) Cerebral vasospasm. Elsevier Science Publishers
33. Yasargil MG, Fox JL (1975) The microsurgical approach to intracranial aneurysms. Surg Neurol 3: 7–14
34. Zubkov YN, Nikiforov BM (1984) Balloon catheter technique for dilatation of constricted cerebral arteries after aneurysmal SAH. Acta Neurochir (Wien) 70: 65–79

Correspondence: J. Paul Muizelaar, M.D., Ph.D., Department of Neurological Surgery, University of California, Davis, 4860 Y Street, suite 3740, Sacramento, CA, USA 95817.

Acta Neurochir (2001) [Suppl] 77: 191–193

Effect of Intra-Arterial Infusion of Papaverine Hydrochloride on Brain Tissue Oxygen Pressure in the Management of Severe Vasospasm Following Aneurysmal Subarachnoid Hemorrhage

R. Reisch[1], **R. Filippi**[1], **H. Böcher-Schwarz**[1], **D. Mauer**[1], **K. Ringel**[2], **P. Stoeter**[2], and **A. Perneczky**[1]

[1] Department of Neurosurgery, Johannes Gutenberg-University, Mainz, Germany
[2] Department of Neuroradiology, Johannes Gutenberg-University, Mainz, Germany

Introduction

Despite considerable advances in diagnostic, surgical and interventional techniques, the overall outcome for patients with aneurysmal subarachnoid hemorrhage remains poor. Concerning perioperative course, cerebral ischaemia is one of the major factors causing secondary brain demage. The aim of all therapeutic interventions is the stabilization and maintance of cerebral blood flow and tissue oxygenation in order to prevent cerebral ischaemia and consecutively brain infarction [1].

To realize this primary goal we introduced a therapeutic management system in our neurosurgical intensive care unit for patients having suffered severe cerebral vasospasm after aneurysmal subarachnoid hemorrhage. In the case of therapy-refracter vasospasm, according to this therapeutic algorithm, intra-arterial papaverin infusion was carried out. Aim of this study was to investigate the effect of intra-arterial infusion of papaverine hydrochloride on brain tissue oxygenation by patients with severe diffuse vasospasm, monitored by polarographic micro-catheter probes.

Keywords: Cerebral vasospasm; intensive care unit; papaverine hydrochloride; subarachnoid hemorrhage.

Material and Methods

During a one year period from January to December 1998, 39 patients underwent surgical and 10 patients interventional treatment after aneurysmal subarachnoid hemorrhage in our department. In all patients, the aneurysm was treated within 24 hours after hemorrhage to avoid rebleeding and allow agressive critical care therapy. Postoperatively, all patients were observed in our neurosurgical intensive care unit.

In the postoperative course standard medical management and monitoring according to international guidelines were used. Aim of the conventional interventions was at first the prevention of cerebral vasospasm with stabilization of vital parameters and continuous application of calcium-channel antagonists. Non-invasive transcranial Doppler (TCD) ultrasound recordings were carried out every day. The clinical presentation of patients was strongly monitored, neurological deterioration was characterized by focal deficit or depression of level of consciousness; other causes such as rebleeding, hydrocephalus, and metabolic disturbances were excluded.

After the completed diagnosis of symptomatic vasospasm with neurological deterioration and increase of cerebral blood flow velocity on TCD findings, the preventive interventions were maximized, hypertension, hypervolemia and haemodilution were induced with volumen-expansion and catecholamine medication.

In the case of severe symptomatic vasospasm refractory to this conventional therapy, early intubation and artificial ventilation was carried out to maintain optimal oxygenation and controlled CO2 elimination. In order to measure cerebral oxygenation we introduced a polarographic Clarcke-type microcatheter (GMS, Kiel, Germany), in the white matter of the frontal region and monitored continuously the brain tissue oxygen partial pressure (PtiO2). The catheter was placed in the hemisphere suffering from vasospasm. The PtiO2 catheter functions as a revoxode: the oxygen diffuses from the brain tissue through the polyethylene wall into its inner electrolyte fluid. Here oxygen transforms at a negatively polarized precious metal electrode to OH ions. The current from the oxygen reduction is the raw signal of the sensor [3, 4].

In the case of reduced brain tissue oxygenation (PtiO2 $<$ 20 mmHg) and increased blood flow velocity (Vm $>$ 160 cm/sec in the middle cerebral artery), despite of maximized conventional critical care therapy, 5 patients underwent diagnostic angiography. In all patients angiography showed severe diffuse vasospasm. Intra-arterial papaverine therapy was instituted immediately, using a microcatheter placed in the internal carotid artery just distal from the ophtalmic segment. Papaverine was mixed with normal saline at a concentration of 0.5%. Papaverine was injected by slow continuous pump infusion over 120 minutes in total doses of 300–600 mg. Posttreatment angiography was performed to assess the effects of treatment in all cases. During the whole procedure PtiO2 was monitored continuously. Pre- and postinfusion value of cerebral blood velocity was also recorded.

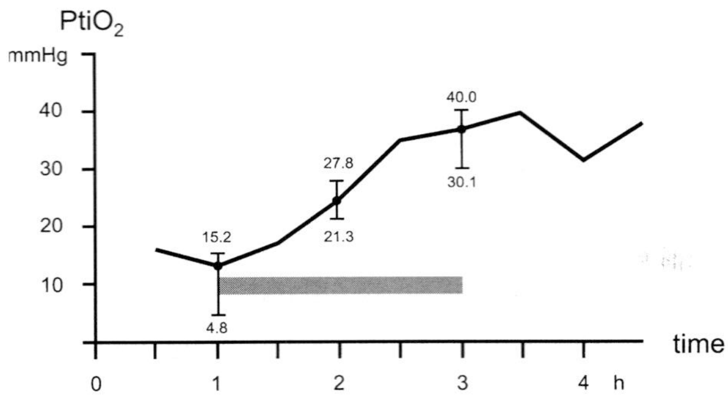

Fig. 1. Graph showing the change of mean PtiO2 value during papaverine infusion in five cases. Note the unbroken improvement of cerebral oxygenation during the procedure. After papaverine infusion during transportation of patient, PtiO2 value showed temporary decrease but stabilization after optimized ventilation and medication in the intensiv care unit. Gray line: papaverine infusion

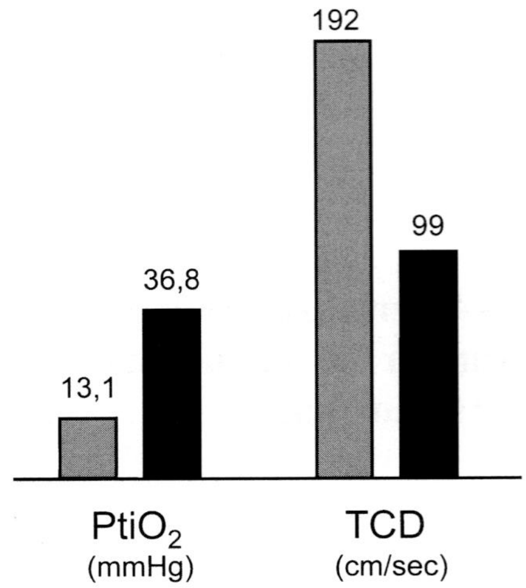

Fig. 2. Bar graph showing the mean PtiO2 level and blood flow velocity values in the middle cerebral artery before and after angioplasty for five patients. ▨ Before papaverine infusion, ■ after papaverine infusion

Results and Discussion

Maintance of cerebral oxygen supply is one of the most important therapeutic goal in neurosurgical intensive care by patients who have suffered aneurysmal subarachnoid hemorrhage [1, 5]. Numerous therapies have been propsed for this condition but have achieved only limited success. There is agreement among authors that preventive interventions are essential including application of calcium channel antagonist nimodipine. Concerning interventional therapy, first of all intra-arterial infusion of papaverine hydrochloride, opinions vary [2, 5, 6, 7].

In our five cases, during intra-arterial infusion of papaverine, PtiO2 value increased unbroken from the mean value of 13.1 to postinfusion mean value of 36.8 mmHg, verified the stabilization of cerebral oxygen supply (Fig. 1). Cerebral blood flow velocity, measured in the middle cerebral artery, decreased in doppler recordings from a preinfusion value of 192 to a mean value of 99.3 cm/sec after papaverine injection (Fig. 2).

The results of this preliminary study show that intra-arterial papaverine infusion benefits cerebral oxygenation, monitored by PtiO2 microcatheter probes. All of our patients experienced improvement in the brain tissue partial oxygen pressure and decreasing of blood flow velocity. After intervention patients were further artificially ventilated to maintain optimal oxygenation and were aggressively managed to increase cerebral perfusion. Under these conditions improvements in tissue oxygen metabolism and perfusion were long lasting, no patients required repeated treatment for recurrent vasospasm. There were no side effects due to infusion of papaverine and no complications due to implantation of the PtiO2 catheter.

Conclusion

According to our therapeutic algorithm, the patients were primarily treated by aggressive critical care management. As ultima ratio, by observed cerebral ischaemia, interventional therapy was carried out. During intra-arterial infusion of papaverine, all of our paients experienced an improvement in the brain tissue, partial oxygen pressure, and decreasing of blood flow velocity.

We strongly believe, that combination of surgical, aggressive critical care and interventional therapy can be successful by management of severe symptomatic vasospasm. Further data collections and prospective trials are required to evaluate the effectiveness of this management with invasive monitoring of cerebral oxygenation in terms of short- and long-term outcome in patients with severe vasospasm following aneurysmal subarachnoid haemorrhage.

References

1. Al-Yamany M, Wallace MC (1999) Management of cerebral vasospasm in patients with aneurysmal subarachnoid hemorrhage. Intensive Care Med 25(12): 1463–1466
2. Clouston JE, Numaguchi Y, Zoarski GH, Aldrich EF, Simard JM, Zitnay KM (1995) Intraarterial papaverine infusion for

cerebral vasospasm after subarachnoid hemorrhage. AJNR 16: 27–38

3. Dings J, Meixensberger J, Jäger A, Roosen K (1998) Clinical experience with 118 brain tissue oxygen partial pressure catheter probes. Neurosurgery 43: 1082–1095
4. Filippi R, Reisch R, Mauer D, Perneczky A (1999) Brain tissue pO2 related to SjvO2, ICP and CPP in severe brain injury. Neurosurg Rev 23: 94–97
5. Kaku Y, Yonekawa Y, Tsukahara T, Kazekawa K (1992) Superselective intra-arterial infusion of papaverine for the treatment of cerebral vasospasm after subarachnoid hemorrhage. J Neurosurg 77: 842–847
6. Kassel NF, Helm G, Simmons N, Phillips CD, Cail WS (1992) Treatment of cerebral vasospasm with intra-arterial papaverine. J Neurosurg 77: 848–852
7. Numaguchi Y, Zoarsky GH, Clouston JE, Zagadaro MT, Simard JM, Aldrich EF, Sloan MA, Maurer PK, Okawara SH (1997) Repeat intra-arterial papaverine for recurrent cerebral vasospasm after subarachnoid hemorrhage. Neuroradiology 39: 751–759

Correspondence: Dr. R. Reisch, Department of Neurosurgery, Johannes Gutenberg-University, Langenbeckstr. 1, D-55131 Mainz, Germany.

Acta Neurochir (2001) [Suppl] 77: 195–197

Long Term Follow up of Angioplasty for Cerebral Vasospasm

J. Srinivasan, A. Moore, J. Eskridge, H. R. Winn, and **D. W. Newell**

Department of Neurological Surgery, Washington, USA

Introduction

Cerebral angioplasty has been reported to be useful for the treatment of symptomatic cerebral vasospasm following subarachnoid hemorrhage [3]. Recent data indicates that angioplasty may be effective in preventing the development of vasospasm [7]. However, the long-term effects of cerebral angioplasty on the human cerebral circulation are not known. In the coronary circulation, complications of angioplasty for atherosclerotic disease include restenosis in 30% of vessels, occlusion of the vessel, transient loss of vascular reactivity, and long-term endothelial dysfunction [4]. In atherosclerotic vessels, angioplasty induces vascular injury and initiates intimal hyperplasia, deposition of extracellular matrix, and ultimately results in vessel remodeling. Although no clinical case reports of delayed complications of cerebral angioplasty have been reported, there has also been no assessment of these patients with regard to their intracranial circulation. The goal of this study was to perform a late evaluation of patients using transcranial Doppler (TCD) to study vascular integrity and function.

Keywords: Vasospasm; angioplasty; transcranial Doppler.

Materials and Methods

Twenty-eight patients who underwent cerebral angioplasty for vasospasm between 1989 and 1998 were reevaluated at an average of 44 months (range 26–71) following angioplasty. The average age of the patient at follow-up was 48 years $\pm$ 10 years. The group was composed of 7 men and 21 women. Follow-up included history, neurologic evaluation, and a standard transcranial Doppler examination of all intracranial vessels.

Transcranial Doppler examinations were performed using standard techniques (Fujioka, 1992). The highest velocity in each vessel segment was recorded. Distal internal carotid artery (ICA) velocities were measured by transorbital or transtemporal TCD sonography, and middle cerebral artery (MCA) and anterior cerebral artery (ACA) velocities were measured by transtemporal TCD. The vertebrobasilar system was assessed by the suboccipital window at the foramen magnum. Both cervical ICA's were insonated at the angle of the mandible. The ratio of the MCA velocity to the ipsilateral cervical ICA velocity (intracranial/extracranial ratio) is defined as the Lindegaard ratio and allows for correction of systemic factors such as hyperdynamic flow or low flow due to severe spasm [5].

A subgroup of 20 patients underwent assessment of cerebral autoregulation in both middle cerebral artery territories using Transcranial Doppler. In one patient, the left MCA territory was excluded because of hyperostosis of the temporal bone and poor vessel insonation. A detailed description of the methodology used to calculate the dynamic autoregulatory response has been published elsewhere, including the equations which describe the computer model used to obtain the autoregulatory index (ARI) [8]. A series of hypothetical response curves is drawn, with ARI values ranging from 0 (no autoregulation) to 9. The actual response is examined and the "best fit" with the model is taken as the ARI. The higher the ARI, the more rapid and efficient is the autoregulatory response [8].

Results were analyzed using the Student's t test. Differences were considered significant at the $p < 0.05$ level. Because of the small numbers, not all results could be analyzed for statistical significance.

A total of 84 vessels were treated originally by angioplasty: 41 MCA's, 4 ACA's, 24 ICA's, 3 posterior cerebral arteries (PCA), 7 vertebral arteries (VA), and 8 basilar arteries (BA).

Results

Clinical

At follow-up examination, clinical outcome data was available on 21 patients. Seven of the remaining patients had their TCD examinations performed early during the course of our study, and no clinical data was recorded. Of the 21 patients, 15 had a good outcome by the Glasgow outcome scale, and 6 had a moderate disability. There were no patients with new strokes, TIA's, or new neurologic deficits. Eight of the 21 patients had hypertension, 2 had diabetes, 4 had hypercholesterolemia, and 9 were smokers. None of the patients had cardiac or peripheral vascular disease.

Table 1. *Transcranial Doppler Velocities in Treated Vessels*

Artery	Time of study	Velocity ± SD cm/sec	p value vs. pre-angioplasty
Middle cerebral	pre-angioplasty	210 ± 46	–
	immediate post-PTA	122 ± 48	<0.0001
	delayed post-PTA	76 ± 21	<0.0001
	late follow-up	61 ± 17	<0.0001
Internal carotid	pre-angioplasty	100 ± 38	–
	immediate post-PTA	74 ± 27	0.006
	delayed post-PTA	66 ± 26	0.0006
	late follow-up	46 ± 9	<0.0001
Basilar	pre-angioplasty	137 ± 41	–
	immediate post-PTA	88 ± 40	0.04
	delayed post-PTA	58 ± 32	0.002
	late follow-up	48 ± 16	0.001
Vertebral	pre-angioplasty	122 ± 63	–
	immediate post-PTA	85 ± 26	0.2
	delayed post-PTA	51 ± 26	0.02
	late follow-up	41 ± 12	0.01

Standard transcranial Doppler examinations were performed prior to angioplasty (Pre-angioplasty), immediately after angioplasty (Immediate post-PTA), upon resolution of vasospasm but prior to discharge from hospital (Delayed post-PTA), and at Late follow-up, an average of 44 months after angioplasty. PTA = percutaneous transluminal angioplasty. The average velocity in each artery is reported in cm/sec and the significance of the velocity as compared to the pre-angioplasty value is stated in the last column (p values were calculated using Students' t-test).

TCD Exam Results

A comparison of velocities recorded by transcranial Doppler performed immediately by pre and post-angioplasty, prior to discharge from the hospital and at late follow-up are shown in Table 1. All patients had significant elevation of their velocities just prior to angioplasty indicative of severe vasospasm. There was a reduction in the velocity immediately postangioplasty and a further reduction prior to discharge. At late follow-up, normal velocities were recorded in all vessels. No individual patient had an abnormal elevated velocity consistent with stenosis, and there were no vessel occlusions. In addition, no abnormally low cerebral blood flow velocity was recorded. Velocities at long term follow-up, when compared to historical controls, are not significantly different; however, because these were not age-matched controls, some vessel velocities fell outside the standard deviation of normal control values. This is shown in Table 1 and Fig. 1.

Assessment of Autoregulatory Function

The dynamic autoregulation studies revealed that the average ARI value was normal in both the treated and untreated MCA territories. No single territory had a low ARI value when compared to the range for historical controls. This indicates that no MCA territory had hemodynamically significant vascular disease (Table 2).

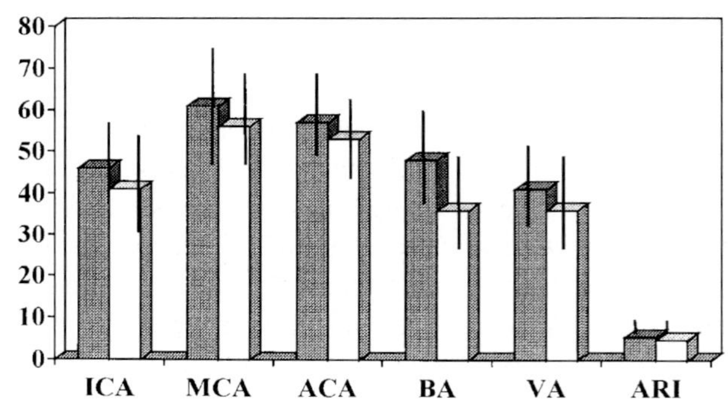

Fig. 1. The average TCD velocities at follow-up are compared to historical controls. No significantly abnormal velocities were recorded in any vessel; the range was greater than that of the historical controls but the patients were not age-matched. The control values for velocities were obtained from Adams [1] and for ARI from Tiecks [8]. ▩ Patients, □ Control

Discussion

Significant delayed vascular disease has been shown in the coronary and carotid circulations following angioplasty for atherosclerosis. The vascular injury induced by angioplasty initiates a reaction in the vessels that leads to poor vessel remodeling and frequent restenosis. In the cerebral circulation, vasospasm in-

Table 2. *Assessment of Autoregulatory Capacity by TCD*

MCA territory	Autoregulatory index (ARI)
Angioplasty	5.41 ± 1.27
Untreated	5.86 ± 1.57
Historical control	4.7 ± 1.0

Autoregulation was tested using dynamic autoregulation testing by transcranial Doppler. The calculation of the autoregulatory index (ARI) is described in the materials and methods section in the text. In general, an ARI value greater than 3.7 is considered normal [8]; all patients at follow-up at normal ARI values in both treated and untreated MCA territories. Because of the small number of patients, a statistical comparison to historical controls could not be calculated.

duces endothelial cell vacuolation, tight junction disruption, and altered permeability [2]. Although there is significant smooth muscle cell contraction, vacuolization, and necrosis, there does not appear to be proliferation of smooth muscle cells in this disease. There is collagen deposition in the adventitia, and intimal thickening begins late during the course of vasospasm and persists for several weeks after the period of clinical vasospasm. Following angioplasty of these vessels, there is flattening of the endothelial layer with patchy denudation with straightening and stretching of the smooth muscle cells. Resolution of these changes begins approximately two weeks after angioplasty, and in a canine model, is often complete within six weeks [2]. Of importance, in cerebral vasospasm, the pressure used to dilate the artery during angioplasty is only 0.5 atmospheres, whereas in the coronary circulation the pressure is between 4 and 8 atmospheres [3]. In our patient population, where atherosclerosis played a minimal role in the disease process, cerebral angioplasty did not have any detrimental long-term effects. In particular, we did not find any vessel stenoses or occlusions, and all vessels appeared to have normal cerebral blood flow velocities. Further, these patients did not have any clinical evidence of progressive cerebrovascular occlusive disease.

In animal models, vasospasm alone mildly reduces vessel reactivity to constricting and relaxing agents for two to three weeks [2]. Angioplasty on vasospastic vessels results in a dramatic decrease in reactivity to pharmacologic agents for approximately two to three weeks. In humans, where vascular reactivity is measured at the arteriolar level, Manno *et al.* reported that 53% of patients with vasospasm had impaired autoregulation [6]. These patients had not undergone angioplasty, so it is unclear whether angioplasty would have further impaired autoregulation. In studying dynamic autoregulation in the MCA territories at follow-up, autoregulatory ability is preserved in the treated territories. This indicates an intact cerebral circulation, with no evidence of a low-flow state secondary to hemodynamically significant proximal vessel disease. We have shown here that cerebral autoregulation in both treated and untreated territories improves following vasospasm, and does not remain impaired on a long-term basis.

Conclusion

Cerebral angioplasty for vasospasm appears to have no delayed consequences for the treated vessels. Although angioplasty for atherosclerotic disease has been shown to have long-term negative effects in the coronary and carotid circulations, this is not the case in the cerebral circulation. This is the first published follow-up of multiple patients who have undergone angioplasty, and it provides reassurance that this technique, as well as being effective, does not have any lasting detrimental effects on the vessels.

References

1. Adams RP, Nichols FT, Hess DC (1992) Normal values and physiologic variables. In: Newell DW, Aaslid R (eds) Transcranial Doppler. Raven Press, New York, pp 41–48
2. Chan PDS, Findlay MF, Vollrath B, Cook DA, Grace M, Chen MH, Ashforth RA (1995) Pharmacological and morphological effects of in vitro transluminal balloon angioplasty on normal and vasospastic canine basilar arteries. J Neurosurg 83: 522–530
3. Eskridge JM, McAuliffe W, Song JK, Deliganis AV, Newell DW, Leis DH, Mayberg MR, Winn HR (1998) Balloon angioplasty for the treatment of vasospasm: results of the first 50 cases. Neurosurgery 42: 510–516
4. Golino P, Chiariello M (1991) New approaches to the prevention of thrombotic restenosis after angioplasty or thrombolysis. J Cardiovasc Pharmacol 17 [Suppl] 5: S41–S47
5. Lindegaard KF, Nornes H, Bakke S, Sorteberg W, Nakstad (1988) Cerebral vasospasm after subarachnoid haemorrhage investigated by means of transcranial Doppler ultrasound. Acta Neurochir (Wien) [Suppl] 42: 81–84
6. Manno EM, Gress DR, Schwamm LH, Diringer MN, Ogilvy CS (1998) Effects of induced hypertension on transcranial Doppler ultrasound velocities in patients after subarachnoid hemorrhage. Stroke 29: 422–428
7. Muizelaar JP, Zwienenberg M, Rudisill NA, Hecht ST (1999) The prophylactic use of transluminal balloon angioplasty in patients with Fisher Grade 3 subarachnoid hemorrhage: a pilot study. J Neurosurg 91: 51–58
8. Tiecks FP, Lam AM, Aaslid R, Newell DW (1995) Comparison of static and dynamic cerebral autoregulation measurements [see comments]. Stroke 26: 1014–1019

Correspondence: J. Srinivasan, University of Washington, Department of Neurological Surgery, 700 9th Avenue, 3rd Floor, Seattle, Washington, 98104, USA.

Treatment of Clinical Vasospasm and Neuroprotection

Acta Neurochir (2001) [Suppl] 77: 201–204

Effect of Fasudil HCl, a Protein Kinase Inhibitor, on Cerebral Vasospasm

M. Shibuya[1], **T. Asano**[2], and **Y. Sasaki**[3]

[1] Chukyo Hospital, Nagoya, Tokyo, Japan
[2] Asahi Chemical Industry Co, Tokyo, Japan
[3] Department of Pharmacology, Kitasato University, Tokyo Japan

Introduction

Fasudil HCl (HA1077, AT877, Eril) was first introduced as a unique vasodilator and intracellular calcium antagonist. It dilated spastic basilar artery by the intravenous injection on day 7 in a two-hemorrhage canine model of chronic cerebral vasospasm. Effectiveness of Fasudil on symptomatic and angiographic vasospasm, cerebral infarction by spasm and clinical outcome had been shown by a double blind trial in patients. Now, it is widely used in Japan in patients with aneurysmal subarachnoid hemorrhage. Current and approved use of Fasudil (30 mg iv 3 times a day for 14 days) ameliorates risk of spasm by about 50%.

The mechanism of Fasudil's effect on cerebral vasospasm has become clearer. Fasudil inhibits several protein kinases involved in the development of cerebral vasospasm: 1) Myosin light chain kinase, final common pathway of smooth muscle contraction, 2) protein kinase C which activates contraction of smooth muscle cells by phosphorylating calponin, protein kinase C also stimulates production of free radicals by activating NADPH oxidase in the polymorphonuclear leukocytes, 3) Rho kinase which inhibits dephosphorylation of activated myosin light chain by myosin phosphatase.

Our recent findings suggest that myosin light chain is double phosphorylated (Ser^{19} and Thr^{18}) in abnormal contraction of the smooth muscle cells. Fasudil inhibited this double phosphorylation more specifically which may explain the unique spasmolytic effect of Fasudil.

Keywords: Cerebral vasospasm; calcium antaponist; Fasudil HCl.

In spite of the progress of treatment there still remain patients who suffer from cerebral ischemia due to chronic cerebral vasospasm after subarachnoid hemorrhage. Although calcium entry blockers have been widely used in western countries, we believe from the results of animal experiments that they are not effective enough for the treatment. Fasudil HCl has a unique effect on vasodilation and brain protection by inhibiting several protein kinases involved in contraction of smooth muscle cells and production of free radicals. Fasudil had been tried in humans since 1987 and approved as an antivasospasm drug in 1995. In this paper, the history of development of Fasudil is reviewed and our current hypothesis on the mechanism of vasospasm is discussed.

Fasudil HCl

Fasudil HCl [HA1077, AT877, Eril, Hexahydro-1-(5 isoquinolinesulfonyl)-1H-1,4-diazepine hydrochloride] is a novel and potent vasodilator. It is water soluble and relatively stable under the light. pH of the water solution is 6.0. Fasudil is quickly metabolized in the body with a biological half life of about 25 min. One of its metabolites in human and rats, but not in dogs, hydroxy-fasudil (M3), also has a vasodilating effect with a half life of about 8 hours.

In Vitro Study

Dog basilar artery strip contracted by a calcium ionophore A23187 (10^{-6} M) could not be relaxed by

Table 1. *Effect of Fasudil in Clinical Studies*

Number of patients	Double blind trial (ref 14) Control 136	Fasudil 129	Imprvd	Comparison with historical control (ref 15) Control 893	Fasudil 494	Imprvd
Symptomatic spasm	50%	35%	30%	30%	20%	33%
Angiographic spasm	62	38	39	39	28	28
Cerebral infarction	38	16	58	–	–	
ADL independent	74	88	19	69	74	7

Higher percentage of patients with symptomatic and angiographic spasm in the double blind trial compared with that of the study with historical control on the right side is due to the fact that patients with severer subarachnoid hemorrhage were preferentially entered in the double blind trial. Better ADL is due to the fact that poor results by other causes than spasm were excluded in the double blind study.

calcium entry blockers such as verapamil, diltiazem or nicardipine, while it was completely relaxed by the addition of 10^{-5} M of Fasudil [13]. In the rabbit aorta strip Fasudil competitively inhibited contraction induced by the addition of Ca^{++} in the incubation media with a pA_2 of 6.71. In the normal saline with Ca^{++} in the incubation media both verapamil and Fasudil inhibited contraction induced by the addition of prostaglandine $F_2\alpha$, while, in a calcium free solution, only Fasudil inhibited the contraction [2]. These data suggest that Fasudil is not a calcium entry blocker but it inhibits action of calcium inside smooth muscle cells.

In Vivo Study

In a dog two-hemorrhage model of vasospasm after subarachnoid hemorrhage, only Fasudil HCl (0.5–10 mg/kg/30 min) dilated the spastic basilar artery by the intravenous injection on day seven after the the first hemorrhage. The dilatation lasted for about two hours. Hypotension by this dose of Fasudil was mild. On the other hand calcium entry blocker (nicardipine) did not dilate the spastic artery even with high doses causing hypotension [17].

Effectiveness of prophylactic use of Fasudil was also shown in the same dog model. Either three mg/kg of Fasudil or saline in control dogs was given intravenously over 30 min two times a day for 7 days [9]. In saline treated dogs, angiographic vasospasm was clearly seen. Histological section of the basilar artery of this group showed typical features such as contraction, corrugation, thickening of the arterial wall with invasion of many inflammatory cells around the artery. Scanning electron microscopic study of the endothelial surface showed a rough surface of corrugation with a marked attachment of the blood cell components: WBC, platelets and RBC. However, Fasudil treated dogs showed marked reduction of angiographic spasm and smooth endothelial surface with few blood cells attached to the endothelial surface on scanning electron microscope [10]. Those inflammatory cells in and around the spastic artery are considered to play important rolls in the development of the spasm by producing free radicals such as superoxide anion.

Effectiveness of Fasudil in Clinical Studies

After phase I and II study, effect of fasudil was examined in a double blind trial in patients with subarachnoid hemorrhage who were operated on within 3 days after the ictus. In order to see the effect of Fasudil on vasospasm, patients with severer subarachnoid hemorrhage among patients with Hunt & Hess grades 1–4 were selected. A total of 287 patients were entered. They were evenly distributed between the placebo and the Fasudil groups. Thirty mg of Fasudil in 2 ml of saline or saline alone (placebo) were dissolved in a 100 ml of saline and injected over 30 min three times a day for 14 days. Fasudil significantly decreased symptomatic spasm from 50 to 35%. Angiographic spasm was decreased from 62% to 38%. Cerebral infarction by spasm as seen on CT scan as a low density area was also decreased from 38% to 16%. Poor outcome due to spasm was decreased from 26% to 12% ($P < 0.05$) [14]. Similar effect of Fasudil on spasm was seen in about 500 patients after it had been commercialized in 1995 when compared with those of 900 patients who had been treated without Fasudil in 1993–4 (Table 1) [15]. Fasudil is now used in the majority of the patients with aneurysmal subarachnoid hemorrhage in Japan.

Effect of Intraarterial Injection of Fasudil

Although the incidence of vasospasm has been significantly decreased by the prophylactic use of Fasudil, there are still patients who develop vasospasm. Intraarterial injection of Fasudil is tried for such patients. Usually 30 mg of Fasudil is diluted in 20 ml of saline and injected in divided doses through the angiographic catheter in the carotid or vertebral arteries. The injection must be done slowly while under blood pressure monitoring. Intraarterial injection of Fasudil is effective in dilating the spastic artery and ameliorating signs of spasm in about half of those patients. The effect is similar to those of papaverine. To our impression Fasudil is superior to papaverine because there were no side effects such as blindness or occlusion of the injected artery which had been reported with papaverine [16].

Our Current Hypothesis of Vasospasm and the Mechanism of Fasudil's Effect

Effect of Fasudil on spasm is now considered to be by the inhibition of several protein kinases: Myosin light chain kinase (MLCK) [3], Protein kinase C [5, 11] and most importantly Rho kinase (Table 2) [7, 18]. MLCK induces smooth muscle cell contraction by increased intracellular calcium which activates calmodulin and MLCK. MLCK also plays a role in the migration of inflammatory cells into the field of spasm [10]. The inflammatory cells produce free radicals by the activation of NADPH oxidase which is activated by protein kinase C. Actually, Fasudil has inhibited production of free radicals by human neutrophils [1].

Table 2. *Ki Values of Fasudil*

Enzyme	Ki (μM)	References
Myosin light chain kinase (MLCK)	36	(3, 11)
Protein kinase C	3.3	(5, 11)
Rho kinase	0.36	(18)

Protein kinase C activates contraction of smooth muscle cells by phosphorylating actin-binding protein calponin. Phosphorylation of calponin neutralizes a supression state of actin-activated myosin Mg-ATP ase. Thus inhibition of protein kinase C by Fasudil leads to relaxation of smooth muscle cells.

Recently it was found that Fasudil strongly inhibited Rho kinase which could be a key enzyme in spasm. Activated MLC by calmodulin – MLCK is dephosphorylated by MLC phosphatase. This phosphatase is down regulated by Rho kinase. Thus, the inhibition of Rho kinase by Fasudil activates MLC phosphatase which leads to a relaxation of smooth muscle cells. In addition, it was found that MLC was phosphorylated in two locations (diphosphorylated: Ser^{19}, Thr^{18}) in abnormal contraction such as interleukin induced spasm in the coronary artery [6, 12] and hemorrhage induced spasm of the femoral artery in dogs [4]. Fasudil inhibited the production of this

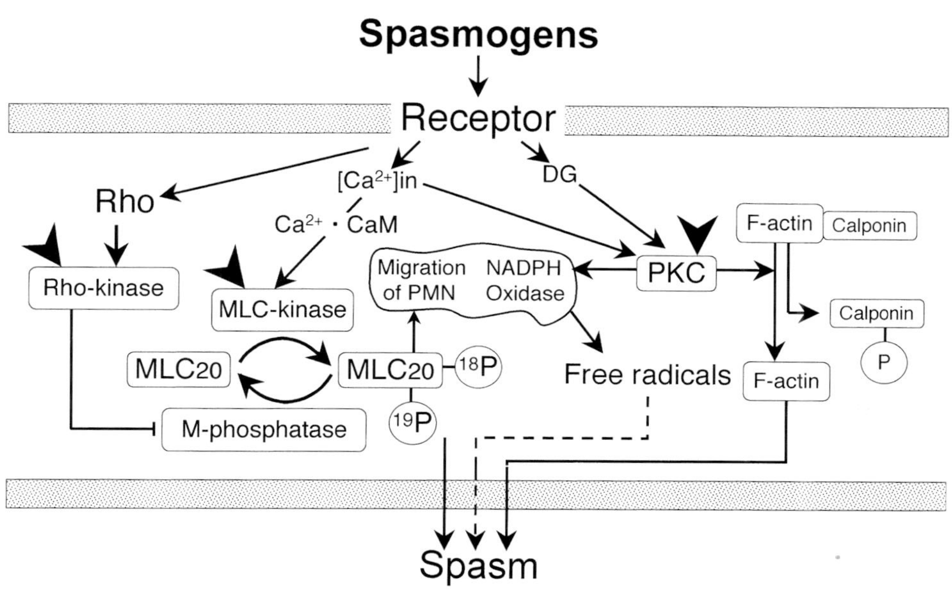

Fig. 1. Arrow heads indicate inhibition by Fasudil. *CaM* Calmodulin, *DG* diacyl glycerol, *M* myosin, *MLC* myosin light chain, *P* phosphate, *PKC* protein kinase C, *PMN* polymorphonuclear leukocyte

diphosphorylated MLC more specifically than monophosphorylated MLC [6]. These experimental data suggest that the most important mechanism of the effect of Fasudil on vasospasm may be the inhibition of Rho kinase (Fig. 1) [7, 8].

References

1. Arai M, Sasaki Y, Nozawa R. (1993) Inhibition by the protein kinase inhibitor HA1077 of the activation of NADPH oxidase in human neutrophils. Biochem Pharmacol 46: 1487–1490
2. Asano T, Ikegaki I, Satoh S, Suzuki Y, Shibuya M, Takayasu M, Hidaka H (1990) Mechanism of action of a novel anti-vasospasm drug, HA1077. J Pharmacol Exp Ther 241-1033-1040
3. Asano T, Suzuki Y, Tsuchiya M, Satoh S, Ikegaki I, Shibuya M, Suzuki Y, Hidaka H (1989) Vasodilator actions of HA1077 in vitro and in vivo putatively mediated by the inhibition of protein kinase. Br J Pharmacol 98: 1091–1100
4. Harada T, Seto M, Sasaki Y, London S, Luo Z, Mayberg M (1995) The time course of myosin light-chain phosphorylation in blood induced vasospasm. Neurosurgery 36: 1178–1182
5. Hidaka H, Inagaki M, Kawamoto S *et al* (1984) Isoquinolinesulfonamides, novel and potent inhibitor of cyclic nucleotide dependent protein kinase and protein kinase C. Biochemistry 23: 5036–5041
6. Katsumata N, Shimokawa H, Seto M *et al* (1997) Enhanced myosin light chain phosphorylation as a central mechanism for coronary artery spasm in a swine model with Interleukin 1β. Circulation 96: 4357–4363
7. Nagumo H, Sasaki Y, Ono Y *et al* (2000) Rho kinase inhibitor HA-1077 prevents Rho-mediated myosin phosphatase inhibition in smooth muscle cells. Am J Physiol Cell Physiol 278: C57–C65
8. Sasaki Y, Shibuya M, Hidaka H (1999) Antispastic Therapeutic, HA1077 (Eril). In: Kohama K, Sasaki Y (eds) Molecular mechanisms of smooth muscle contraction. Molecular Biology Intelligence Unit 5 RG Landes Co. Austin, Texas, pp 119–132
9. Satoh S, Suzuki Y, Harada T *et al* (1992) Possible prophylactic potential of HA1077, a Ca^{2+} channel antagonist and vasodilator, on chronic cerebral vasospasm. Eur J Pharmacol 220: 243–248
10. Satoh S, Yamamoto Y, Toshima Y *et al* (1999) Fasudil, a protein kinase inhibitor, prevents the development of endothelial injury and neutrophil infiltration in a two-hemorrhage canine subarachnoid model. J Clin Neurosci 6: 394–399
11. Seto M, Sasaki Y, Hidaka H *et al* (1991) Effect of HA1077, a protein kinase inhibitor, on myosin phosphorylation and tension in smooth muscle. Eur J Pharmacol 195: 267–272
12. Seto M, Sasaki Y (1999) Diphosphorylation of myosin light chain and spastic contraction of smooth muscle. In: Kohama K, Sasaki Y (eds) Molecular mechanism of smooth muscle contraction. Molecular Biology Intelligence Unit 5 RG Landes Co. Austin, Texas, pp 97–106
13. Shibuya M, Suzuki Y, Takayasu M *et al* (1988) The effect of an intracellular calcium antagonist HA1077 on delayed cerebral vasospasm in dogs. Acta Neurochir (Wien) 90: 53–59
14. Shibuya M, Suzuki Y, Sugita K *et al* (1992) Effect of AT877 on cerebral vasospasm after subarachnoid hemorrhage. Results of a prospective placebo-controlled double blind trial. J Neurosurg 76: 571–577
15. Shibuya M, Oosuka K, Suzuki Y *et al* (1999) Clinical and angiographic effect of Fasudil HCl (AT877) on cerebral vasospasm In: Dorsch N (Ed) Cerebral vasospasm VI, Proceeding of the VIth International Conference on Cerebral Vasospasm Sydney 1997, pp 261–263
16. Tachibana E, Harada T, Shibuya M *et al* (1999) Intraarterial infusion of Fasudil hydrochloride for treating vasospasm following subarachnoid hemorrhage Acta Neurochir (Wien) 141: 13–19
17. Takayasu M, Shibuya M, Suzuki Y *et al* (1986) The effect of HA compound calcium antagonists on delayed cerebral vasospasm in dogs. J Neurosurg 65: 80–85
18. Uehata M, Ishizaki T, Satoh H *et al* (1997) Calcium sensitization of smooth muscle mediated by a Rho-associated protein kinase in hypertension. Nature 389: 990–994

Correspondence: Masato Shibuya, M.D., Chukyo Hospital, Nagoya 457-8510 Japan.

Acta Neurochir (2001) [Suppl] 77: 205–207

Combined Administration of Fasudil Hydrochloride and Nitroglycerin for Treatment of Cerebral Vasospasm

Y. Tanaka[1], T. Masuzawa[1], M. Saito[1], T. Yamada[1], A. Ebihara[1], H. Iwasa[2], and S. Mori[2]

[1] Department of Surgical Neurology, Jichi Medical School, Japan
[2] Department of Neurosurgery, Omiya Medical Center, Jichi Medical School, Japan

Introduction

We examined the Ca^{2+} sensitivity of vascular smooth muscle in experimental cerebral vasospasm in canine basilar artery. From the results of our experiments we concluded that the increase in this Ca^{2+} sensitivity may be one of the most important factors in cerebral vasospasm [1, 2, 4]. Therefore, we considered that treatment to decrease Ca^{2+} sensitivity might be effective for the prevention of cerebral vasospasm. Based on this consideration, we examined a new therapy of combined administration of fasudil hydrochloride and nitroglycerin for cerebral vasospasm that decreases the Ca^{2+} sensitivity of vascular smooth muscle.

Keywords: Fasudil hydrochloride; nitroglycerin; vasospasm.

Materials and Methods

Fifty patients who were operated on in our hospitals within 72 hours after subarachnoid hemorrhage from August 1996 to August 1999 were investigated. They were divided into two groups, one given a single administration of fasudil and the other a combined administration of fasudil and nitroglycerin. There were 25 patients in each group and no differences between the two groups regarding gender, age, neurological grade, or CT classification of subarachnoid hemorrhage (Fig. 1). The incidence of delayed ischemic neurological deficit (DIND), outcome, and complications were investigated. DIND was diagnosed based on the deterioration of neurological symptoms when other causes were excluded by radiological and biochemical studies.

The protocol of the combined administration group is as follows: Normotensive normovolemic therapy and cisternal or ventricular drainage were performed as basic treatment. If blood pressure fell below 120, dopamine or dobutamine was given. Fasudil hydrochloride was administered intravenously at 90 mg/day for 14 days after the clipping operation. Continuous intravenous administration of nitroglycerin (0.5–1.0 μg/kg/min) was performed for 14 days after the clipping operation.

Protocol of the single administration group is as follows: Hypertensive normovolemic therapy and cisternal or ventricular drainage was performed as basic treatment. Blood pressure was maintained over 150 by administration of dopamine or dobutamine. Fasudil hydrochloride was given in the same manner as in the combined administration group.

Results

DIND occurred in 24% of the combined administration group and in 60% of the single administration group. There was a significant difference in the incidence of DIND between the two groups ($P < 0.01$). The outcome of the combined administration group was good recovery in 92% and moderate disability in 8%, while in the single administration group the outcome was good recovery in 68%, moderate disability in

Materials	Fasudil + nitroglycerin	Fasudil
(1) No. of cases	25 (M 9, F16)	25 (M 9, F16)
(2) Age (yrs.)	55.8 ± 10.2	56.9 ± 11.5
(3) Neurological grade (Hunt&Kosnik)		
Grade I:	3	5
II:	7	8
III:	10	7
IV:	5	5
(4) Location of aneurysm		
ACA	11	8
ICA	6	5
MCA	5	12
VA	3	0
(5) CT classification (Fisher)		
Group II	2	6
III	23	16
IV	0	3

Fig. 1. The clinical features of the patients

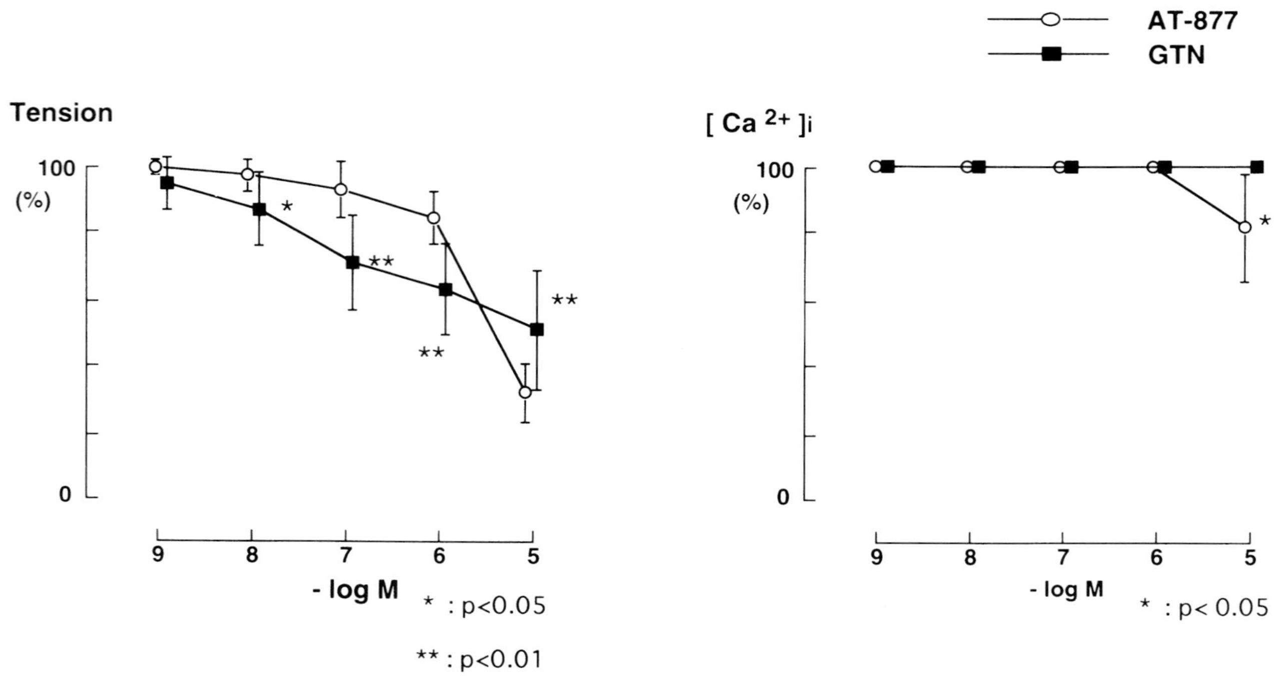

Fig. 2. The concentration-inhibition curve for fasudil hydrochloride (AT-877) or nitroglycerin (*GTN*) on thromboxane A_2-induced contraction in experimental vasospasm. The left side shows change in muscle tension and the right side the change in the cytosolic Ca^{2+} concentration ($[Ca^{2+}]i$). 100% represents the tension and $[Ca^{2+}]i$ before administration of AT-877 or GTN

20%, severe disability in 4%, and death in 8% of the patients. There was a significant difference in outcome between the two groups ($P < 0.05$).

The complications of combined administration therapy are as follows. There were 4 cases of mild hypotension (BP < 120), but the systolic blood pressure could easily be maintained above 120 with the administration of dopamine or dobutamine. No other complications were found.

Discussion

We investigated the Ca^{2+} sensitivity of cerebrovascular smooth muscle in cerebral vasospasm with simultaneous recording of muscle tension and cytosolic Ca^{2+} concentration, using Ca^{2+} indicator fura-2 [1, 4]. Our experimental results suggest that vasospasm increases basal Ca^{2+} sensitivity and also augments the effects of receptor agonists to increase Ca^{2+} sensitivity [1]. Accordingly, we consider the increase in Ca^{2+} sensitivity in vascular smooth muscle to be one of the most important mechanisms of cerebral vasospasm and that treatment to decrease the Ca^{2+} sensitivity may be effective for the prevention of vasospasm. Based on this consideration, we investigated the inhibitory effect of fasudil hydrochloride and nitroglycerin in experimental vasospasm in canine basilar artery [3]. The experimental results are as follows. Cumulative addition of fasudil or nitroglycerin showed a concentration-dependent inhibition in muscle tension with a slight decrease in cytosolic Ca^{2+} concentration (Fig. 2). These results suggest that the main mechanism responsible for the inhibitory effect of fasudil and nitroglycerin is a decrease in Ca^{2+} sensitivity. The inhibitory effect of the combined administration of fasudil and nitroglycerin on muscle tension was stronger than that of the single administration of fasudil. However, there was no significant difference in the change in cytosolic Ca^{2+} concentration between the two groups (Fig. 3). These results suggest that the combined administration of fasudil and nitroglycerin augments the inhibitory effect on muscle tension and also acts to decrease Ca^{2+} sensitivity in the contractile elements.

From our experiments we concluded that treatment decreasing Ca^{2+} sensitivity might be effective for the prevention of cerebral vasospasm. Based on this consideration, we originated a new therapy, the combined administration of fasudil hydrochloride and nitroglycerin. This treatment decreased the occurrence of

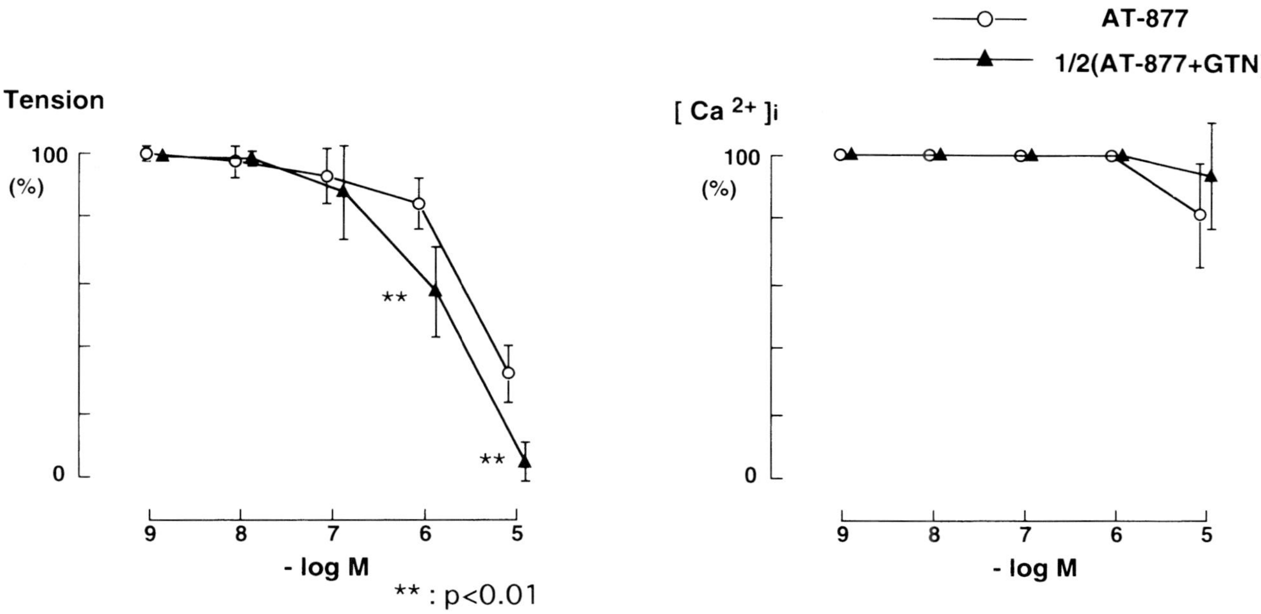

Fig. 3. Comparison of inhibitory effect between single administration of AT-877 and combined administration of AT-877 and GTN on thromboxane A_2-induced contraction in experimental vasospasm. 100% represents the tension and $[Ca^{2+}]i$ before single administration of AT-877 or combined administration of AT-877 and GTN

DIND and improved the prognosis of patients with subarachnoid hemorrhage. Our results suggest that the combined administration of fasudil hydrochloride and nitroglycerin is effective for the prevention of cerebral vasospasm.

Conclusion

The combined administration of fasudil hydrochloride and nitroglycerin is effective for the prevention of cerebral vasospasm.

References

1. Tanaka Y, Saito M, Yamada T, Fujimoto K, Masuzawa T (1998) Change in Ca^{2+} sensitivity of cerebrovascular smooth muscle in experimental chronic cerebral vasospasm. Neurol Med Chir (Tokyo) 38: 459–463
2. Tanaka Y, Shoji H, Saito M, Yamada T, Masuzawa T (1998) Change in Ca^{2+} sensitivity of canine cerebrovascular smooth muscle induced by PKC activator in experimental cerebral vasospasm. Proc Spasm Symp 14: 184–188
3. Tanaka Y, Shoji H, Saito M, Yamada T, Masuzawa T (1996) Inhibitory effect of combined administration of AT-877 and verapamil or nitroglycerin on thromboxane A_2-induced contraction in cerebrovascular smooth muscle in experimental vasospasm. Proc Spasm Symp 12: 276–280
4. Yamada T, Tanaka Y, Fujimoto K, Nakahara N, Shinoda S, Masuzawa T (1994) Relationship between cytosolic Ca^{2+} level and contractile tension in canine basilar artery of chronic vasospasm. Neurosurgery 34: 496–504

Correspondence: Dr. Y. Tanaka, 3311-1 Yakushiji, Minamikawachi-machi, Kawachi-gun, Tochigi, Japan.

Acta Neurochir (2001) [Suppl] 77: 209–211

Clinical Effect of Fasudil Hydrochloride for Cerebral Vasospasm Following Subarachnoid Hemorrhage

H. Masaoka, Y. Takasato, T. Nojiri, T. Hayakawa, H. Akimoto, H. Yatsushige, H. Toumori, Y. Miyazaki, and **M. Honma**

[1] Department of Neurosurgery, National Disaster Medical Center, Tokyo, Japan
[2] The second Department of Surgery, National Disaster Medical Center, Tokyo, Japan
3256 Midori-cho, Tachikawa, Tokyo, Japan

Introduction

Cerebral vasospasm due to subarachnoid hemorrhage still remains a leading cause of morbidity and mortality in patients with ruptured intracranial aneurysms. As the prophylactic measure against vasospasm, we have employed nicardipine and hyperdynamic therapy after surgery and have obtained better outcome in most cases than before. However, these treatments have not completely eliminated the delayed ischemic deficits.

Fasudil hydrochloride, a newly developed vasodilator, has been proven to be effective on cerebral vasospasm. We induced this drug to achieve better results as an additional treatment for vasospasm since 1996. The present study was designed to evaluate the therapeutic effect of Fasudil hydrochloride on the prevention of cerebral vasospasm, in special concern with the occurrence of angiographical vasospasm and outcome.

Keywords: Subarachnoid hemorrhage; cerebral vasospasm; fasudil hydrochloride; effectiveness.

Materials and Methods

85 patients with ruptured intracranial aneurysms were enrolled in this study. All patients underwent early clipping surgery within 48 hours after onset of subarachnoid hemorrhage. They were managed postoperatively in a similar fashion. They all received continuous intravenous administration of high-dose nicardipine (0.1–0.15 mg/kg/hr), dobutamin and intravascular volume expansion with albumin and low molecular-weight dextran as the standard treatment for vasospasm for 14 days.

Angiography was performed in every case on admission and around day 7, which is probably the time of maximal radiological vasospasm. We excluded 11 of these patients from the assessment of the effect on vasospasm because they did not perform the second angiogram since they had died early or showed complications with severe pneumonia. But these 11 patients received the same treatment, and all deaths during the same evaluated period were considered management mortalities, so we added them to the assessment of the final outcome later. The remaining 74 patients were divided into two groups. The control group consisted of 19 cases admitted from Jul. 1995 to Jan. 1996 and was treated without Fasudil. The other was the Fasudil group with 55 cases from Feb. 1996 to Mar. 1998 and was treated with the drug injected 30 mg 3 times a day for consecutive 14 days.

Angiographical vasospasm was quantified by measuring arterial diameters on Towne's projection of internal carotid angiogram. By using the modified Yoshimoto's method [7], arterial diameters were measured at 3 predetermined points, and the ratio of the diameters of the intracranial arteries to the extracranial internal carotid artery was calculated. Diameter ratio $(DR) = (M1 + A1)/C5$. M1, A1 and C5 was the arterial diameter at the narrowest point of each segment. The degree of angiographic vasoapasm was expressed as the relative alteration in the DR for the postoperative angiogram to that for the preoperative ones. Patients' outcome was assessed at discharge according to the Glasgow Outcome Scale. Clinical data were analyzed by a Student t-test and a Mann-Whitney u-test with Stat View II software. A p value of less than 0.05 was considered significant.

Results

The clinical characteristics of all patients of both groups are shown in Table 1. Number of patients was different, but otherwise similar between the two groups. Age, sex and location of aneurysm did not significantly differ between the groups. On admission, all cases were graded according to the scale of Hunt and Kosnik and also classified according to Fisher's CT grading scale. No significant differences were found among the two groups in these gradings. In this series, almost half of all cases were poor clinical grade patients.

Table 1. *Clinical Characteristics of Patients. Control: Patients Treated Without Fasudil Hydrochloride. Fasudil: Patients Treated with Fasudil Hydrochloride*

	Control	Fasudil
No. of patients	19	55
Sex (male/female)	8/11	25/30
Age (years)		
– Mean	57	57
– Range	31–82	29–91
Location of aneurysm		
– ICA	6 (32%)	18 (33%)
– Acom	5 (26%)	22 (40%)
– ACA	0 (0%)	2 (4%)
– MCA	8 (42%)	13 (23%)
Hunt & Kosnik grade on admission		
– Grade 1	2 (11%)	8 (15%)
– Grade 2	8 (42%)	15 (27%)
– Grade 3	0 (0%)	8 (15%)
– Grade 4	8 (42%)	11 (20%)
– Grade 5	1 (5%)	13 (23%)
Fisher's group on admission		
– Group 1	1 (5%)	0 (0%)
– Group 2	4 (21%)	15 (27%)
– Group 3	9 (48%)	27 (49%)
– Group 4	5 (26%)	13 (24%)

Table 2. *The Degree of Angiographical Vasospasm in the Patients Treated Without Fasudil (Control) or with Fasudil (Fasudil)*

	Control	Fasudil
Total	91.6 ± 4.8%	94.4 ± 2.1%
Operative side	87.7 ± 1.3%	90.3 ± 0.9%
Nonoperative side	93.6 ± 1.5%	98.9 ± 1.0%
Hunt & Kosnik grade		
– 1–3	82.4 ± 1.1%	96.7 ± 1.0%
– 4–5	96.9 ± 1.6%	91.8 ± 1.0%

Table 3. *Glasgow Outcome Scale at Discharge in the Patients Treated Without Fasudil (Control) or with Fasudil (Fasudil)*

Glasgow Outcome Score (GOS)	Control	Fasudil
1 (Dead)	4 (18%)	2 (3%)
2 (Vegetative state)	1 (5%)	3 (5%)
3 (Severe disability)	4 (18%)	7 (11%)
4 (Moderate disability)	4 (18%)	18 (29%)
5 (Good recovery)	9 (41%)	33 (52%)
Total	22 (100%)	63 (100%)

Table 2 summarises the result of the degree of angiographical vasospasm. The patients in the Fasudil group tended to have less severe angiographic vasospasm than those in the Control group. But there was no significant difference in the degree of vasospasm between both groups. The effect of Fasudil might be masked by that of nicardipine and hyperdynamic therapy. In the Fasudil group, the patients with good grade had less severe vasospasm than those with poor grade. The effect of Fasudil on angiographical vasospasm was not prominent.

Concerning the incidence of symptomatic vasospasm, neurological deterioration was diagnosed in all patients who developed a new focal deficit that could not be explained by any cause other than vasospasm or worsening of existing deficits or a decreased level of consciousness. Symptomatic vasospasm was observed in 5% of control group and 16% of the Fasudil group transiently, but none of them showed permanent neurological sequelae. In this study, many poor grade patients were included. The diagnosis of neurological deterioration in such cases is often difficult. These results might be different according to observers. Concerning side effect of this drug, hemorrhagic complication occurred in 2 patients, but their final outcome was not worsened.

Table 3 shows the final outcome at discharge. The Fasudil group had a better outcome than the control group even though their Hunt and Kosnik grades and Fisher's CT grading were similar. These differences were statistically significant between both groups. Comparing the final outcome of 2 subgroups according to the preoperative clinical grades, the better outcome was more prominent in the poor grade subgroup than in the good grade one.

Discussion

Fasudil hydrochloride is a newly developed vasodilator. This drug inhibits protein kinase such as myosin light-chain kinase and protein kinase C [2] and has been proven to be effective on cerebral vasospasm [5, 6]. The fasudil group had better final outcome than the control group. There was a functional recovery in 59% of the patients in the control group and in 81% of those in the Fasudil group. Considering that the degree of angiographic vasospasm was more severe in the poor grade patients, these results did not correlate with the finding of angiographic vasospasm.

Recent experimental studies have shown that Fasudil has neuroprotective properties [1, 3]. This drug increases the blood flow of the cerebral cortex and prevents delayed neuronal death. Also this drug inhibits endothelial injury and neutrophil infiltration and so on. The metabolite of Fasudil also has been shown a

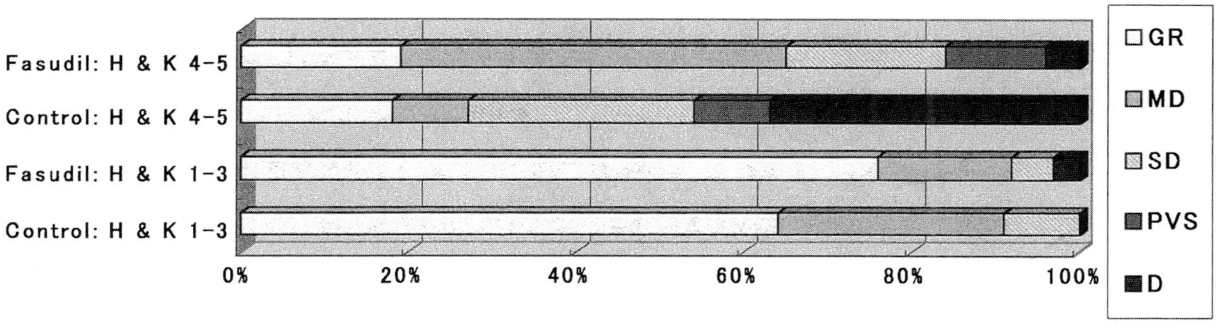

Fig. 1. Glasgow outcome scale at discharge in the patients treated without fasudil (Control) or with fasudil (Fasudil). Comparison of both groups according to the severity of subarachnoid hemorrhage

brain protective effect and its half life in blood is very long [4]. The efficacy of this drug might be due to the pharmacological protection of cerebral tissue rather than prevention of arterial narrowing.

Conclusion

We conclude that fasudil hydrochloride is safe and effective in improving functional outcome of the patients with aneurysmal subarachnoid hemorrhage. Taking into account the results of effect on angiographic vasospasm and the final outcome, this efficacy might be due to pharmacological protection of cerebral tissue rather than prevention of arterial narrowing.

References

1. Arai M, Sasaki Y, Nozawa R (1993) Inhibition by the protein kinase inhibitor HA1077 of the activation of NADPH oxidase in human neutrophils. Biochem Pharmacol 46: 1487–149
2. Asano T, Ikegaki I, Satoh S, Suzuki Y, Shibuya M, Takayasu M, Hidaka H (1987) Mechanism of action of a novel antivasospasm drug, HA1077. J Pharmacol Exp Ther 241: 1033–1040
3. Asano T, Ikegaki I, Saitoh S, Mochizuki D, Hidaka H, Suzuki Y, Shibuya M, Sugita K (1991) Blockade of intracellular actions of calcium may protect against ischemic damage to the gerbil brain. Br J Pharmacol 103: 1935–1938
4. Kazuki S, Tanabe H, Matsukawa M, Sumioka S, Isono N, Yasuda S, Miyamoto T, Ohta T (2000) Time courses in the blood and antivasospasm effects of fasudil hydrochloride and the metabolite in patients with subarachnoid hemorrhage. Jpn J Neurosurg (Tokyo) 9: 146–151
5. Shibuya M, Suzuki Y, Sugita K, Saito I, Sasaki T, Takakura K, Nagata I, Kikuchi H, Takemae T, Hidaka H, Nakashima M (1992) Effect of AT877 on cerebral vasospasm after aneurysmal subarachnoid hemorrhage. J Neurosurg 76: 571–577
6. Takakura K, Sugita K, Kikuchi H, Saitou I, Shibuya M, Suzuki Y, Sasaki T, Takemae T, Nagata I, Nakashima M (1992) Effect of AT-877 on cerebral vasospasm and delayed cerebral ischemic symptoms after aneurysmal trial. Yakuri To Chiryo 20 [Suppl] 20: s1627–1658
7. Yoshimoto Y, Kwak S (1995) Age-related multifactorial causes of neurological deterioration after early surgery for aneurysmal subarachnoid hemorrhage. J Neurosurg 83: 984–988

Correspondence: Dr. H. Masaoka, Department of Neurosurgery, National Disaster Medical Center, Tokyo, Japan.

Acta Neurochir (2001) [Suppl] 77: 213–215

A Novel Drug Delivery System as Prophylaxis for Cerebral Vasospasm

Y. Takanashi[1], **T. Ishida**[2], **T. Meguro**[3], **M. J. Kirchmeier**[2], **T. M. Allen**[2], and **J. H. Zhang**[3]

[1] Department of Neurosurgery, Yokohama City University School of Medicine, Yokohama, Japan
[2] Department of Pharmacology, University of Alberta, Edmonton, Alberta, Canada
[3] Department of Neurosurgery, University of Mississippi Medical Center, Jackson, Mississippi, USA

Introduction

Experimental work has extensively demonstrated that calcium antagonists can reverse established angiographically identified vasospasm when administered by the intrathecal route, despite being ineffective when administered by the peripheral route [3, 5]. However, the effective time in the therapeutic window may be temporary even if bolus application by intrathecal route was feasible. Therefore, externalized ventricular catheter or repeated lumbar puncture is needed to keep a therapeutic drug concentration in the cerebrospinal fluid (CSF), which is troublesome in a clinical setting.

We have devised that a sustained-release form of a protein kinase inhibitor, Fasudil, can maintain a therapeutic concentration in the CSF within a therapeutic window. The purpose of this study was to devise a novel drug delivery system which can be directly applied into the CSF, and then to clarify the preventive effect of liposome-entrapped Fasudil on cerebral vasospasm in a rat model.

Keywords: Cerebral vasospasm; drug delivery systems; fasudil; rat.

Materials and Methods

Preparation of Liposomes

Liposomes were prepared according to the method of Allen [1]. The mean diameter of liposomes which was determined by dynamic light scattering was in the range of 110 ± 10 nm. Fasudil (Sigma Chemical Co., St. Louis, MO) was loaded into the liposomes at a phospholipid (PL): Fasudil ratio of 1:0.4 (w/w) and incubated for 1 hour at 65°C. Spectrophotometry ($\lambda = 320$ nm) finally determined the concentration of the liposome-entrapped Fasudil.

Releasing Property of Liposome-Entrapped Fasudil in Vitro

The in vitro drug-release kinetics of the liposome-entrapped Fasudil was measured in control CSF (Sigma Chemical Co., St. Louis, MO) for 7 days. The concentration of the Fasudil in liposomes was determined by spectrophotometry ($\lambda = 320$ nm) at the various time points.

Experimental Model of SAH and Study Design

Male Sprague-Dawley rats weighing 350–400 g were used for the experiments. Subarachnoid hemorrhage (SAH) in rats was induced by double autologous blood injection via cisterna magna [4]. On day 2 following second blood injection, treated rats (n = 10) received 0.4 mg liposome-entrapped Fasudil via the cisterna magna. Likewise, control rats (n = 10) received drug-free liposomes. The drug-free liposomes contained the same amount of PL as the liposome-entrapped Fasudil. Sham-operated animals (n = 3) were used for normal caliber of rat basilar arteries. On day 7 after SAH, the basilar artery was removed for measurement by light microscopy and the concentration of liposome-entrapped Fasudil in the CSF was examined. Finally, the caliber of each sample was expressed as the percentage to the caliber of the normal basilar artery.

Table 1. *Caliber Change on Rat Basilar Artery**

	Treated group	Control group
Average diameter of rat basilar artery (%)*	86.6 ± 4.8	65.9 ± 7.2†,‡

*When normal caliber rat basilar artery obtained from the sham-operated group is expressed as 100%, caliber of each group is shown as mean ± standard deviation († $P < 0.001$ vs. treated group, ‡ $P < 0.001$ vs. Sham-operated group).

Results

Releasing Property of Liposome-Entrapped Fasudil in Vitro and in Vivo

The release of Fasudil from liposomes in vitro was biphasic. In the first 6 hours at 37°C, approximately 30% of the Fasudil was released from liposomes, and over 7 days, 60% of the contents were gradually released (n = 3). By contrast, most of the Fasudil in vivo was released from liposomes on day 7 after SAH. Mean CSF concentrations of liposome-entrapped Fasudil in rats were 980 ng/ml (n = 7) on day 7.

Evaluation of Vasoconstriction on Basilar Artery

Treatment with 0.4 mg liposome-entrapped Fasudil significantly prevented constriction of rat basilar artery (86.6 ± 4.8%) compared to the control group (65.9 ± 7.2%) (Table 1).

Discussion

We studied in the present experiments that a single intrathecal administration of liposome-entrapped Fasudil significantly ameliorated the vasoconstriction in rat basilar artery and no obvious adverse effect was noted in rat SAH model.

The advantage of using liposomes comes from a sustained release of therapeutically relevant concentrations of the drug over a therapeutic window. A sustained-release preparation of Fasudil, small enough to be administered in the CSF, could continuously deliver drug into the CSF. The relatively slow release of drug from liposomes mimicks some aspects of drug infusion, including a significant decrease in the toxicity of the free drug. Thus, the therapeutic index of Fasudil was increased by virtue of both an increase efficacy and a decrease in systemic toxicity.

Calcium antagonists by intrathecal route for the treatment of cerebral vasospasm could avoid the potential systemic adverse effect such as hypotension. Therefore, it has been reported that intrathecal route of calcium antagonists has been evaluated for the prevention of cerebral vasospasm [3, 5]. However, the effective therapeutic concentration by intrathecal bolus application may be short, so that externalized ventricular catheter or repeated lumbar puncture must be applied to keep a therapeutic drug concentration in the CSF. These frequent or continuous intrathecal administrations are impractical, especially in a clinical setting. Therefore, a single injection of liposome-entrapped Fasudil which can be safely delivered in the CSF might be a novel approach for the treatment of cerebral vasospasm following SAH.

Many works have confirmed that interaction with blood components and the mononuclear phagocyte system affect the clearance and elimination of liposomes in case of intravenous application [2]. As CSF contains a small amount of blood in case of SAH, it is conceivable that the discrepancy in the releasing rate between in vitro and in vivo might be responsible for blood components in the CSF. However, as little is known about the clearance and elimination of liposomes in the CSF, further studies will be needed to elucidate the optimal drug release rate as well as pharmacokinetics of liposomal drugs in the CSF.

Conclusion

Treatment with liposome-entrapped Fasudil by a single intrathecal injection has a considerable vasodilating effect. The liposomal drug functioned as a sustained drug release system resulting in free drug concentration within the therapeutic range. The promising results obtained from the current study represent a major breakthrough in the treatment of cerebral vasospasm following SAH.

References

1. Allen TM, Hansen C (1991) Pharmacokinetics of stealth versus conventional liposomes: effect of dose. Biochim Biophys Acta 1068: 133–141
2. Devine D, Marjan J (1997) The role of immunoproteins in the survival of liposomes in the circulation. Crit Rev Ther Drug Carrier Syst 14: 105–131
3. Gioia A, White R, Bakhtian B, Robertson J (1985) Evaluation of the efficacy of intrathecal nimodipine in canine models of chronic cerebral vasospasm. J Neurosurg 62: 721–728

4. Suzuki H, Kanamaru K, Tsunoda H, Inada H, Kuroki M, Sun H, Waga S, Tanaka T (1999) Heme oxygenase-1 induction as an intrinsic regulation against delayed cerebral vasospasm in rats. J Clin Invest 104: 59–66
5. Voldby B, Petersen O, Buhl M, Jakobsen P, Østergaard R (1984) Reversal of cerebral arterial spasm by intrathecal administration of a calcium antagonist (nimodipine). An experimental study. Acta Neurochir (Wien) 70: 243–254

Correspondence: Yoshihiro Takanashi, M.D., Ph.D., Department of Neurosurgery, Yokohama City University, School of Medicine, 3-9 Fukuura, Kanazawa-ku, Yokohama, Japan, 236-0004.

Acta Neurochir (2001) [Suppl] 77: 217–220

Development of Nicardipine Prolonged-Release Implants for Preventing Vasospasm

H. Kasuya, A. Kawashima, A. Sasahara, H. Onda, and **T. Hori**

Department of Neurosurgery, Tokyo Women's Medical University, Tokyo, Japan

Introduction

The intrathecally-implantable drug-delivery system was developed to maintain an effective concentration of vasodilatory drug in the target cistern for preventing cerebral vasospasm after subarachnoid hemorrhage (SAH), without systemic side effects nor the side effects associated with long-term intrathecal drug administration through indwelling catheters [2, 5]. Nicardipine was selected for the material of this drug delivery system because intrathecal administration of nicardipine has been reported to ameliorate or reverse vasospasm in animal SAH models [3] and has been used widely, effectively, and safely in patients with SAH, especially in Japan [4, 6]. The purpose of this study was to determine the efficacy of nicardipine prolonged-release implant for preventing vasospasm in dogs in a dose-escalating placebo-controlled blind fashion.

Keywords: Cerebral vasospasm; drug delivery system; nicardipine; copoly(lactic/glycolic acid).

Materials and Methods

Development of Nicardipine Prolonged-Release Implants

A rod-shaped pellet (1 mm in diameter, 8–10 mm in length) was prepared by heat compression. Copoly-(lactic/glycolic acid) (PLGA) (PLG1600ML; molecular weight 4000, lactic acid ratio of 0.5) (900 mg) and nicardipine free base (100 mg) was mixed. The dried powder (10 mg) was charged into a Tefron tube (1-mm inner diameter) and compressed. The release of nicardipine from the pellet was examined in buffered saline in a flask. The amount of nicardipine released was analyzed by high performance liquid chromatography (HPLC; Hitachi L6000, Hitachi, Tokyo, Japan).

Canine SAH Model

The dogs received phenobarbital intravenously and were intubated. A 5 French angiographic catheter (Anthron head hunter, Toray Co., Tokyo) was advanced into the internal carotid artery (ICA), under fluoroscopic guidance. Cerebral angiography consisted of one arterial-phase injection of 2 ml iopamidol (Schering Co., Tokyo, Japan). Surgery for the induction of a subarachnoid clot followed as described before [5]. After right frontotemporal craniectomy, 8 pellets with or without nicardipine were placed in the right ICA cistern and Sylvian fissure by operators blinded with regard to the groups. Then, a clot of 0.5 ml/kg autologous arterial blood was carefully placed around the exposed arteries, and the dura was closed.

Eighteen mongrel dogs of either gender, each weighing between 15 and 24 kg, were randomly assigned to one of 3 groups (placebo-treated, low-dose or high-dose nicardipine-treated). Eight placebo pellets were used in placebo ($n = 6$) group; one nicardipine pellet (approximately 0.8 mg nicardipine) and 7 placebo pellets in the low-dose nicardipine ($n = 6$) group; 8 nicardipine pellets (approximately total 8 mg nicardipine) in the high-dose nicardipine ($n = 6$) group.

Repeat Cerebral Angiography, Death, and Pathological Examination

Angiography was repeated on Day 7 and Day 14. Five ml cerebrospinal fluid (CSF) was removed from the cisterna magna for the measurement of nicardipine on Day 7 and Day 14. The animals were sacrificed by the injection of an overdose of pentobarbital on Day 14, after which exanguination and perfusion with 1000 ml of normal saline were performed. For each animal, the calvaria was removed and the brain was taken out.

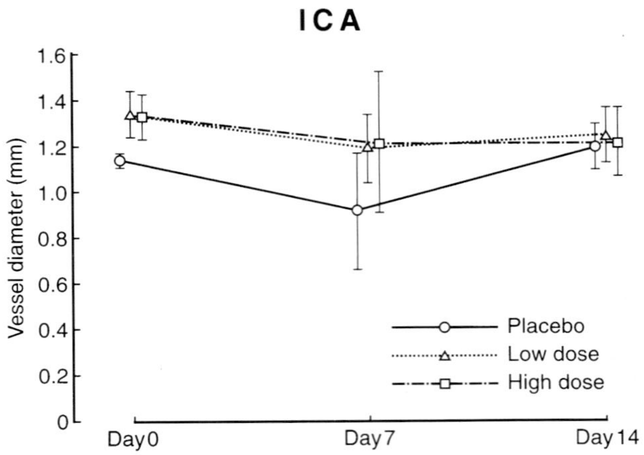

Fig. 1. Time course of change in vessel diameters of the right internal carotid artery (ICA) (mean ± SD) for 3-day periods at Day 0, Day 7, and Day 14 in placebo (n = 6), low-dose (n = 6) nicardipine- and high-dose (n = 6) nicardipine-treated groups

Results

In Vitro Study of Nicardipine Prolonged-Released Implants

In the first 2 days, about 8% of the nicardipine was released per day; in the next 2 days, about 20% per day. The amount of nicardipine released within the first 4 days was 61.9% of the total nicardipine content. After 4 days, the curve for cumulative release was less steep.

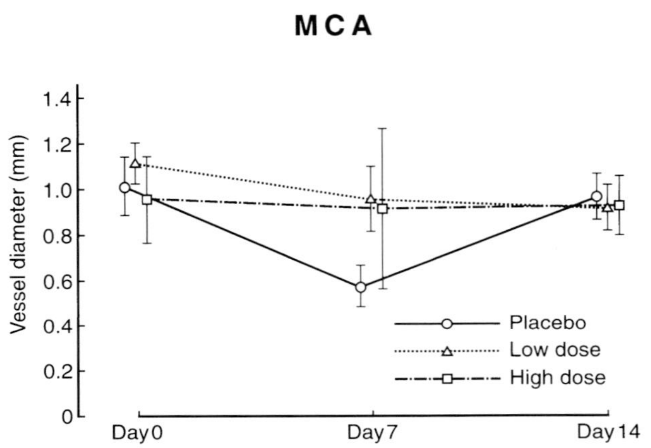

Fig. 2. Time course of change in vessel diameters of the right middle cerebral artery (MCA) (mean ± SD) for 3-day periods at Day 0, Day 7, and Day 14 in placebo (n = 6), low-dose (n = 6) nicardipine- and high-dose (n = 6) nicardipine-treated groups. There was a significant difference (p = 0.0004) in the change over time between the 3 groups

Effect of Nicardipine-Prolonged Implants in the Canine SAH Model

In the placebo-treated group, diffuse arterial narrowing was observed at the intracranial arteries of the clot side (right) on Day 7. This cerebral vasospasm was resolved by Day 14. There was evidence of very mild vasospasm in the nicardipine-treated groups. There were significant differences of the changes over time in vessel diameters of the right middle cerebral artery (MCA) ($p = 0.0004$) (Fig. 1) and the right anterior cerebral artery (ACA) ($p = 0.0037$) (Fig. 2) between the 3 groups. The changes over time in vessel diamter of right ICA (Fig. 3) and left cerebral arteries were not significant between groups.

The percent reduction of vessel diameters on the clot side on Day 7 in the placebo, low-dose nicardipine, and high-dose nicardipine-treated groups was 43%, 14% and 7% at the right MCA. There were significant differences between groups ($p = 0.0319$). There were also significant differences between placebo and low-dose ($p = 0.0247$), and between placebo and high-dose ($p = 0.0074$).

Nicardipine Content of Clot and CSF

There was no difference in the weight of the remaining clot between the placebo, low-dose nicardipine, and high-dose nicardipine-treated groups. No remaining pellets were found at necropsy. The remaining clots of low-dose and high-dose nicardipine-treated groups (average weight, 0.50 g and 0.43 g, respectively) contained a mean amount (0.4 μg and 5.2 μg, respectively) of nicardipine, i.e., the mean concentration in the clots was 9.7×10^{-7} mol/L and 5.1×10^{-6} mol/L, respectively. Nicardipine was not

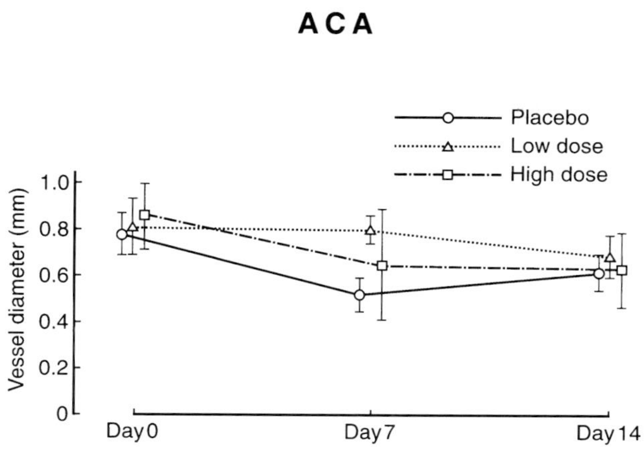

Fig. 3. Time course of change in vessel diameters of the right anterior cerebral artery (ACA) (mean $\pm$ SD) for 3-day periods at Day 0, Day 7, and Day 14 in placebo (n = 6), low-dose (n = 6) nicardipine- and high-dose (n = 6) nicardipine-treated groups. There was a significant difference ($p = 0.0037$) in the change over time between the 3 groups

detected in any CSF samples from the cisterna magna (below 2×10^{-8} mol/L).

Discussion

The main observation of the present study is that intrathecal implantation of nicardipine prolonged-release pellets at the time of SAH production significantly reduced the severity of cerebral vasospasm on Day 7. In the placebo-treated group, diffuse arterial narrowing was observed in the intracranial arteries of the clot side (right) on Day 7. This cerebral vasospasm was resolved by Day 14. There was very little evidence of vasospasm at ICA, MCA and ACA in the nicardipine-treated groups on Day 7 even for low-dose nicardipine implants containing 0.8 mg nicardipine. The clots and pellets were placed mainly in the Sylvian fissure, where the sphenoidal segments of the MCA were exposed. The average percent reduction of vessel diameters on the clot side on Day 7 in the placebo, low-dose, and high-dose groups was 43%, 14% and 7% at the MCA.

Nicardipine has been shown to cause dose-dependent relaxation in herical strips of bovine cerebral arteries contracted with high K^+, with the maximal relaxation being achieved at 10^{-9} mol/L; the maximal relaxation of arteries contracted with oxyhemoglobin was achieved at 10^{-6} mol/L [2]. We have already shown that the mean concentration of nicardipine in the clot on Day 7 was 1.5×10^{-4} mol/L in SAH animals treated with implants containing 8 mg nicardipine [2]. On Day 14, the average concentration in the clots adjacent to cerebral arteries was 9.7×10^{-7} mol/L in the low-dose and 5.1×10^{-6} mol/L in the high-dose nicardipine-treated groups, values which were still higher than the concentration of the maximum relaxation of arteries contracted by high K^+. Though the concentration of nicardipine in the clot adjacent to the arteries does not directly indicate that of the periarterial space, it may be similar to that of the surrounding environment in the limited cistern.

We are now developing PLGA implants with nicardipine for humans, designed to be placed in the cistern of M1 or M2 of the MCA or that of A1 and A2 of the ACA, where vasospasm related to delayed ischemic neurological deficits is most common. Since the materials have a long history of usage in sutures and drug delivery systems with a proven safety profile for parenteral applications [1], this device is concluded to be biocompatible with brain tissue. In the clinical reports of intrathecal nicardipine therapy, 2 mg of nicardipine was injected three times a day, or 4 mg twice a day for an average of 10 days through cisternal drainage [4, 6]. The total amount of nicardipine used in human was 10 times higher than that of the high-dose group in our canine study. PLGA pellets with this amount of nicardipine can be implanted in human SAH patients.

Conclusion

Nicardipine prolonged-release pellets prevented vasospasm in dogs significantly even at low-dose (0.8 mg), while maintaining an appropriate concentration of nicardipine in the clot adjacent to the arteries.

References

1. Athanasiou KA, Niederauer GG, Agrawal CM (1996) Sterilization, toxicity, biocompatibility and clinical applications of polylactic acid/polyglycolic acid copolymers. Biomaterials 17: 93–102
2. Kawashima A, Kasuya H, Shiokawa K, Miyajima M, Izawa M, Takakura K (1998) Efficacy of nicardipine prolonged-release pellet on cerebral vasospasm in dogs. No Shinkei Geka (Jpn) 26: 37–43
3. Pasqualin A, Vollmer DG, Marron JA, Tsukahara T, Kassell NF, Torner JC (1991) The effect of nicardipine on vasospasm in rabbit basilar artery after subarachnoid hemorrhage. Neurosurgery 29: 183–188
4. Shibuya M, Suzuki Y, Enomoto H, Okada T, Ogura K, Sugita K

(1994) Effects of prophylactic intrathecal administrations of nicardipine on vasospasm in patients with severe aneurysmal subarachnoid hemorrhage. Acta Neurochir (Wien) 131: 19–25

5. Shiokawa K, Kasuya H, Miyajima M, Izawa M, Takakura K (1998) Prophylactic effect of papaverine prolonged-release pellets on cerebral vasospasm in dogs. Neurosurgery 42: 109–116
6. Toyota A, Nishizawa Y (1991) Cerebral vasospasm after subarachnoid hemorrhage, and inhibitory effect of nicardipine investigated by means of transcranial Doppler ultrasonography. No Shinkei Geka (Jpn) 19: 1143–1150

Correspondence: Hidetoshi Kasuya, M.D., Department of Neurosurgery, Tokyo Women's Medical University, Kawada-cho 8-1, Shinjuku-ku, Tokyo 162, Japan 162-8666.

Acta Neurochir (2001) [Suppl] 77: 221–223

Inhibition of Overexpression of Endothelin-1 by an RNA Synthesis Inhibitor, Doxorubicin, in the Rat Vasospasm Model

T. Mima and **M. G. Mostafa**

Department of Neurosurgery, Kochi Medical School, Kochi, Japan

Introduction

There are three isoforms of endothelin (ET) such as ET-1, ET-2, and ET-3, and the vascular endothelium expresses only ET-1 binding to ET receptor type A of adjacent vascular smooth muscle cells of the vessel wall and causes a potent and sustained contraction [1, 5, 7, 8]. Cerebral vasospasm after subarachnoid hemorrhage (SAH) remains one of the major decisive factors in the clinical course of SAH patients and ET-1 has been identified as one of the causative substances [5, 8].

It has been reported that a non-specific RNA synthesis inhibitor, dactinomycin (actinomycin-D), aimed to suppress de novo synthesis of peptides including ET-1, almost completely prevented cerebral vasospasm in the dog two-hemorrhage model [6], and that ET receptor antagonists and ET-converting-enzyme blockers attenuated cerebral vasospasm in various animal SAH models [8]. However, the spasm-preventive effect of dactinomycin [6] seems to be much more potent than that of ET receptor antagonists or ET-converting-enzyme blockers so far tested. Considering the possibility of clinical use of RNA synthesis inhibitors, which have been used as anti-cancer drugs for long time, we previously examined the therapeutic dose and timing of administration of dactinomycin and other RNA synthesis inhibitors and found that doxorubicin (DOX) is more effective than dactinomycin [2]. In the present study, by a method of reverse transcription polymerase chain reaction (RT-PCR), we investigated whether mRNA of ET-1 is effectively inhibited by DOX.

Keywords: Endothelin-1; doxorubicin; RNA synthesis inhibitor; RT-PCR.

Materials and Methods

All experiments were conducted according to the guidelines for the care and use of animals at Kochi Medical School, Kochi, Japan. We used the rat femoral artery vasospasm model that has been reported to have a similar time course and morphological characteristics of cerebral vasospasm after SAH [3]. Male Wistar rats (Charles River, Japan) weighing 300–400 g were used. Under pentobarbital anesthesia (50 mg/kg), a 1-cm segment of the right femoral artery was covered with a Silastic cuff and 0.1 ml of fresh autologous whole blood without heparin was injected into the cuff (day 0). We used the left femoral artery without any surgical manipulation as an internal control. Diameter changes were measured as follows. Animals were fixed by intracardial perfusion with 4% paraformaldehyde and 1% glutaraldehyde in phosphate buffer. Both sides of femoral arteries were cross-sectioned at three locations: close to the proximal end, at the mid point, and close to the distal end. The caliber at the major and the minor axis of each cross-section were measured in a blinded fashion by separate observers and the sum of caliber readings of the spasm side were divided by that of the control side.

First, we examined the natural time course of vasospasm using time points of day 4 ($n = 7$), day 7 ($n = 9$), day 10 ($n = 8$), and confirmed that day 7 shows the most severe vasoconstriction (Fig. 1). In this study, therefore, we used the time point of day 7 to see the effect of DOX on vasospasm. We estimated 0.6 mg/kg of DOX as a clinical dose in anti-cancer therapy. To examine dose-response of DOX on prevention of vasospasm, the rats were divided into four groups: vehicle ($n = 9$), DOX 0.06 mg/kg ($n = 6$), DOX 0.2 mg/kg ($n = 8$), and DOX 0.6 mg/kg ($n = 10$). The drugs were injected intraperitoneally on day 1.

For RT-PCR analysis for mRNA of ET-1, the animals were divided into two groups: vehicle ($n = 5$) and DOX 0.6 mg/kg ($n = 5$). We injected the drug intraperitoneally on day 1 and measured the mRNA level of rat ET-1 and that of the rat beta-actin as an internal control on day 7. Nucleotide sequences of oligoprimers for rat ET-1 mRNA and beta-actin were designed as follows. ET-1 forward: 5-AAG CCC TTC TAG GTC TAA GC-3 (bases 442–462). ET-1 reverse: 5-GGC CTC CAA CCT TCT T-3 (bases 685–701). beta-actin forward: 5-GAG GCC CAG AGC AAG AGA GG-3 (bases 169–188). beta-actin reverse: 5-TAC ATG GCT GGG GTG TTG AA-3 (bases 379–398). Bilateral femoral arteries were freshly removed and the total RNA was isolated by the acid guanidinium thiocyanate-phenol-chloroform method. The reverse transcription of total RNA to complementary deoxyribonucleic acid (cDNA) and subsequent

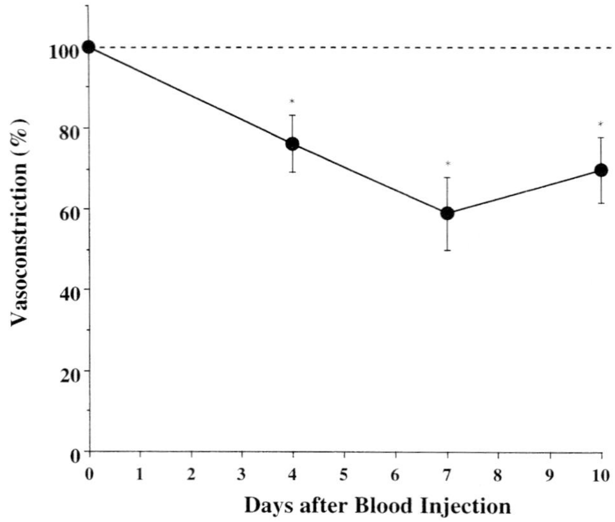

Fig. 1. Natural time course of vasospasm. The luminal diameter was most severely narrowed on day 7 ($p < 0.01$ vs. day 4, $p < 0.05$ vs. day 10). * $p < 0.01$ vs. day 0

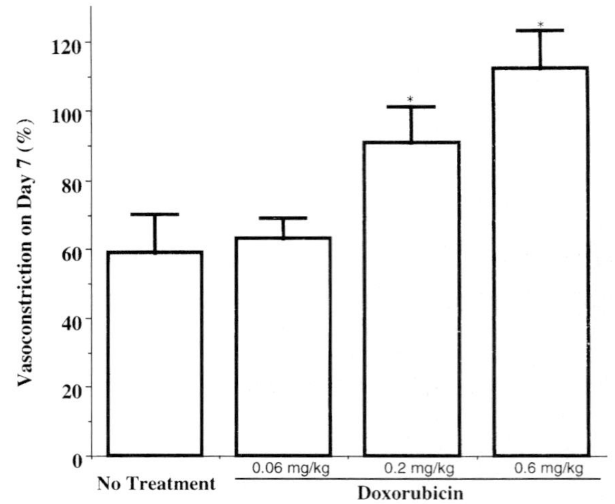

Fig. 2. Dose response of doxorubicin effect on prevention of vasospasm on day 7. A clinical dose (0.6 mg/kg) or one third of the clinical dose (0.2 mg/kg) injected on day 1 significantly prevented vasospasm compared with no treatment (vehicle injection). * $p < 0.001$ vs. no treatment

PCR was performed using Takara RNA PCR kit (Takara Biochemicals, Tokyo, Japan). cDNA was synthesized from 1 μg of total RNA in a 20 μl reaction volume, following the standard reverse transcription protocol. Resultant cDNA was amplified by PCR in a final volume of 50 μl, according to the manufacturer's PCR protocol with Taq DNA polymerase (Takara Biochemicals, Tokyo, Japan). The PCR was performed as follows: 30 seconds at 94 degree C, 30 seconds at 58 degree C and 1.5 minutes at 72 degree C for 35 cycles.

Results

Dose-response of DOX on prevention of vasospasm: The clinical dose (0.6 mg/kg) of DOX completely prevented vasospasm ($p < 0.001$ vs. vehicle) and even showed slight vasodilation (Fig. 2). One third, but not one tenth, of the clinical dose significantly attenuated vasospasm.

RT-PCR analysis for mRNA of ET-1: A band of 260 base pairs corresponding to rat ET-1 was not visible in the control side of the artery but slightly expressed in the spasm side in vehicle group (Fig. 3). DOX inhibited expression of ET-1 mRNA in the spasm side. However, a house keeping gene used as an internal marker, beta-actin mRNA, was expressed equally in both sides of the arteries in both vehicle and DOX groups (Fig. 3).

Discussion

The present study has demonstrated that a nonspecific RNA synthesis inhibitor, DOX, significantly prevented vasospasm when more than one third of the clinical dose was administered. Furthermore, this phenomena coincided with the result that aberrant expression of ET-1 mRNA in the vasospasm-destined artery was effectively inhibited by DOX.

Recently, it was reported that antisense prepro ET-1 oligonucleotide treatment inhibited expression of mRNA of prepro ET-1 and reduced vasospasm in the dog two-hemorrhage model [4]. However, the reduction of vasospasm was not statistically significant and combination therapy with cisternal administration of recombinant tissue plasminogen-activator achieved an almost complete reduction of vasospasm [4]. In contrast, intravenous injection of dactinomycin alone in the dog two-hemorrhage model [6] and intraperitoneal injection of DOX alone in the rat vasospasm model in this study as well as in our previous report [2] resulted in complete reversal of vasospasm. Regarding this difference in efficacy, one of the possible reasons is that systemic administration of RNA synthesis inhibitors may be more effective than cistern administration of the antisense prepro ET-1 oligonucleotide in inhibition of aberrant expression of ET-1. Another possibility is that since the pathogenesis of cerebral vasospasm is multifactorial, DOX might inhibit aberrant expression of not only ET-1 but also other proteins and peptides that are involved in the process of vasospasm such as protein kinase C, myosin light chain kinase, and Rho associated kinase. Contrary to this advantage, DOX

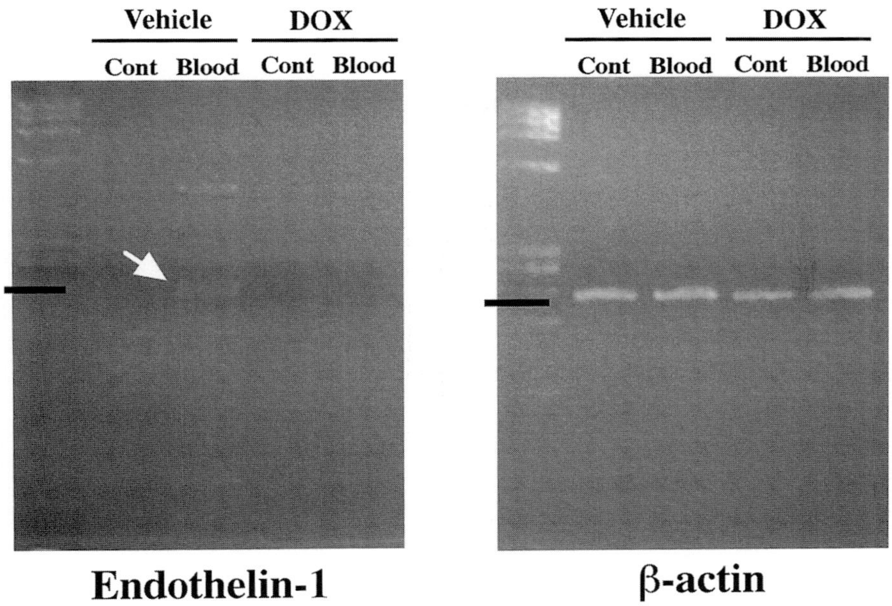

Fig. 3. RT-PCR of rat endothelin-1 and beta-actin. With no treatment (*No-Treat*), endothelin-1 (260 base pairs) is slightly expressed in spasm side of the femoral artery surrounded with blood (*Blood*) as indicated by an arrow but not in the control side (*Cont*). Doxorubicin treatment (*DOX*) inhibited endothelin-1 expression in the spasm side of the artery (*Blood*). beta-actin (230 base pairs) is equally expressed in both the spasm side (*Blood*) and control side (*Cont*) and DOX did not decrease the expression level in both sides

may simultaneously have the disadvantage of suppressing molecules related to arterial dilating function: nitric oxide, prostacyclin, and contraction-prohibiting proteins such as calponin and h-caldesmon.

Conclusion

An RNA synthesis inhibitor, DOX, effectively inhibited aberrant expression of ET-1 in the vasospasm-destined artery in the rat cerebral vasospasm model. DOX might be potent enough to inhibit induction of a small number of mRNAs but not a large number of mRNAs such as house-keeping genes.

References

1. Mima T, Yanagisawa M, Shigeno T, Goto K, Takakura K, Masaki T (1989) Endothelin acts in feline and canine cerebral arteries from the adventitial side. Stroke 20: 1553–1556
2. Mima T, Mostafa MG, Mori K (1997) Therapeutic dose and timing of administration of RNA synthesis inhibitors for preventing cerebral vasospasm after subarachnoid hemorrhage. Acta Neurochir [Suppl] (Wien) 70: 65–67
3. Okada T, Harada T, Barkh DH, Mayberg MR (1990) A rat femoral artery model for vasospasm. Neurosurgery 27: 349–356
4. Ohkuma H, Parney I, Megyesi J, Ghahary A, Findlay JM (1999) Antisense preproendothelin-oligoDNA therapy for vasospasm in a canine model of subarachnoid hemorrhage. J Neurosurg 90: 1105–1114
5. Shigeno T, Mima T (1990) A new vasoconstrictor peptide, endothelin: profiles as vasoconstrictor and neuropeptide. Cerebrovasc Brain Metab Rev 2: 227–239
6. Shigeno T, Mima T, Yanagisawa M, Saito A, Goto K, Yamashita K, Takenouchi T, Matsuura N, Yamasaki Y, Yamada K, Masaki T, Takakura K (1991) Prevention of cerebral vasospasm by actinomycin-D. J Neurosurg 74: 940–943
7. Yanagisawa M, Kurihara H, Kimura S, Tomobe Y, Kobayashi M, Mitsui Y, Yazaki Y, Goto K, Masaki T (1988) A novel potent vasoconstrictor peptide produced by vascular endothelial cells. Nature 332: 411–415
8. Zimmermann M, Seifert V (1998) Endothelin and subarachnoid hemorrhage: an overview. Neurosurgery 43: 863–876

Correspondence: Tatsuo Mima, Department of Neurosurgery, Kochi Medical School, Nankoku City, Kochi 783-8505, Japan.

Acta Neurochir (2001) [Suppl] 77: 225–227

Effects of High Cervical Spinal Cord Stimulation (CSCS) on Regional Cerebral Blood Flow after Induced Subarachnoid Haemorrhage in Rats

H. Ebel[1], **G. Semmelmann**[1], **K. Schomäcker**[2], **A. Balogh**[3], **M. Volz**[1], **J. Funke**[1], **H. Schicha**[2], and **N. Klug**[1]

[1] Department of Neurosurgery, University of Cologne, Germany
[2] Department of Nuclear Medicine, University of Cologne, Germany
[3] Department of Neurosurgery, Debrecen University, Debrecen, Hungary

Introduction

Cerebral vasospasm is the most frequent cause of morbidity and mortality in patients after SAH. The direct measurement of regional cerebral blood flow (rCBF) is a valuable adjunct for monitoring SAH patients. Single photon emission computed tomography (SPECT) with ^{99m}Tc-HMPAO is an adequate technique for the measurement of CBF [9, 10]. It measures the net effect of vasospasm on cerebral perfusion. ^{99m}Tc-HMPAO is a radioactive agent crossing the blood-brain barrier. It is trapped within the brain with flow-dependent distribution. Decreased cerebral uptake of ^{99m}Tc-HMPAO in cerebrovascular disease has been shown to correspond well with the results of other methods [3]. Despite a wide variety of treatment modalities no definitive treatment prevents vasospasm. Spinal cord stimulation (SCS) has been accepted to improve microcirculatory parameters in patients with critical limb ischemia [1]. Furthermore, it was proven that cervical spinal cord stimulation increases cerebral blood flow in normal conditions [4]. With reference to these findings, we investigated the effects of high cSCS on rCBF after induced SAH by means of ^{99m}Tc-HMPAO.

Keywords: Subarachnoid haemorrhage; spinal cord stimulation; ^{99m}Tc-HMPAO; cerebral vasospasm.

Material and Methods

The experiments were carried out on 24 Wistar rats, randomly divided into three groups [group I: baseline measurement; group II: SAH; group III: SAH and cSCS]. All animals were anaesthesized by intraperitoneal application of nembutal. Animals were positioned prone on a heating blanket to ensure physiological temperature. Femoral vein was catheterized for fluid infusion, and ^{99m}Tc-HMPAO application, femoral artery for MABP monitoring. The head was fixed in a stereotactic frame, laminectomy of C1 and C2 was performed. The cisterna magna was stereotactically punctured and in 16 animals SAH was induced by injecting 0.5 ml autologous blood. 48 hours after induction of SAH anaesthesia was repeated and 14.8 MBq ^{99m}Tc-HMPAO (37 MBq = 1 mCi/ml) was administered intravenously. In group III the radioactivity was administered after 3 hours of cSCS (n = 8). The microelectrodes were applied onto the epidural surface at the level of C1 and C2 (Fig. 1). The intensity of the stimulating current, rectangular pulses of 50 Hz with an impulse width of 200 μs was adjusted close to the treshold for producing motor effects (3.5 V to 4.8 V). This intensity was selected to submaximally recruit the low-treshold, large-diameter fibers without activating thin high-threshold fibers. To rule out an influence of mean arterial blood presssure on rCBF, blood pressure was measured continuously during the stimulation period. All animals were sacrificed 30 minutes after application. The ^{99m}Tc activities were determined separately in blood, cerebrum and cerebellum and related to a radioactivity-standard. The cerebellum/blood- and cerebrum/blood-ratios were calculated using the corresponding radioactivity concentrations, expressed as % of applied radioactivity per gram tissue. Values are expressed as mean ± standard deviation. The extraction-rates were compared using a non-parametrical Wilcoxon-test, with $p < 0.05$ considered statistically significant.

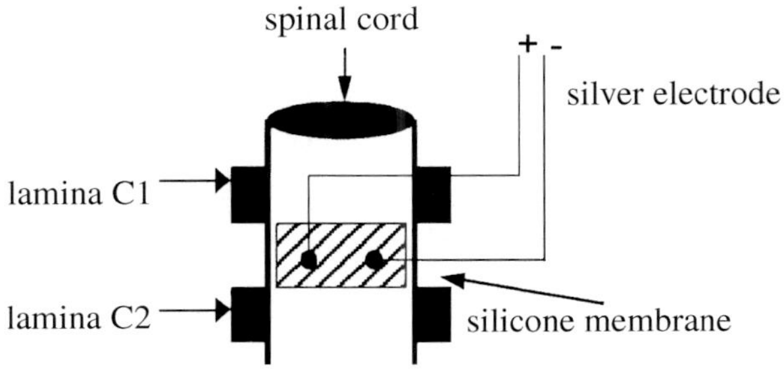

Fig. 1. Schematized depiction of the dorsal aspect of the spinal cord after laminectomy (*C1/C2*) showing the electrodes in place

Table 1. *Statistical Analysis (Wilcoxon Rank Sum W Test)*

Groups	Cerebellum/blood	Cerebrum/blood
Group I/II	0.0019	0.0030
Group II/III	0.0070	0.0104
Group I/III	0.5737	1.000

significant = $p < 0.05$

Results

The following mean values were calculated for the cerebellum/blood ratio: group I: 1.06, SD 0.21; group II: 0.66, SD 0.21; group III: 1.00, SD 0.37. Comparing the mean values a highly significant difference could be found between group II and III (p = 0.007) and between group I and II (p = 0.0019). No significance was found comparing group I and III (p = 0.5737) (Table 1, Fig. 2). The mean values calculated for the cerebrum/blood ratio were as follows: group I: 0.89, SD 0.11; group II: 0.67, SD 0.13; group III: 0.86, SD 0.23. The following differences were significant: group II/group III (p = 0.0104) and group I/group II (p = 0.0030). The comparison of group I with group III revealed no significance (p = 1,000) (Table 1, Fig. 2). Before the stimulation was started the mean of the MABP amounted to 74.3 ± 16.6 mmHg. No significant changes in blood pressure were obtained during the stimulation period.

Discussion

Beside sympathetic and aminergic fibres, extraparenchymal cerebral arteries are also innervated by perivascular nerves, releasing dilating transmitters such as substance P (SP) and calcitonin gene-related peptide (CGRP) [7]. The depletion of the dilating transmitters after SAH appears to participate in the development of vasospasm [5]. Four sources of cerebrovascular CGRP have been described: 1. the ophthalmic and 2. the maxillary division of the trigeminal ganglion, 3. the internal carotid miniganglion and finally 4. the upper cervical dorsal root ganglia (C1–C3), which served as target for the electrical stimulation [5, 7].

First reports on changes in cerebral haemodynamics by SCS date back to Hosobuchi [4]. In 1989, Matsui examined the effects of cSCS after middle cerebral artery occlusion in cats. The high cSCS reduced the rate of deaths within 24 hours after the occlusion. A drastic prevention of infarct progression was found in the group of stimulated animals. The authors conclude that the results provide a clinical application of cSCS for stroke patients, although no evident mechanism of action was obtained [8]. In 1995 Linderoth *et al.* proved that preemptive spinal cord stimulation reduces ischemia in an animal model of vasospasm, especially if the treatment was initiated before the ischemic period. A depression of sympathetic activity and the

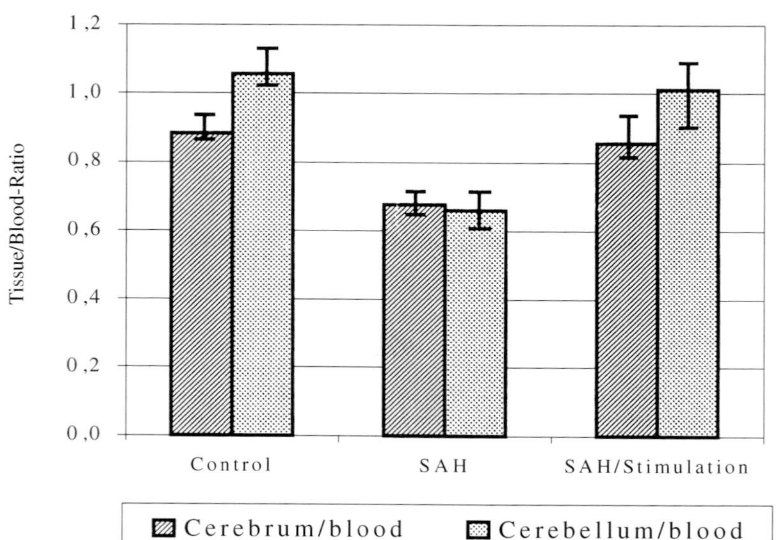

Fig. 2. Tissue/Blood-ratios (Mean ± SD) of the 3 groups

local release of vasoactive substances could be responsible for the efficacy of the spinal cord stimulation [6]. As could be demonstrated cSCS enhances cerebral and cerebellar blood flow after SAH in rats.

SPECT perfusion studies have been investigated for the use of identifying patients with SAH who are at risk of vasospasm and permanent ischemia. Naderi *et al.* reported that brain SPECT with ^{99m}Tc-HMPAO is an accessible technique demonstrating varying degrees of regional cerebral hypoperfusion in patients with delayed ischemic deficits due to vasospasm [9]. In another retrospective study of 16 patients the sensivity of SPECT for the detection of vasospasm was 89% and the specifity was 75% [10]. Consequently, rigorous comparison of SPECT and CT findings is essential to avoid misinterpretation of SPECT abnormalities due to other pathology. Thus, SPECT is a valuable adjunct for the measurement of cerebral perfusion after SAH.

Conclusion

The results of this study show a significant decrease of radioactivity extraction by cerebellum and cerebrum after experimentally induced SAH in rats which must be interpreted as a global hypoperfusion. After induced SAH the electrical stimulation of the upper cervical spinal cord enhances regional cerebral and cerebellar blood flow in rats without any alterations in MABP. Regarding experimental findings the disturbance of the cerebral autoregulation after SAH is limited to a few minutes [2]. Thus, it must be concluded that the increase of regional cerebral blood flow induced by cSCS is independent of an altered cerebral autoregulation. Possibly cSCS constitutes a new approach treating the disturbed rCBF flow after SAH.

References

1. Augustinsson LE, Carlsson CA, Holm J, Jivegard L (1985) Epidural electrical stimulation in severe limb ischemia. Ann Surg 202: 104–110
2. Brinker T, Seifert V, Dietz H (1992) Cerebral blood flow and intracranial pressure during experimental subarachnoid haemorrhage. Acta Neurochir (Wien) 115: 47–52
3. Büll U, Stirner H, Braun H, Kreiten K, Ferbert A (1987) SPECT with ^{99m}Tc-HMPAO and ^{99m}Tc-pertechnetate to assess regional cerebral blood flow (rCBF) and blood volume (rCBV). Preliminary results in cerbrovascular disease and interictal epilepsy. Nucl Med Comm 8: 519–524
4. Hosobuchi Y (1986) Electrical stimulation of the cervical spinal cord increases cerebral blood flow in humans. Appl Neurophysiol 48: 372–376
5. Juul R, Aakhus S, Björnstad K, Gisvold SE, Brubakk AO, Edvinsson L (1994) Calcitonin gene-related peptide (human α-CGRP) counteracts vasoconstriction in human subarachnoid haemorrhage. Neurosci Lett 170: 67–70
6. Linderoth B, Gheradini G, Ren B, Lundeberg T (1995) Preemptive spinal cord stimulation reduces ischemia in an animal model of vasospasm. Neurosurgery 37: 266–272
7. Liu-Chen LY, Mayberg MR, Moskowitz MA (1983) Immunohistochemical evidence for a substance P containing trigeminovascular pathway to pial arteries in cats. Brain Res 268: 162–166
8. Matsui T, Hosobuchi Y (1989) The effects of cervical spinal cord stimulation (cSCS) on experimental stroke. Pace-Pacing-Clin-Electrophysiol 12: 726–732
9. Naderi S, Özgüven MA, Bayhan H, Gökalp H, Erdogan A, Egemen N (1994) Evaluation of cerebral vasospasm in patients with subarachnoid hemorrhage using single photon emission computed tomography. Neurosurg Res 17: 261–265
10. Powsner RA, O'Tuama LA, Jabre A, Melhem ER (1998) SPECT imaging in cerebral vasospasm following subarachnoid hemorrhage. J Nucl Med 39: 765–769

Correspondence: Dr. med. Heinrich Ebel, Neurochirurgische Klinik, Universität zu Köln, Joseph-Stelzmann-Str.9, D-50924 Köln, Germany.

Acta Neurochir (2001) [Suppl] 77: 229–230

Vasodilating Effect of Spinal Cord Stimulation for Cerebral Vasospasm

M. Shinonaga and **Y. Takanashi**

Department of Neurosurgery, Hiratsuka Kyousai Hospital, Kanagawa, Japan

Introduction

The cerebral vasospasm is still a major problem in the treatment of subarachnoid hemorrhage (SAH). Many therapeutic means are used for the treatment of cerebral vasospasm including triple H therapy, administration of calcium channel blocker, intraarterial injection of papaverine, intrathecal injection of t-PA, intraluminal angioplasty, etc. We have been trying a new method – spinal cord stimulation (SCS)- for the treatment of cerebral vasospasm [12]. SCS is widely used for pain control, and for peripheral vascular disease [2, 11]. It is also used for the treatment of angina pectoris [1]. The effect of SCS for cerebral blood flow is unclear. We studied the vasodilating effect of SCS for cerebral vasospasm in measuring cerebral blood flow (CBF).

Keywords: Cerebral blood flow; cerebral vasospasm; spinal cord stimulation.

Materials and Methods

12 cases of SAH with ruptured aneurysm were studied. Hunt and Kosnik grade was 2 to 4. Eearly clipping operation was performed. Cerebral vasospasm was prevented by irrigation of the clot in the cistern during surgery, HHH therapy, administration of calcium channel blocker, intravenous injection of fusadil hydrochloride and SCS.

SCS Treatment

Just after clipping operation, under endotracheal general anesthesia the patient was placed prone. 3 cm midline skin incision was made on the upper thoracic area. SCS electrode (Medtronic 3487A) was inserted into the epidural space through the epidural needle by loss of resistance methods. The tip of the electrode was placed midline at C2 level. Electrical stimulation continued for about three weeks. The rate of stimulation was 50 to 100 Hz, amplitude was 2 to 5 volts.

Measurement of CBF

CBF was measured with cold Xe CT scan for 5 minutes inhalation of Xe gas. CBF was measured at 8 ROI before and during SCS treatment.

Results

Table 1 shows the clinical outcome evaluated with Glasgow Outcome Score. The results of outcome was good recovery in eight cases, moderately disability in two cases and severe disability in two cases. No complication was experienced in SCS treatment. CBF was measured in eight cases. The change of CBF is shown in Table 2. CBF increased in four cases, and decreased in one case. In three cases change of CBF remained within 10%.

Illustrative Case

The patient was a 46 year old female. She was admitted to our hospital with sudden onset of coma. On admittance to our hospital her breathing was ataxic. CT scan showed severe SAH. Hunt & Kosnik grade was 4. After neck clipping of right MCA aneurysm, SCS electrode was placed. From day 5 to day 20 SCS treatment was continued. Regional CBF in right MCA territory, where massive

Table 1. *Clinical Characteristic of 12 Cases with Severe SAH*

Case no	Age	Sex	H&K grade	Aneurysm	Outcome
1	57	F	4	A com.	good recovery
2	46	F	4	rt. MC	good recovery
3	71	F	2	rt. MC	good recovery
4	62	F	3	A com.	moderate disability
5	56	M	2	A com.	good recovery
6	63	F	3	rt. MC	good recovery
7	45	M	3	rt. PC	moderate disability
8	69	F	4	lt. IC-PC	severe disability
9	71	M	2	A com.	good recovery
10	40	F	2	rt. MC	good recovery
11	56	M	2	lt. MC	good recovery
12	62	M	3	A com	severe disability

Table 2. *CBF Change Measured by Xe CT Scan preSCS and During SCS*

Case	AC Territory		MC Territory		PC Territory		Basal ganglia	
	pre	during	p	d	p	d	p	d
KT	17.8	19.3	21.8	23.4	12.4	18.1	28.4	37.5
MI	19.9	18.2	26.3	37.0	27.8	36.6	37.1	30.4
SA	23.3	22.6	36.6	33.6	29.0	28.9	35.8	36.7
EW	23.7	24.3	30.4	30.1	24.5	23.0	32.7	29.0
RY	18.9	21.5	32.1	31.4	25.8	37.5	37.8	43.1
HN	20.2	19.5	23.8	32.4	23.7	25.0	19.7	27.9
SI	23.2	28.4	44.2	44.9	40.9	35.2	36.3	35.3
MS	23.0	12.2	34.0	15.9	35.6	15.2	29.7	19.0

clot was noted at operation, increased from 17.0 to 19.3 ml/100 mg/min. She was discharged from hospital without any deficit on day 24.

Discussion

In most cases of severe SAH, CBF usually decreases during the first 2 weeks by cerebral vasospasm [7, 8]. Adequate prevention of vasoconstriction brings good clinical outcome. But no definite vasodilating method for cerebral vasospasm is used. SCS is widely used for pain control [2] SCS has vasodilating effects and is used for treatment of peripheral vascular disease [3, 11]. The effect of SCS for CBF is not well studied. Hosobuchi, Brosata and Meglio *et al.* reported that SCS increased CBF [3, 4, 5, 6, 9] The exact mechanism of SCS is not clarified. Reduction of the sympathetic nervous system is suspected. We tried SCS for the treatment of cerebral vasospasm. In half the cases CBF increased, and the clinical outcome was satisfactory. SCS is a simple, easy and safe method. In severe cases of SAH, SCS is worthy of prevention and treatment of cerebral vasospasm.

Conclusion

SCS prevented severe vasospasm after SAH. CBF increased in half the cases by SCS. SCS is one of the treatment modalities for late vasospasm after SAH. SCS might be useful for other cerebral ischemic disease.

References

1. Anderson C, Hole P, Oxhoj H (1995) Spinal cord stimulation as a pain treatment for angina pectoris. The Pain Clin 8: 333–339
2. Barolat G (1995) Current status of epidural spinal cord stimulation. Neurosurg Qu 5: 98–124
3. Broseta J, Garcia-March G, Sanchez MJ, Goncales J (1985) Influence of spinal cord stimulation on peripheral blood flow. Appl Neurophysiol 48: 367–370
4. Brosete J, Sanchez-Ledesma MJ, Silvia J *et al* (1992) High cervical spinal cord electric stimulation in brain infarction. Acta Neurochir (Wien) 117: 95–96
5. Hosobuchi Y (1985) Electric stimulation of the cervical spinal cord increases cerebral blood flow in humans. Appl Neurophysiol 48: 372–376
6. Hosobuchi Y (1991) Treatment of cerebral ischemia with electrical stimulation of the cerebral spinal cord. Pace 14: 122–126
7. Ishii R (1979) Regional cerebral blood flow in patient with ruptured intracranial aneurysms. J Neurosurg 50: 587–594
8. Matsuda M, Shiino A, Handa J (1990) Sequential changes of cerebral blood flow after aneurysmal subarachnoid hemorrhage. Acta Neurochir (Wien) 105: 98–106
9. Meglio M, Cioni B, Visocchi M, Nobili F, Rodriguez C, Rosadini G, Chiappini F, Sandric S (1991) Spinal cord stimulation and cerebral haemodynamics. Acta Neurochir (Wien) 111: 43–48
10. North RB, Kidd DH, Zuhurak M, James CS, Long DM (1993) Spinal cord stimulation for chronic intractable pain: Experience over two decades. Neurosurgery 32: 384–395
11. Tallis RC, Sedgwick EM, Hardwidge C, Garfield JS (1983) Spinal cord stimulation in peripheral vascular disease. J Neurol Neurosurg Psychiatry 46: 478–484
12. Takanashi Y, Shinonaga M (2000) Spinal cord stimulation for cerebral vasospasm as prophylaxis. Neurologia Medico-chir 40: 352–357

Correspondence: Dr. M. Shinonaga, Department of Neurosurgery, Hiratsuka Kyousai Hospital, 9-11 Oiwake, Hiratsuka, Kanagawa, Japan 254-8502.

Hemodynamic Therapy and Neuroprotection

Acta Neurochir (2001) [Suppl] 77: 233–235

Metaanalysis of Trials of Tirilazad Mesylate in Aneurysmal SAH

N. W. C. Dorsch[1], **N. F. Kassell**[2], **M. S. Sinkula**[3], and **the Participants**

[1] Department of Neurosurgery, Westmead Hospital, New South Wales, Australia
[2] University of Virginia, Charlottesville, USA
[3] Pharmacia & Upjohn, Kalamazoo, USA

Introduction

Tirilazad mesylate is the first of the new generation of 21-aminosteroid drugs [1] to come into clinical use. The steroid molecule was modified to remove the usual steroid side effects, and by the addition of a large amine molecule to the 21 carbon. It is a potent inhibitor of iron-dependent lipid peroxidation and free radical scavenger.

Experimental studies suggested that tirilazad is effective in some situations of cerebral ischaemia, and in preventing delayed vasospasm after subarachnoid haemorrhage (SAH) [7]. Several trials in head injury and ischaemic stroke have shown no effectiveness. A phase II pilot study in North American centres confirmed its safety in aneurysmal SAH, although the probable most effective dose was not certain. This led to the design of two large multi-centre phase II/III trials, one in North America and one in other countries, which were followed by two other studies on female patients only.

Keywords: Aneurysmal subarachnoid haemorrhage; tirilazad mesylate; metaanalysis; clinical grades IV and V.

Material and Methods

The four major studies have been reported already [3–6]. The results of each trial will be summarised in turn. All were essentially the same in basic design – they were carried out on adult patients with SAH due to a saccular aneurysm, with exclusion of other causes of SAH such as mycotic or traumatic aneurysm or arteriovenous malformation. Patients in all clinical grades, measured on a modified WFNS Scale (where motor GCS score was estimated on the worst rather than on the best limb) were eligible. Treatment had to start within 48 hours of the last haemorrhage, and to continue to the end of the tenth day. Nimodipine was used as background treatment in all patients. Early surgery was recommended but not mandatory, and other management was left to the treating surgeon. There were restrictions on the use of other steroids or calcium antagonists. Patients were excluded if they had severe neurological, psychiatric or other disease, or were pregnant or breastfeeding.

All studies were double-blind and vehicle-controlled, with a block randomisation system for each centre. Results were analysed on an intent-to-treat basis for all patients who were randomised and received at least one dose of test substance. Statistical analysis was with appropriate tests for the main endpoints of incidence of symptomatic vasospasm, death rate at three months, and overall outcome based on the five point Glasgow Outcome Scale (Good Recovery 1, Death 5). Where more than one dose level of tirilazad was compared with vehicle, a Bonferroni correction for multiple testing was included. Safety data and side effects were also analysed.

An integrated analysis of the results of the four studies, with particular reference to patients in clinical grades IV and V, follows.

Results

The first trial [4] was in over 1000 patients in 42 centres in Europe and Australasia, with intravenous nimodipine as background treatment. Three doses of tirilazad, 0.6, 2.0 and 6.0 mg/kg/day, were tested against drug vehicle, with roughly equal numbers of patients in each of the four groups. No effect was seen from the lower doses. In the 6 mg/kg/day (TIR6) group there was no decrease in the incidence of angiographic or transcranial Doppler vasospasm, but symptomatic vasospasm, the primary endpoint for the study, was considerably less than in those receiving drug vehicle (VEH), with 18% compared with 26% in controls ($P = 0.047$, which did not reach the required value of 0.016). The overall death rate at three months postSAH was significantly lower (12% versus 21%, $P = 0.008$, odds ratio (OR) 0.51, 95% confidence interval (CI) 0.32–0.84). The proportion making a good recovery, Glasgow Outcome Scale (GOS) 1, was higher at 63% compared with 53% ($P = 0.015$).

On further analysis it was found that the improvement was in male patients only – death rate for men was 27% control and 3% treated (P < 0.001), and for women was the same 18% in both groups. Males who were admitted in grade IV or V also had a lower death rate (VEH 10 of 19 cases, TIR6 none of 15; P < 0.001) and a higher proportion of favourable outcomes (GOS 1 or 2).

A parallel trial was run in centres in Canada and the USA [3], the main differences being that there were only two treated groups (TIR2 and TIR6), and that oral rather than intravenous nimodipine was used as background treatment; the principal endpoint for this study was three month mortality. Only a trend towards a reduced death rate was seen, with 13% for TIR6 and 16% for VEH (P = 0.48). The difference was again only in males, where death rate was 9% and 13% respectively; in grade IV and V patients one of 20 Tir patients and four of 12 VEH died (P = 0.05). A possible explanation for the difference from the first trial is the much greater use of anticonvulsants in North America; phenytoin in particular affects metabolism and decreases the availability of tirilazad.

Two further studies were done later in females only, each with only two groups, one receiving tirilazad vehicle and one tirilazad 15 mg/kg/day (TIR15). In one study in Europe, Australasia and South Africa [5], there was a highly significant reduction in the incidence of symptomatic vasospasm, which affected 25% TIR15 and 34% VEH patients (P = 0.005). A parallel increase in the use of therapeutic HHH therapy was seen in the vehicle group, with 24% compared with 18% for TIR (P = 0.02). Outcome was the same in both groups, with death rates 18% in each. Again, a trend was noted towards a lower death rate in poorgrade patients, with 32% for TIR15 and 37% in VEH patients.

A similar study was done in units in the USA, Canada and Mexico [6], with the principal endpoint of death rate in grades IV and V. The incidence of vasospasm was similar and overall death rates were 13% TIR and 15.6% VEH, while the death rate in poorgrade patients was for TIR15 24.6%, significantly less than for VEH (43.4% dead; P = 0.016).

Metaanalysis

When patients from all four studies are combined, including males receiving TIR6 and females TIR15, the overall results showed a better outcome (death rate for TIR 13.4% of 994 patients, for VEH 17.3% of 956, P = 0.024, OR 0.75, 95%CI 0.59–0.96). Important differences were seen mainly in patients who entered the studies in WFNS grade IV or V. For this group the combined death rate was 25.0% of 220 entered patients for TIR and 39.9% of 233 receiving vehicle (P = 0.001, OR 0.56, 95%CI 0.37–0.86). Time to treatment was also important, most of the effect being seen in those entered within 24 hours of SAH (death rates 15.7 and 55.2% respectively, P < 0.001, OR 0.15, 95%CI 0.07–0.33). The results for males and females separately are shown in Table 1.

Table 1. *Outcome in Grade IV/V Patients*

	Tirilazad (M6, F15)		Vehicle
Males number	35		31
Percent dead	3		42
		P = 0.0001	
Good outcome percent	26		10
Females number	185		202
Percent dead	29		40
		P = 0.03	
Good outcome percent	28		22

The technique of shift analysis was used to look at changes in outcome category between the two groups, with four categories of good, moderate deficit, severe deficit, and vegetative plus dead, and the assumption that any shift was by one level only. Respective percentages of pooled poorgrade patients in the vehicle group were 20.7, 19.4, 18.1 and 41.8%. If one assumes an upward shift of 30% of patients from each level to the next, the calculated values would be 26.7, 19.0, 25.0 and 29.3%. Actual proportions in the tirilazad group were 27.9, 16.4, 26.0 and 29.7%, very close to those calculated.

Discussion

The different effect in men and women is important. It was shown [2] that with similar doses of tirilazad a higher blood level is achieved in males, the difference being especially marked in young premenopausal women. Such sex differences had not been seen before in drug trials.

The results in the first female trial were interesting, with much less vasospasm but no effect on outcome. The increased use of therapeutic or "rescue" HHH, a treatment known to be effective against vasospasm, may account for the lack of a difference in outcome between control and treated groups.

The similar design of these four trials, in spite of variations in the doses used and in the principal endpoints, is reasonable justification for a metaanalysis. This is important especially when the treatment is useful only in a subgroup of the whole population, especially if the trends are similar between studies; the numbers of the subgroup in each study may be too small for statistical significance, leading to a type II error, which is avoided when all the trials are combined.

The technique of shift analysis is useful in demonstrating that there was an overall trend towards improvement of outcome across the whole spectrum of the GOS. It also explains the observed increase with treatment in the proportion with a severe deficit (TIR 26%, VEH 18%) – a large number who would have been vegetative or dead (42% of VEH patients) have "moved up" to the severe category, while fewer who would have been severe (18% of VEH) have moved up out of that category.

References

1. Braughler JM, Pregenzer JF, Chase RL, Duncan LA, Jacobsen EJ, McCall JM (1987) The 21-aminosteroids: potent inhibitors of lipid peroxidation for the treatment of central nervous system trauma. J Biol Chem 262: 10438–10440
2. Fleishaker JC, Hulst-Pearson LK, Peters GR (1995) Effect of gender and menopausal status on the pharmacokinetics of tirilazad mesylate in healthy subjects. Am J Therapeut 2: 553–560
3. Haley EC Jr, Kassell NF, Apperson-Hansen C, Maile WH, Alves WM, the Participants (1997) A randomized, double-blind, vehicle-controlled trial of tirilazad mesylate in patients with aneurysmal subarachnoid hemorrhage: a cooperative study in North America. J Neurosurg 86: 467–474
4. Kassell NF, Haley EC Jr, Apperson-Hansen C, Alves WM, the Participants (1996) Randomized, double-blind, vehicle-controlled trial of tirilazad mesylate in patients with aneurysmal subarachnoid hemorrhage: a cooperative study in Europe, Australia, and New Zealand. J Neurosurg 84: 221–228
5. Lanzino G, Kassell NF, Dorsch NWC, Pasqualin A, Brandt L, Schmiedek P, Truskowski LL, Alves WM, the Participants (1999) Double-blind, randomized, vehicle-controlled study of high dose tirilazad mesylate in women with aneurysmal subarachnoid hemorrhage, part I. A cooperative study in Europe, Australia, New Zealand, and South Africa. J Neurosurg 90: 1011–1017
6. Lanzino G, Kassell NF, the Participants (1999) Double-blind, randomized, vehicle-controlled study of high dose tirilazad mesylate in women with aneurysmal subarachnoid hemorrhage. Part II. A cooperative study in North America. J Neurosurg 90: 1018–1024
7. Vollmer DG, Kassell NF, Hongo K, Ogawa H, Tsukuhara T (1989) Effect of the non-glucocorticoid 21-aminosteroid U-74006F on experimental cerebral vasospasm. Surg Neurol 31: 190–194

Correspondence: N. W. C. Dorsch FRACS, Department of Neurosurgery, Westmead Hospital, Hawkesbury Road, New South Wales 2145, Australia.

Acta Neurochir (2001) [Suppl] 77: 237–241

Triple H Therapy after Aneurysmal Subarachnoid Hemorrhage. A Review

B. Romner and **P. Reinstrup**

Neurointensive Care Unit, Department of Neurosurgery, University Hospital of Lund, Sweden

Introduction

Outcome in patients with aneurysmal subarachnoid hemorrhage (SAH) have improved over the past two decades with advances in neurosurgery and neurocritical care, including an emphasis on early aneurysm clipping to prevent rebleeding. However, cerebral ischemia related to vasospasm remains an important cause of morbidity and mortality, despite the beneficial effects of the calcium channel blocker nimodipine.

Excessive natriuresis and intravascular volume contraction occur frequently after SAH and have been implicated as risk factors for delayed cerebral ischemia related to vasospasm [20, 21]. SAH causes progressive reduction of cerebral blood flow (CBF) for up to 3 weeks and can result in loss of the normal capacity to autoregulate [13].

Experimental studies indicate that volume expansion can improve CBF in ischemic regions independent of perfusion pressure because of beneficial effects on cardiac output and blood rheology [16], and uncontrolled case series [1, 7, 18] have reported that hypervolemic therapy can reverse ischemic deficits in symptomatic patients. Accordingly, postoperative hypervolemic therapy is now routinely performed at most medical centers, on the assumption that this intervention may augment CBF, prevent delayed ischemia, and improve clinical outcome [20]. However, both increases [14, 17] and decreases [25] in CBF have been reported after volume expansion in SAH patients, and CBF measurements in hypervolemic and normovolemic subjects have never been directly compared.

Keywords: Subarachnoid hemorrhage; vasospasm; triple H therapy; clinical outcome evaluation; review.

Material

A literature review was performed (MEDLINE) to identify articles dealing with hyperdynamic therapy (triple H) management in SAH during the period of 1978 to 2000. Twelve clinical studies reporting different strategies using triple H as *prophylaxis* or *treatment* for cerebral vasospasm are presented in this review. The different studies presented in the results are divided in pro's and con's regarding the effect of different hyperdynamic therapy protocols. Only three studies [4, 9, 12] are designed as controlled, prospective and randomized.

Methods

Various protocols for triple H therapy have been proposed. To prevent delayed ischaemic neurological deficits (DIND), some centers use triple H as a prophylactic treatment in all cases of aneurysmal SAH, while most centers initiate triple H therapy only in patients demonstrating symptoms of DIND. Hyperdynamic therapy consists of hemodilution, hypervolemia, and hypertension. An explanation of the different corner-stones in triple H follows below.

Isovolemic Hemodilution (H)

The purpose of isovolemic hemodilution is an increase in CBF. A decrease in blood viscosity will theoretically result in increased perfusion. Hematocrite (hct) is a major indicator of blood viscosity and a decrease to approximately 33–35% is desired, which is considered to balance optimal viscosity and maximal oxygen delivery to the brain. To achieve this, the blood volume to be withdrawn is calculated from the hct value, and this amount is simultaneously replaced with colloid solutions. There are no changes in systemic arterial blood pressure, central venous pressure, pulmonary wedge pressure, or raised intracranial pressure. Thus, isovolemic hemodilution can be used more safely in elderly patients, and in patients with cardiovascular disease [6, 8]. Experimentally, both cerebral oxygen transport and cerebral oxygen metabolism in dogs with global ischemia were highest at hct 0.31 [23].

Hypervolemic Hemodilution (HH)

Hypervolemia is achieved by infusion of colloids. Hypervolemia is supposed to increase regional CBF throughout the brain but particularly in areas that have lost cerebral autoregulation. In dysfunctional ischemic regions, local flow may become directly proportional to alterations in cardiac output in the presence or absence of similar changes in blood pressure. The increased blood flow to acutely ischemic areas is believed to rescue reversibly ischemic and malfunctioning brain tissue from infarction. However, the hypervolemic hemodilution treatment is not without risks, as it may result in cardiac overload, pulmonary edema, cerebral edema, and increased intracranial pressure [6, 22, 24].

Hypertensive Hypervolemic Hemodilution (HHH)

Induced hypertension in addition to hypervolemic hemodilution after aneurysmal occlusion is suggested to improve the rheology of blood flow in the microcirculation. A vasopressor, usually dopamine, is administered until systolic blood pressure reaches 160 to 180 mm Hg, elevating the perfusion pressure and presumably increasing local CBF above the ischemic threshold. Addition of a vasopressor to hypervolemic hemodilution contributes synergistically to elevate and sustain the elevation of CBF. Potential risks besides those desribed above are cardiac arrythmias and myocardial infarction [2, 7, 17, 20, 21].

Results

The following 12 studies evaluating the effects of hyperdynamic therapy in aneurysmal subarachnoid hemorrhage are summarized in Table 1.

Prospective Randomized Studies

Lennihan *et al.* [9] evaluated the effect of hypervolemic therapy on cerebral blood flow after SAH in a randomized controlled trial including 82 patients. In this study, a stratified treatment randomization including number of days since SAH and postoperative Hunt-Hess grade was made, while other factors that have been predictive of delayed ischemia, such as to quantify the amount of SAH on admission computed tomography (CT) scan or analyze transcranial Doppler (TCD) data was not taken into account. CBF values (xenon-133 clearance) in hypervolemic and normovolemic subjects were compared. Hypervolemic patients received significantly more fluid and had higher pulmonary artery diastolic and central venous pressures than normovolemic patients. There was no difference in mean global CBF during the treatment period between the groups. Symptomatic vasospasm occurred in 20% of patients in each group and was associated ($p = 0.04$) with reduced minimum regional CBF values. In summary, they found that hypervolemic therapy after aneurysm clipping did not result in increased CBF compared with normovolemic therapy.

Egge *et al.* [4] designed a prospective randomized study including 32 patients. The patients were treated after SAH and clipping of an aneurysm following two different protocols. Sixteen patients received hypervolemic fluid therapy according to the HHH model, the other 16 received normovolemic fluid therapy aiming at a well balanced fluid state day by day. They were not able to uncover differences between the two groups regarding cerebral vasospasm, neither clinical nor on the TCD recordings. When evaluating the regional cerebral perfusion by means of single photon emission computed tomography (SPECT) analysis, no differences were seen between the two groups. The clinical outcomes at one year follow-up were equal in both groups. From an economical point of view the hyperdynamic therapy fell out more expensive. Furthermore, more complications (hemorrhagic diathesis and postoperative hematomas) were seen in this group.

Mayer *et al.* [12] reported a study of 43 patients with aneurysmal SAH treated with one or two different fluid protocols. For one group of patients, albumin

Table 1. *Summary of 12 Studies Evaluating the Effects of Hyperdynamic Therapy after Aneurysmal Subarachnoid Hemorrhage*

Study (reference no.)	Year	Prospective	Randomized	n	Prophylactic or treatment	Hyperdynamic therapy		
Lennihan *et al.* [9]	2000	yes	yes (stratified)	82	prophylactic	Hd	Hv	–
Egge *et al.* [4]	2000	yes	yes (stratified)	32	prophylactic	Hd	Hv	Ht
Mayer *et al.* [12]	1998	yes	yes (stratified)	43	prophylactic	Hd	Hv	–
Solomon *et al.* [20]	1988	yes	no	56	prophylactic	Hd	Hv	Ht
Origitano *et al.* [17]	1990	yes	no	43	prophylactic	Hd	Hv	Ht
Solomon *et al.* [21]	1988	yes	no	47	prophylactic	Hd	Hv	–
Yamakami *et al.* [25]	1987	yes	no	35	prophylactic	Hd	Hv	–
Mori *et al.* [14]	1995	yes	no	98	treatment	Hd	Hv	Ht
Shimoda *et al.* [22]	1993	no	no	94	treatment	Hd	Hv	–
Darby *et al.* [2]	1994	no	no	13	treatment	Hd	–	Ht
Awad *et al.* [1]	1987	yes	no	42	treatment	Hd	Hv	Ht
Muizelaar *et al.* [15]	1986	no	no	4	treatment	Hd	Hv	Ht

N Number of patients in study, *Hd* hemodilution, *Hv* hypervolemia, *Ht* hypertension.

was given in sufficient amounts to maintain the central venous pressure at about 8 mm Hg. In the second group, the CVP was maintained at approximately 5 mm Hg. Supplemental 5% albumin solution given to maintain CVP of >8 mm Hg prevented sodium and fluid losses but did not have an impact on blood volume. Blood volume declined by 10% in both groups. Pulmonary edema requiring diuresis occurred in one patient in the hypervolemia group.

Prospective Non-Randomized Studies

Awad *et al.* [1] assessed the incidence and clinical course of symptomatic vasospasm following SAH using a uniform management protocol. Out of 118 consecutive patients, 42 (35.6%) developed characteristic signs and symptoms of clinical vasospasm with angiographic verification of spasm in 39 cases. All patients with clinical vasospasm received hypervolemic hemodilution therapy aiming for a hematocrit of 33–38%, a central venous pressure of 10–12 mm Hg (or a pulmonary wedge pressure of 15–18 mm Hg), and a systolic arterial pressure of 160–200 mm Hg (120–150 mm Hg for unclipped aneurysms) for the duration of clinical vasospasm. At the end of hypervolemic hemodilution therapy, 47.6% had become neurologically normal, 33.3% had a minor neurologic deficit, and 19% had a major neurologic deficit or were dead. There were three instances of cardiopulmonary deterioration (7%), all of which were in patients without Swan-Ganz catheters, and all resolved with appropriate diuresis. One patient rebled and died while on hypervolemic therapy. The authors conclude that early surgery and aggressive management of clinical vasospasm with hypervolemic hemodilution therapy can be accomplished with minimal morbidity.

Solomon *et al.* [20] presented 56 patients who had bled within 7 days before admission. Urgent aneurysm surgery was performed within 24 hours after presentation. All patients were then treated with prophylactic volume expansion therapy and induced hypertension until day 14 after SAH. Overall, 41 patients (73%) returned to their premorbid occupations without neurological deficit. They conclude that delayed cerebral ischemia after SAH can be effectively minimized with prophylactic volume expansion therapy.

Origitano *et al.* [17], claimed triple-H therapy to be a safe and effective modality for elevating and sustaining CBF after SAH, and in combination with early aneurysm surgery, triple-H therapy minimized delayed ischemia and improved outcome. In 43 patients with SAH, a protocol for prophylactic triple-H therapy was utilized. Mean hemoglobin and hematocrit were lowered, hypervolemic treatment was given, as well as intravenous infusion of dopamine to maintain systolic blood pressure at 150 to 175 mm Hg in patients with clipped aneurysms. Serial CBF measurements were performed using the xenon-133 inhalation technique to maximize therapy. Thirty-six of the 43 patients (84%) were discharged capable of an independent lifestyle, while 2 patients developed delayed ischemia and infarction.

Solomon *et al.* [21] used prophylactic volume expansion therapy for the prevention of delayed cerebral ischemia after early aneurysm surgery in 47 consecutive patients with ruptured intracranial aneurysms. Their preliminary observations indicated not only that the incidence of cerebral ischemia was not increased but that it appeared to be substantially reduced.

Mori *et al.* [14], reported 98 patients who underwent early craniotomy for aneurysm clipping surgery after SAH. Fifty-one patients (52%) developed symptomatic vasospasm. Circulating blood volume and CBF were measured periodically. Cardiac output and pulmonary capillary wedge pressure were also measured using a Swan-Ganz catheter. They observed a progressive reduction in hemispheric CBF in patients who developed symptomatic vasospasm, which improved after volume expansion with albumin and dextran. The authors conclude that hypervolemic hemodilution therapy decreases hematocrit level and red cell aggregability while increasing cardiac output.

Yamakami *et al.* [25] performed 55 pairs of regional CBF measurements using the xenon-133 inhalation method before and after volume expansion in 35 patients with ruptured cerebral aneurysms. In patients with symptomatic vasospasm, CBF decreased significantly after volume expansion, while in patients without symptomatic vasospasm, volume expansion produced no change in CBF. The results of their study suggest that increasing the intravascular volume above normal by volume expansion does not increase CBF nor reverse symptomatic vasospasm.

Retrospective Non-Randomized Studies

Muizelaar *et al.* [15] presented a series of 43 patients operated on for ruptured anterior circulation aneurysms. Five patients (11.6%) developed clinical signs of cerebral ischemia postoperatively. In four of those patients, the diagnosis of "vasospasm" was made with measurements of CBF (xenon-133 inhalation or intravenous injection). Treatment with induced arterial hypertension with phenylephrine was instituted. Within one hour, the CBF measurement was repeated to document the effect of treatment. With treatment the average hemispherical blood flows increased in all four cases. There was also an immediate and obvious positive clinical effect in all patients.

Shimoda *et al.* [22], reported 112 out of 323 patients who did develop a delayed ischemic deficit after SAH. Hypervolemic therapy was instituted only after the onset of an ischemic deficit. 94 patients were managed with hypervolemic therapy (47 with a conventional regimen and 47 with an "optimum" regimen). Among the patients who received hypervolemic therapy, 68 patients (72%) experienced no intracranial complication, 18 (19%) exhibited aggravation of the brain edema, and eight (9%) developed a hemorrhagic infarction. The authors conclude, that hypervolemic therapy may be very harmful in the early phase after SAH. They found optimum hypervolemic therapy to be more successful than conventional hypervolemic therapy.

Darby *et al.* [2], evaluated retrospectively, the effects of dopamine-induced hypertension on local CBF in 13 patients suspected of suffering clinical vasospasm after aneurysmal SAH. They found that dopamine-induced hypertension led to increased CBF in ischemic (<25 mL/100 g per minute), noninfarcted territories without producing an increase in mean global CBF.

Discussion

Cerebral vasospasm following aneurysmal subarachnoid hemorrhage is the most important cause of morbidity and mortality amongst patients suffering such a hemorrhage besides an eventual rebleeding and the bleeding itself. Therefore, during the last decades great efforts have been taken both clinically and scientifically to find effective therapeutical measures useful in this clinical battlefield.

Previous studies have given us reason to believe that 70–90% of patients with SAH within one or two weeks will experience some narrowing of the greater cerebral arteries revealed by angiography. Not all of them will have detectable clinical deficits, but some 30% will have symptoms varying from light headache with perhaps some dizziness to hemiparalysis and even death. These DIND typically hit the patients within 7–14 days after the SAH. Symptoms may evolve gradually over days as the lumen of the arteries in question narrows, blood flow subsides and autoregulatory mechanisms grow inefficient. The perfusion of greater or lesser parts of the brain then sinks below critical values and therefore transient or permanent neurological deficits may develop. DIND often develops much faster, within hours or less.

In a recent rewiev over hyperdynamic therapy, Pritz [19] presented practical aspects on the treatment of cerebral vasospasm. Successful medical treatment of neurological symptoms due to vasospasm requires vigilance, an accurate diagnosis, and prompt intervention. The results of TCD, routinely performed at regular intervals after SAH, coupled with neurologic decline in the absence of electrolyte and/or cardiovascular pulmonary abnormalities, should suggest that these symptoms stem from vasospasm. CT will exclude cerebral edema, hydrocephalus, stroke due to vessel occlusion, and hematoma as the cause of these deficits. Cerebral angiography will document the vessels affected by vasospasm as well as satisfactory aneurysm clipping and vessel patency.

Several reports from uncontrolled studies described resolution of deficits from vasospasm following elevation of blood pressure, volume expansion, and/or hemodilution [1, 7, 10, 15] with improved outcome relative to vasospasm compared with historical controls. However, the efficacy of triple H therapy has not been demonstrated in controlled trials, and studies of cerebral blood flow after initiation of therapy have been equivocal [11]. In addition, studies have not been performed to determine which component of this therapy is most important. Only a proportion of patients with vasospasm respond to triple H therapy, with stroke and death rates from vasospasm approaching 15% in the series with the best outcome [1, 15]. Initiation of triple H therapy is associated with significant risk, including cardiac failure, electrolyte abnormalities, cerebral edema, bleeding abnormalities, and rupture of an unsecured aneurysm [10]. Patients receiving this treatment are usually monitored in an intensive care setting with a Swan-Ganz catheter, arterial lines, and frequent serum electrolyte determinations. In many protocols measurements of left ventricular end-diastolic pressure and cardiac output are used to optimize hemodynamics according to the Starling curve [10]. An uncontrolled series suggested that therapy may be more effective if initiated prophylactically before the onset of symptoms, preferably after clipping of the aneurysm [20]. Treatment is usually continued beyond the period of risk for vasospasm or until reduction of vasospasm by clinical and TCD parameters.

Triple H therapy remains the mainstay of management of delayed ischemic neurological deterioration after SAH although in therapy resistant cases angioplasty may have a role in the future. Clinicians should be aware however, that despite strong evidence of reversal of neurological deficit there is no evidence of improved morbidity or mortality from triple H therapy [3]. Indeed the reduced need for triple H therapy in the nicardipine arm of the Cooperative Aneurysm Study without any difference in outcome could be interpreted as the strongest evidence so far against it [5]. A large multicenter clinical trial comparing high dependency care in patients following aneurysmal SAH, with and without deliberate triple H therapy, with patient outcome as the primary endpoint and the incidence of symptomatic vasospasm as the secondary endpoint is now essential to establish whether the additional cost of triple H therapy can be justified.

References

1. Awad IA, Carter LP, Spetzler RF, Medina M, Williams Jr FC (1987) Clinical vasospasm after subarachnoid hemorrhage: response to hypervolemic hemodilution and arterial hypertension. Stroke 18: 365–372
2. Darby JM, Yonas H, Marks EC, Durham S, Snyder RW, Nemoto EM (1994) Acute cerebral blood flow response to dopamine-induced hypertension after subarachnoid hemorrhage. J Neurosurg 80: 857–864
3. Dearden NM (1998) Triple H therapy in the management of cerebral vasospasm. Eur J Anaesthesiol 15 [Suppl] 17: 70–79
4. Egge A, Sjoholm H, Solberg T, Ingebrigtsen T, Romner B (2000) Triple-H therapy in aneurysmal SAH. A clinical randomized study. 7th International Conference on Cerebral Vasospasm, Interlaken, Switzerland (abstract)
5. Haley EC, Kassell NF, Torner JC (1993) A randomised controlled trial of high dose intravenous nicardipine in aneurysmal subarachnoid hemorrhage: a report of the co-operative aneurysm Study. J Neurosurg 78: 537–547
6. Heros RC, Korosue K (1989) Hemodilution for cerebral ischemia. Stroke 20: 423–427
7. Kasell NF, Peerless SJ, Durward QJ, Beck DW, Drake CG, Adams Jr HP (1982) Treatment of ischemic deficits from vasospasm with intravascular volume expansion and induced arterial hypertension. Neurosurgery 11: 337–343
8. Korosue K, Ishida K, Matsuoka H, Nagao T, Tamaki N, Matsumoto S (1988) Clinical, hemodynamic, and hemorheological effects of isovolemic hemodilution in acute cerebral infarction. Neurosurgery 23: 148–153
9. Lennihan L, Mayer SA, Fink ME, Beckford A, Paik MC, Zhang H, Wu YC, Klebanoff LM, Raps EC, Solomon RA (2000) Effect of hypervolemic therapy on cerebral blood flow after subarachnoid hemorrhage: a randomized controlled trial. Stroke 31: 383–391
10. Levy M, Gianotta S (1991) Cardiac performance indices during hypervolemic therapy for cerebral vasospasm. J Neurosurg 75: 27–31
11. Mayberg MR, Batjer HH, Dacey R, Diringer M, Haley EC, Heros RC, Sternau LL, Torner J, Adams Jr HP, Feinberg W, Thies W (1994) Guidelines for the management of aneurysmal subarachnoid hemorrhage. A statement for healthcare professionals from a special writing group of the Stroke Council, American Heart Association. Stroke 25: 2315–28
12. Mayer SA, Solomon RA, Fink ME, Lennihan L, Stern L, Beckford A, Thomas CE, Klebanoff LM (1998) Effect of 5% albumin solution on sodium balance and blood volume after subarachnoid hemorrhage. Neurosurgery 42: 759–768
13. Messeter K, Brandt L, Ljunggren B, Svendgaard NA, Algotsson L, Romer B, Ryding E (1987) Prediction and prevention of delayed ischemic dysfunction after aneurysmal subarachnoid hemorrhage and early operation. Neurosurgery 20: 548–553
14. Mori K, Arai H, Nakajima K, Tajima A, Maeda M (1995) Hemorheological and hemodynamic analysis of hypervolemic hemodilution therapy for cerebral therapy for cerebral vasospasm after aneurysmal subarachnoid hemorrhage. Stroke 26: 1620–1626
15. Muizelaar JP, Becker DP (1986) Induced hypertension for the treatment of cerebral ischemia after subarachnoid hemorrhage: direct effect on cerebral blood flow. Surg Neurol 25: 317–325
16. Ohtaki M., Tramner BI (1993) Hyperdynamic therapy for focal cerebral ischemia of rats: use of colloidal volume expansion and dobutamine. Surg Neurol 40: 131–137
17. Origitano TC, Wascher TM, Reichman OH, Anderson DE (1990) Sustained increased cerebral blood flow with prophylactic hypertensive hypervolemic hemodilution ("triple-H" therapy) after subarachnoid hemorrhage. Neurosurgery 27: 729–739
18. Pritz MB, Giannotta SL, Kindt GW, McGillicuddy JE, Prager RL (1978) Treatment of patients with neurological deficits associated with cerebral vasospasm by intravascular volume expansion. Neurosurgery 3: 364–368
19. Pritz MB (1997) Treatment of cerebral vasospasm due to aneurysmal hemorrhage: past, present, and future of hyperdynamic therapy. Neurosurg Qu 7: 273–285
20. Solomon RA, Fink ME, Lennihan L (1988) Early aneurysm surgery and prophylactic hypervolemic hypertensive therapy for the treatment of aneurysmal subarachnoid hemorrhage. Neurosurgery 23: 699–704
21. Solomon RA, Fink ME, Lennihan L (1988) Prophylactic volume expansion therapy for the prevention of delayed cerebral ischemia after early aneurysm surgery. Arch Neurol 45: 325–332
22. Shimoda M, Oda S, Tsugane R, Sato O (1993) Intracranial complications of hypervolemic therapy in patients with a delayed ischemic deficit attributed to vasospasm. J Neurosurg 78: 423–429
23. Tu Y-K, Kuo MF, Liu H-M (1997) Cerebral oxygen transport and metabolism during graded isovolemic hemodilution in experimental global ischemia. J Neural Sci 150: 115–122
24. Wood JH, Simeone FA, Kron RE, Snyder LL (1984) Experimental hypervolemic hemodilution: physiological correlations of cortical blood flow, cardiac output, and intracranial pressure with fresh blood viscosity and plasma volume. Neurosurgery 14: 709–723
25. Yamakami I, Isobe K, Yamaura A (1987) Effects of intravascular volume expansion on cerebral blood flow in patients with ruptured cerebral aneurysms. Neurosurgery 21: 303–309

Correspondence: Bertil Romner, M.D., Ph.D., Department of Neurosurgery, University Hospital of Lund 221 85 Lund, Sweden.

Acta Neurochir (2001) [Suppl] 77: 243–246

Triple "H" Therapy does not Increase Cerebral Blood Flow after Induced Subarachnoid Hemorrhage in Pigs. Results of a Pilot ^{99m}TC-HMPAO-Single Photon Emission Computed Tomography Study

M. Dueck[1], **H. Ebel**[2], **M. Volz**[2], **J.-Y. Lee**[2], and **G. Semmelmann**[2]

[1] Department of Anesthesiology, University of Cologne, Cologne, Germany
[2] Department of Neurosurgery, University of Cologne, Cologne, Germany

Introduction

The so-called triple "H" therapy (THT) is routinely used to treat or to prevent cerebral vasospasm after subarachnoid hemorrhage (SAH). The three H's stand for hypervolemia, hemodilution and hypertension. Although no prospective, randomized, controlled clinical study really demonstrates a better outcome after SAH, there is a widespread use of THT. On the other hand literature reports complications like pulmonary edema, myocardial ischemia and cerebal edema and even animal studies are controversial.

After reaching a significant increase of cerebral blood flow (CBF) after induced SAH by electrical stimulation of the Gasserian ganglion in a SPECT perfusion study [2] we used the same protocol to assess the effect of THT in pigs.

Keywords: Subarachnoid hemorrhage; hypertensive-hypervolemic-hemodilutional therapy; cerebral blood flow; cerebral vasospasm.

Material and Methods

The protocol was fully approved by the Institutional Animal Care and Use Committee at University of Debrecen, Hungary and is in accordance with the Hungarian Association for Laboratory Animal Science guidelines for the care and use of laboratory animals.

Six domestic pigs (Duroc-Mongolica), weighing 29 to 37 kg, were randomly divided into two groups [control group I: SAH, no THT (n = 3); experimental group II: SAH and THT (n = 3)]. The first part of the experiment consisted of a native SPECT in all animals (groups I and II).

The main experiment was carried out at least 48 hours after the native SPECT (half-life ^{99mc}Tc-HMPAO: 6 hours). Tracheotomy and femoral cutdown for insertion of an arterial line and a pulmonary artery catheter (PAC) were performed. The arterial line was used for continuous monitoring of mean arterial blood pressure (MAP). The PAC was inserted to monitor cardiac output (CO), pulmonary wedge pressure (PWP) and central venous pressure (CVP), for fluid infusion and for drug administration.

Anesthesia was performed with fentanyl, midazolam and pancuronium and controlled ventilation was started. Blood gas analyses were done every 30 minutes. Arterial partial oxygen pressure was maintained between 90 and 130 mm Hg and endexpiratory carbon dioxide pressure ($etCO_2$) was continuously monitored to keep arterial pCO_2 constant at about 40 mm Hg (ranging from 36 to 44 mm Hg). Temperature was kept at $38 \pm 1\,°C$.

A parenchymal pressure sensor was calibrated and inserted into the right frontoparietal parenchyma at 8 mm depth. A pterional craniotomy was performed to place a 19-gauge catheter into the suprasellar cistern. Dura was closed in watertight fashion.

After baseline measurement for 10 minutes SAH was induced by injecting 10 ml autologous arterial non-heparinized blood through the cisternal catheter within 20 seconds. 30 minutes after SAH induction THT was applied for 30 minutes in the experimental group II. Intravascular volume expansion was achieved with infusion of 6% hetastarch and epinephrine was administered to elevate MAP. During THT $etCO_2$ was kept constant.

The radioactivity (^{99mc}Tc-HMPAO) was injected 30 minutes after starting THT. In the control group radioactivity was applied after the same time interval.

On average 68 minutes after administration of ^{99mc}Tc-HMPAO brain SPECT studies were performed using a four-headed dedicated brain emission computer tomograph. The animals were kept ventilated during the SPECT. Uptake values were expressed as the percentage of the injected radioactivity present in the whole brain at the time of acquisition.

All animals were sacrificed. The brains were removed and fixed in formalin for macroscopic documentation and histological examination.

Results

Intracranial Pressure (ICP)

Mean ICP of both groups was 5.7 mm Hg (5–8 mm Hg) before SAH induction. During bolus blood

Table 1. *Hypervolemic Effects of THT*

Animal	Baseline CVP [mm Hg]	CVP during THT (Δ CVP; %) [mm Hg]	Baseline PWP [mm Hg]	PWP during THT (Δ PWP, %) [mm Hg]	Volume hetastarch [ml]
1 (Group I)	(5)		(9)		
2 (Group I)	(6)		(7)		
3 (Group II)	8	14 (+6; +75%)	8	14 (+6; +75%)	750
4 (Group I)	(6)		(7)		
5 (Group II)	4	13 (+9; +225%)	8	16 (+8; +100%)	800
6 (Group II)	6	8 (+2; +33%)	8	12.5 (+4.5; +56%)	700
Mean (Group II)	6	11.7 (+5.7; 95%)	8	14.2 (+6.2; 78%)	750

Table 2. *Cardiovascular Effects of THT*

Animal	Baseline MAP [mm Hg]	MAP during THT (Δ MAP; %) [mm Hg]	Baseline CO [l/min]	CO during THT (Δ CO, %) [l/min]
1 (Group I)	(96)		(2.3)	
2 (Group I)	(91)		(2.8)	
3 (Group II)	83	146 (63; +75%)	2.5	9.0 (6.5; +260%)
4 (Group I)	(80)		(2.1)	
5 (Group II)	85	131 (46; +54%)	2.3	6.1 (3.8; +165%)
6 (Group II)	74	143 (69; +93%)	2.7	7.0 (4.3; +159%)
Mean (group II)	80.7	140 (59.3; +73%)	2.5	7.4 (4.9; +196%)

application short term increases in ICP with a mean maximum of 75.3 mm Hg (13–129 mm Hg) followed by rapid decreases could be observed in both groups. Animal 1 (control group) showed only a slight increase from 5 to 13 mm Hg.

Hemodynamic Effects of Triple "H" Therapy (THT)

Mean CVP of group II was 6 mm Hg and mean PWP was 8 mm Hg before THT. Infusion of 6% hetastarch produced a CVP of 11.7 mm Hg (mean), whereas PWP was elevated to 14.2 mm Hg (mean). Thus, the induction of the hypervolemic state was effective with a mean CVP increase of 5.7 mm Hg and a mean PWP increase of 6 mm Hg. The mean volume of hetastarch required to reach the higher CVP and PWP values was 750 ml (Table 1).

Baseline MAP of 80.7 mm Hg was elevated to 140 mm Hg (mean), an increase of 73% over control values. Simultaneously, CO increased from a baseline value of 2.5 l/min to a mean of 7.4 l/min, a difference of 196% (Table 2).

Single Photon Emission Computed Tomography (SPECT)

Mean uptake of radioactivity, expressed in % of applied radioactivity/kg brain weight at the time of acquisition, was 0.64 in native SPECT (both groups). After induction of SAH mean uptake in control group (group I) was 0.52 and 0.42 in group II. Each animal of the THT group showed a decrease in uptake. The same effect was seen in animals 2 and 4 of the control group, whereas animal 1 (control group) showed an increase of the uptake of radioactivity (Table 3).

Discussion

Delayed neurological deterioration following SAH is attributed to cerebral vasospasm. In the presence of this vasospasm cerebral autoregulation is thought to be impaired and consequently, CBF becomes pressure dependent. The rationale behind THT is to increase MAP, raise CO and decrease blood viscosity in order to improve CBF in ischemic areas with impaired autoregulation [3, 6].

Table 3. *Uptake of Radioactivity*

Animal	Native SPECT [%/kg tissue weight]	Uptake after SAH and THT [%/kg tissue weight]	Uptake after SAH (no THT) [%/kg tissue weight]
1 (Group I)	0.52		0.58
2 (Group I)	0.69		0.46
3 (Group II)	0.59	0.44	
4 (Group I)	0.59		0.51
5 (Group II)	0.75	0.44	
6 (Group II)	0.66	0.37	
Mean	0.63	0.42	0.52

Against this theoretical background the decrease in uptake of ^{99m}Tc-HMPAO in the treatment group, demonstrating a decrease of CBF, is an unexpected result. There are two crucial questions concerning our study: 1) Which phenomenon did we really study? 2) Is SPECT an accessible technique to assess CBF after SAH?

1) Several animal models have been used to study the pathophysiological mechanisms and the effects of different treatments of cerebral vasospasm after SAH. We used an animal model established by McCormick [4]. The induction of SAH resulted in a significant deposition of blood in the supratentorial basal cisterns and cortical surfaces and the histological examination revealed red blood cells in the subarachnoid. This produced the expected decrease of ^{99m}Tc-HMPAO uptake in animals 2 and 4 (control group). Only animal 1 showed a slight increase from 0.52 to 0.58 accompanied by a very small increase of ICP during induction of SAH. Because all animals of the treatment group demonstrated a clear increase of ICP, we conclude that the induction of SAH was significant in the THT group.

The animal model we used only simulates acute conditions after SAH and therefore can only lead to statements concerning the early phase of SAH. According to Oropello [6] the ischemic injury of the first minutes after SAH may play a more important role than the later vasospasm.

2) Probably, delayed neurological deficits after SAH are not simply caused by vasospasm but are multifactorial (embolization, thrombosis, reperfusion injury) [6]. SPECT perfusion studies demonstrate that SPECT facilitates the detection of this early state of hypoperfusion [1, 5].

After reaching a significant increase of uptake of ^{99m}Tc-HMPAO by stimulation of the Gasserian ganglion [2] we expected the same effect after THT. On the contrary, our study revealed a slight decrease of uptake of ^{99m}Tc-HMPAO. This decrease has to be interpreted as a reduction of CBF in the early phase after SAH under THT.

We cannot differentiate whether the observed hypoperfusional state is due to epinephrine, to hetastarch or to both. Maybe, the choice of catecholamine alters the efficacy of THT. At least, the use of other treatment protocols (norepinephrine or dopamine instead of epinephrine) does not lead to a better complication rate [6].

Conclusion

In our study THT, carried out with epinephrine/hetastarch, slightly decreased CBF after induced SAH in pigs. In view of its severe potential complications and the lack of clear evidence of its efficacy, the use of THT as a routine treatment of cerebal ischemic injury after SAH has to be questioned. If applied, THT implies cardiovascular monitoring (PAC) to minimize potential side effects.

References

1. Facco E, Munari M, Behr AU, Baratto F, Zucchetta P, Bui F, Cesaro S, Giron GP (1998) Assessment of brain perfusion in coma and comparison between SPECT and CT scan data: Preliminary report. Neurolog Res [Suppl] 1(20): S40
2. Ebel H, Semmelmann G, Volz M, Lee J, Dueck M (2001) Effects of electrical stimulation of the Gasserian ganglion on regional cerebral blood flow after induced subarachnoid hemorrhage in pigs evaluated by ^{99m}Tc-HMPAO. Min Inv Neurosurg (in press)
3. Kassell NF, Peerless SJ, Durward QJ, Beck DW, Drake CG, Adams HP (1982) Treatment of ischemic deficits from vasospasm with intravascular volume expansion and induced arterial hypertension. Neurosurgery 11: 337–343
4. McCormick JM, McCormick PW, Zabramski JM, Spetzler RF

(1993) Intracranial pressure reduction by a central α-2 adrenoreceptor agonist after subarachnoid hemorrhage. Neurosurgery 32: 974–979

5. Masdeu JC, Brass LM (1995) SPECT imaging of stroke. J Neuroimag 5: S14–S22
6. Oropello JM, Weiner L, Benjamin E (1996) Hypertensive, hypervolemic, hemodilutional therapy for aneurysmal subarachnoid hemorrhage. Is it efficacious? No Crit Care Clin 12: 709–730

Correspondence: Dr. Michael Dueck, Department of Anesthesia, Joseph-Stelzmann-Str. 9, D-50924 Cologne, Germany.

Acta Neurochir (2001) [Suppl] 77: 247–250

Cerebral Vasospasm after Subarachnoid Hemorrhage: Hypertensive Hypervolemic Hemodilution (Triple-H) Therapy According to new Systemic Hemodynamic Parameters

N. Krayenbühl, T. Hegner, Y. Yonekawa, and **E. Keller**

Department of Neurosurgery, University Hospital Zurich, Switzerland

Introduction

Hypertensive hypervolemic hemodilution (triple-H) therapy is effective in reversing delayed ischemic deficits (DID) from cerebral vasospasm (CVS) [1, 6]. The most frequent severe complication of triple-H therapy is volume overload with consecutive pulmonary edema [1, 6, 10]. Monitoring of mean arterial pressure (MAP), central venous pressure (CVP) and pulmonary artery occlusive wedge pressure (PAOP) are conventionally used to control triple-H therapy, although their limitations to estimate intravascular volume state are well recognized [8]. Moreover, pulmonary artery catheterization as an invasive method is controversially discussed in literature [2]. Recently an alternative method, based on transpulmonary double-indicator dilution, has been established for assessment of intravascular volume [5]. Global enddiastolic volume (GEDV) and intrathoracic blood volume (ITBV) have been reported to reflect the intravascular volume status more adequately than CVP and PAOP. Also, extravascular lung water (EVLW) is a reliable predictor for early pulmonary edema [5]. With the development of a transpulmonary single thermodilution, the method became even easier to apply as bedside-monitoring on the ICU [9]. In addition the system allows continuous estimation of cardiac output (CO) by femoral arterial thermodilution calibrated pulse contour analysis [4].

We hypothesized that measurements, based on estimation of intracardiac volumes, may be more sensitive to control hypervolemia during triple-H therapy in patients with normal myocardial function than the conventionally used filling pressures CVP and PAOP. Therefore, the aim of the present study was to establish the new bedside monitoring technique in the environment of a neurosurgical intensive care unit and to examine its clinical value to guide triple-H therapy.

Keywords: Subarachnoid hemorrhage; vasospasm; triple-H therapy; intrathoracic blood volume.

Materials and Methods

From May 1999 to May 2000 27 patients with aneurysmal SAH and triple-H therapy were prospectively studied. The study was approved by the Ethics Committee of the University of Zurich (E-015/99). Triple-H therapy was induced when transcranial Doppler (TCD) blood flow velocities increased (middle cerebral artery mean blood flow velocities > 120 cm/sec or increase > 30 cm/sec within 24 hours) and/or the patient developed deficits from CVS. Surgery to clip the ruptured aneurysm was performed as soon as scheduling permitted (mean day 2). Patients with impaired cardiac function, peripheral occlusive arterial disease or coagulation disorders were excluded. Before the patients developed signs of CVS daily fluid balance was aimed to be positive adjusting fluid intake by intravenous infusion of crystalloids. Triple-H therapy was induced by administration of colloid and crystalloid infusion. Dopamine, dobutamine and norepinephrine were adjusted to maximize cardiac function. Excessive natriuresis and diuresis was inhibited with fludrocortisone 0.2 mg/day. If patients with DID showed no neurological improvement or worsened within an hour after starting the triple-H therapy, angiography and treatment with percutaneous angioplasty and/or superselective papaverine infusion into the spastic vessels were performed, after exclusion of hypoxia, electrolyte imbalance and hydrocephalus. Patients, in whom symptomatic CVS persisted or reoccurred immediately after the above mentioned intervention, were treated with barbiturate coma and/or hypothermia according to our standardized treatment regimen.

Before initiation of triple-H therapy, a 13 cm long 4-F arterial catheter with a thermistor embedded in its wall (PV-2015L13, Pulsion Medical Systems, Munich) was inserted in the femoral artery and connected to the pulse contour analysis computer (PICCO Pulsion Medical Systems, Munich). Arterial thermodilution was performed with a 10 ml ice cold ringer lactate bolus rapidly injected into a 12 Gauge central venous line. MAP, heart rate, temperature, CO and systemic vascular resistance SVR were monitored continuously.

Thermodilution with calibration of CO and determination of GEDV, ITBV and EVLW were regularly performed every six hours. During unstable hemodynamic conditions (arrhythmias, varying heart rate and MAP) additional thermodilution measurements were performed. Continuous CO was determined by an algorithm for pulse contour analysis, which involves measuring the area under the systolic portion of the arterial pulse wave (A_{syst}) from the end of diastole to the end of the ejection phase. Dividing A_{syst} by the empirically determined characteristic aortic impedance (Z_{AO}) provides a measure of stroke volume. The latter multiplied with the heart rate (HR) yields the CO (CO [l/min] $= HR \times A_{syst} \times Z_{AO}^{-1}$) [4]. The calibration of the actual characteristic aortic impedance for the individual patients was obtained by three subsequent determinations of CO by arterial thermodilution.

In addition to the conventional parameters (MAP > 105 mmHg, CVP 8–12 mmHg, hematocrit 28–32%) triple-H therapy was estimated to be most effective if the following target values (calculated in indices) were reached: (Cardiac index) CI > 4 l/min/m^2, (intrathoracic blood volume index) ITBVI 1000–1200 ml/m^2 and (extravascular lung water index) EVLWI < 10 ml/kg. The reoccurrence rate of symptomatic CVS after percutaneous angioplasty/papaverine and the incidence of pulmonary edema were analyzed. Hydrostatic pulmonary edema was defined as the chest x-ray showing signs of pulmonary congestion (perihilar haze, poorly outlined pulmonary vessels, subpleural edema) in the absence of specific signs of pneumonia or hypoalbuminemia.

Results

In 27 patients with signs of CVS 615 measurements during triple-H therapy were obtained. No complications associated with the measurement method were observed. Patient characteristics are listed in Table 1. In one patient instead of elevated TCD blood flow velocities CVS could not be localized in angiography. Nevertheless, this patient developed DID and cerebral perfusion was assumed to be compromised in small vessels. Therefore triple-H therapy was continued but no angioplasty or papaverine infusion was performed. The mean value of the 615 measurements in all 27 patients was 105 ($\pm$9,9 SD) mmHg for MAP, 11 ($\pm$3,9 SD) mmHg for CVP, 4,5 ($\pm$0,9 SD) l/min/m^2 for CI, 1102 ($\pm$261 SD) ml/m^2 for ITBVI and 8 ($\pm$3,4 SD) for EVLWI. The values were in the therapeutic range as shown in Table 2. In 53%, 54%, 19%, 63% respectively 26% of the measurements target values were not reached and led to therapeutic implications (further volume expansion, administration of vasopressor agents or diuretics). In 10 of 27 patients more than 50% of the defined target values for MAP and CVP were reached. Only in one of these 10 patients with MAP and CVP within the therapeutic range target values for CI, ITBVI and EVLWI were reached simultaneously. 16 of 27 patients (59%) developed DID (table 3). From these 16 patients 12 were treated with angioplasty and/or papaverine infusion. Papaverine instillation was not performed in four patients with progressive deficit because of acute internal carotid artery (ICA) spasm during angiography (one patient), severe carotid stenosis (one patient), or unstable hemodynamic or respiratory conditions not allowing transport of the patients (two patients). CVS after instillation of papaverine reoccurred in seven patients (26%) (table 3). Four patients were treated with papaverine for a second time. Pulmonary edema occurred in one patient and responded well to administration of diuretics. Elevated EVLWI correlated with the signs of pulmonary congestion in the chest x-ray films. Complications related to the method, like local infection, bleeding or occurance of femoral pseudoaneurysms did not occur.

Table 1. *Patient Characteristics*

GENDER	
Number of patients	
Male	8
Female	19
Age mean (range)	56 (31–76)
HUNT & HESS GRADE	
Number of patients	
I	3
II	13
III	2
IV	7
V	2
Localization of ruptured aneurysm	
Number of patients	
ICA	4
AcoA	10
Percallosal artery	2
Anterior choroidal artery	1
MCA	7
Localization of vasospasm in angiography	
Number of patients	
ICA unilateral	1
ACA	
unilateral	3
bilateral	1
MCA	
unilateral	7
bilateral	5
MCA unilateral + ACA unilateral	8
MCA unilateral + ACA bilateral	1
CVS not localized	1
Number of measurements	
All patients	615
Per patient, mean (SD)	23 ($\pm$11)
Measurement period	
Number of days, mean (SD)	6.5 ($\pm$2.4)

ICA Internal carotid artery; *ACoA* anterior communicating artery; *ACA* anterior cerebral artery; *MCA* middle cerebral artery.

Table 2. *615 Measurements of Systemic Hemodynamic Parameters During Triple-H Therapy: Target Values and Number of Measurements Within Therapeutic Range*

Parameter[in]	Target values (%)	Number of values in therapeutic range (%) N = 615	Number of values not therapeutic range N = 615
MAP	>105 mmHg	326 (53%)	289 (47%)
CVP	8–12 mmHg*	329 (54%)	286 (46%)
CI	>4 $l/min/m^2$	497 (81%)	118 (19%)
ITBVI	1000–1200 ml/m^2	225 (37%)	390 (63%)
EVLWI	<10 ml/kg	455 (74%)	160 (26%)

* In mechanically ventilated patients positive endexpiratory pressure as PEEP (mmHg) ×0.5 was added to CVP target values. *N* Total number of measurements.

Table 3. *Outcome of 27 Patients with Vasospasm and Triple-H Therapy*

	Number of patients (%) N = 27
Treatment with triple-H therapy	27 (100%)
Symptoms of DID	16 (59%)
Treatment with additional angioplasty and/or superselective papaverine infusion	12 (44%)
Reoccurrance of CVS after first angioplasty/papaverine	7 (26%)
Incidence of pulmonary edema	1 (<0.5%)
Permanent DID with disability from CVS	2 (7%)
Death from CVS	0 (0%)

N Total number of patients; *Triple-H* hypertensive hypervolemic hemodilution; *DID* delayed ischemic deficit; *CVS* cerebral vasospasm.

Discussion

615 valuable measurements with the methodology were obtained. No procedural complications were observed. The new monitoring system, less invasive than pulmonary artery catheterization, seems to be safe and easy to perform in neurosurgical ICU patients.

Triple-H therapy diminishes disability from CVS [1, 6]. Pulmonary edema is the most severe complication of triple-H therapy and occurs in 17 to 23% [6, 10]. Reliable assessment of intravascular volume status is essential during triple-H therapy. Numerous reports have demonstrated limitations of filling pressures as guides for monitoring of intravascular volume [5, 7]. CVP is influenced by right ventricular function and other factors that alter resistance, compliance and impedance of the venous system, whereas PAOP is altered particularly in the mechanically ventilated patient by intrathoracic and intraabdominal pressure [8]. Compared to literature, the incidence of pulmonary edema was very low in our patients with the new monitoring strategy. Treatment with angioplasty and papaverine was often successful, probably because of sustained effective triple-H during and after the procedure [3]. Determination of ITBV and EVLW are based on estimation of intracardiac volumes. Therefore, the technique is more sensitive to control intravascular volume status and allows detection of even small changes in volume load in patients with normal myocardial function [7]. This suggests, supported by our first experiences, that the new monitoring system might be the optimal instrument to guide triple-H therapy. However, some limitations of the method have to be considered. The diagnostic value of monitoring GEDV and ITBV is reduced in patients with impaired ventricular function [7]. In heart failure left ventricular compliance is reduced and with volume loading, increases of cardiac filling pressures might be relatively more pronounced and sensitive than changes in ventricular size.

Conclusion

With the small number of patients studied we cannot properly analyze the importance of MAP, CO, ITBV and EVLW as independent factors to guide triple-H therapy. Larger populations will allow multivariate analysis and definition of optimal target values for the systemic hemodynamic parameters.

The new monitoring system to estimate CO, ITBV and EVLW may be most suited to guide triple-H therapy. It is less invasive than pulmonary artery catheterization and reflects intravascular volume status more reliably than conventional filling pressures. The method seems to be safe and easy to perform in the

ICU environment. Further studies in larger populations are needed to define the optimal target values in triple-H therapy for the most effective regimen.

References

1. Awad IA, Carter LP, Spetzler RF (1986) Clinical vasospasm after subarachnoid hemorrhage: response to hypervolemic hemodilution an arterial hypertension. Stroke 18: 365–372
2. Dalen JE, Bone RC (1996) Is it time to pull the pulmonary artery catheter? JAMA 276: 916–918
3. Fandino J, Kaku Y, Schuknecht B, Valavanis A, Yonekawa Y (1998) Improvement of cerebral oxygenation patterns and metabolic validation of superselective intraarterial infusion of papaverine for the treatment of cerebral vasospasm. J Neurosurg 89: 93–100
4. Goedje O, Hoeke K, Lichtwarck-Aschoff M, Falt Chauser A, Lamm P, Reichart B (1999) Continuous cardiac output by femoral arterial thermodilution calibrated pulse contour analysis: Comparison with pulmonary arterial thermodilution. Crit Care Med 27: 2407–2412
5. Hoeft A, Schorn B, Weyland A, Scholz M, Buhre W, Stepanek E, Allen SJ, Sonntag H (1994) Bedside assessment of intravascular volume status in patients undergoing coronary bypass surgery. Anesthesiology 81: 76–86
6. Kassell NF, Peerless SJ, Duward QJ, Beck DW, Drake CG, Adams HP (1982) Treatment of ischemic deficits from vasospasm with intravascular volume expansion and induced arterial hypertension. Neurosurg 11: 337–343
7. Mundigler G, Heinze G, Zehetgruber M, Gabriel H, Siostrzonek P (2000) Limitations of the transpulmonary indicator dilution method for assessment of preload changes in critically ill patients with reduced left ventricular function. Crit Care Med 28: 2231–2237
8. Raper R, Sibbald WJ (1986) Misled by the wedge? The Swan-Ganz catheter and left ventricular preload. Chest 89: 427–434
9. Sakka SG, Ruhl CC, Pfeiffer UJ, Beale R, McLuckie A, Reinhart K, Meier-Hellmann A (2000) Assessment of cardiac preload and extravascular lung water by single transpulmonary thermodilution. Intensive Care Med 26: 180–187
10. Solenski NJ, Haley Jr EC, Kassell NF (1995) Medical complications of aneurysmal subarachnoid hemorrhage: a report of the multicenter, cooperative aneurysm study. Crit Care Med 23: 1007–1017

Correspondence: Niklaus Krayenbühl M.D., Department of Neurosurgery, University Hospital Zürich, Frauenklinikstr. 10, 8091 Zürich, Switzerland.

Acta Neurochir (2001) [Suppl] 77: 251–254

Antiischemic Therapy of Severe Prolonged Vasospasm after Aneurysmal SAH: Effects on Quality of Life

I. Kreitschmann-Andermahr, B. O. Hütter, and **J. M. Gilsbach**

Department of Neurosurgery, University Hospital, University of Technology Aachen, FRG

Introduction

The in-between broad acceptance of early surgery and improved intensive care management have led to a significant reduction of vasospasm associated morbidity and mortality within the last 25 years. However, the large body of publications concerned with the prevention and treatment of vasospasm still denote its role as one of the major complications in the postoperative management after aneurysmal subarachnoid hemorrhage (SAH). Next to purely mechanical measures such as balloon dilatation of vasospastic vessels and intraarterial papaverine infusion, which as of now lack verification by means of larger controlled clinical trials, established medical treatment concepts focus on pharmacological approaches such as the calcium antagonist nimodipine and hypervolemic hemodilution and hypertension ("Triple-H" therapy). The present study was concerned with the question whether "aggressive" sustained hypertension as one of the components of "Triple-H" has additional benefit for the patients with severe and prolonged vasospasm that is reflected in their later quality of life. Health-related quality of life (HQOL) was chosen as an outcome parameter because it covers substantial areas of the patients' daily life not assessed by conventional outcome scales such as the Glasgow Outcome Scale (GOS), which is merely reduced to the level of physical function.

Keywords: SAH; vasospasm; triple-H therapy; quality of life.

Patients and Methods

A series of 780 consecutive patients with spontaneous aneurysmal SAH proven by CT-scan and/or lumbar puncture with four vessel angiography demonstrating no other vascular malformation than an aneurysm as the bleeding source were treated in our department between 1990 and 1997. Of these, 91 (11.6%) developed severe and prolonged vasospasm defined as mean blood flow velocities measured by transcranial Doppler (TCD) exceeding 160 cm/sec with a duration of blood flow velocities greater than 120 cm/sec for at least five days. Thirty-nine of these patients received a conventional regimen based on normovolemic hemodilution, maintenance of normal to slightly elevated blood pressure values and bed rest during the period of dopplersonographic vasospasm, while in the other 52 patients an aggressive treatment regimen of TCD-guided catecholamine-induced hypertension was additionally employed as soon as blood flow velocities exceeded a threshold value of 120 cm/sec [6]. All of the surviving patients and their life-companions were invited by mail to fill out the Aachen Life Quality Inventory (ALQI), a self-report and proxy-rating questionnaire based on the modified German version of the Sickness Impact Profile [5]. The ALQI was developed especially for the use in patients with brain damage. It measures sickness-related complaints in the following 11 areas of life: activation, mobility, house-work, work, free-time activities, ambulation, autonomy, social contact, family relations, communication and intellectual capacity. The 117 items enable the calculation of 11 subscale impairment scores, a summary score of total impairment (Total score), a Psycho-social summary score and a Physical score. The subscale "Work" is not included into the Total score because of methodological problems. The proxy-rating version of the ALQI was developed in order to account for the problem of decreased introspection in some patients with brain damage. For both ALQI versions, the degree of internal consistency can be regarded as excellent to satisfactory for the summary scores as well as for the individual subscales [5].

The HQOL study sample comprises the 71/91 (78%) patients who returned the questionnaires, 41 of whom had received the aggressive hypertensive treatment (catecholamine group) while in 30 the conventional treatment concept had been employed (here termed control group). There were 19 men and 52 women in the study sample. Table 1 gives an overview of the clinical parameters in both groups.

The only significantly different clinical parameter between the two groups was the highest mean blood flow velocity measured by TCD which was significantly higher in the catecholamine group. Both groups were furthermore comparable in terms of the severity of the bleeding (Fisher CT-grading system; Chi-square $p = 0.31$) as well as the clinical state on admission (Hunt & Hess; Chi-square $p = 0.57$).

Table 1. *Clinical Characteristics in Both Groups*

	Control group		Catechol. Group		t-test
	Mean	(SD)	Mean	(SD)	p
Age (years)	46.3	(10.9)	44.4	(12.7)	0.53 ns
Delay SAH/follow-up (months)	27.9	(4.9)	28.6	(4.6)	0.54 ns
Max. blood flow velocity (TCD)	184.1	(26.4)	202.3	(32.3)	0.01*
Duration of vasospasm (days)	12.4	(5.4)	11.7	(4.3)	0.56 ns

Table 2. *Neurological Parameters in 91 Patiens with Severe and Prolonged Vasospasm*

Entire collective	Control group (n = 39)		Catechol. Group (n = 52)		p
Delayed neurological deficits	22	(56%)	20	(38%)	<0.01*
Vasospastic infarctions	13	(33%)	17	(33%)	0.98 ns
Fatalities due to vasospasm[#]	5	(13%)	3	(6%)	0.18 ns
Pat. discharged GOS IV[#]	9	(23%)	4	(8%)	0.056*

[#] Small N permutation test Holm procedure; Beta error p = 0.10 [10].

Results

In the entire collective of the 91 patients with severe and prolonged vasospasm, there were no differences in terms of fatalities caused by vasospasm and the number of vasospastic infarctions between the conventionally treated patients (n = 39) and the catecholamine patients (n = 52). However, in the latter group significantly less delayed neurological deficits were observed and significantly less patients were discharged in a vegetative state (GOS = IV). For an overview of these neurological parameters in both groups see Table 2.

Neurological outcome as assessed by the GOS was not statistically different between the two treatment groups in those patients who returned the ALQI (Chi-square p = 0.53). Only one patient (2%) in the catecholamine group rated GOS = IV at discharge had been able to return the questionnaire, whereas the majority of the other patients had been in a good neurological state at discharge (GOS I and II: 26 patients (34%) in the control group and 32 patients (45%) in the catecholamine group).

Because the clinical parameter "maximally increased mean blood flow velocities" proved to be significantly different in these patients between the control and the catecholamine group, an analysis of covariance (ANCOVA) was performed in order to control for the effect of the different increased mean blood flow velocities. HQOL as assessed by the ALQI served as the dependent variable. However, neither in the subscales of the ALQI nor in one of the ALQI summary scores, a significant difference between the patients who had received the conventional treatment and the catecholamine patients emerged in terms of self-assessed HQOL. Furthermore, no significant effect of the covarivate "maximally increased mean blood flow velocities" was observed in any of the subscales or sum scores of the ALQI for the self-rated quality of

Table 3. *Self-Rated HQOL in n = 71 Patients after Severe and Prolonged Vasospasm*

ALQI subscales	Control group Mean	Catechol. group Mean	ANCOVA p
Activation	4.2	2.4	>0.05 ns
Mobility	1.0	1.2	>0.05 ns
House-work	2.8	3.2	>0.05 ns
Social contact	2.3	2.7	>0.05 ns
Family relations	1.2	1.1	>0.05 ns
Ambulation	1.9	1.6	>0.05 ns
Free-time activities	3.3	3.2	>0.05 ns
Communication	0.8	0.6	>0.05 ns
Autonomy	0.1	0.3	>0.05 ns
Cognition	6.9	6.2	>0.05 ns
Psycho-Social score	12.0	10.2	>0.05 ns
Physical score	12.8	12.6	>0.05 ns
ALQI Total score	24.8	22.8	>0.05 ns

No single effect of the covariate "maximally increased mean blood flow velocities".

Table 4. *Proxy-Rated HQOL in n = 71 Patients after Severe and Prolonged Vasospasm*

ALQI subscales	Control group Mean	Catechol. group Mean	ANCOVA+ p	COV+ P
Activation	2.0	2.1	>0.05 ns	*
Mobility	0.8	1.0	>0.05 ns	*
House-work	2.9	3.1	>0.05 ns	ns
Social contact	2.8	2.4	>0.05 ns	ns
Family relations	1.2	1.7	>0.05 ns	*
Ambulation	1.5	1.6	>0.05 ns	ns
Free-time activities	3.8	2.8	>0.05 ns	ns
Communication	0.7	0.8	>0.05 ns	ns
Autonomy	0.2	0.3	>0.05 ns	ns
Cognition	5.7	5.9	>0.05 ns	ns
Psycho-Social score	12.0	10.2	>0.05 ns	*
Physical score	11.0	12.0	>0.05 ns	ns
ALQI Total score	21.7	22.0	>0.05 ns	ns

* Covariate "maximally increased mean blood flow velocities"; $p<0.05$.
+ Main effect of group (catecholamine vs. conventionally treated).

life. Table 3 provides the details of the results of the ALQI self-rating version between the two groups.

In close correspondence to the self-rated HQOL, in the proxy-rating version of the ALQI, no significant differences between the catecholamine and the control group emerged in terms of later quality of life (Table 4). However, in the ALQI subscales "Activation", "Family relations" and "Mobility" as well as the ALQI Psycho-social score, a significant unfavorable effect on HQOL by the covariate "maximally increased mean blood flow velocities" became evident.

Discussion

It was the aim of the present study to assess the effect of induced sustained hypertension on HQOL by means of TCD-guided continuous catecholamine administration in an 8 year series of patients with severe and prolonged vasospasm after aneurysmal SAH. While several older studies reported on an improved neurological outcome under "Triple-H" therapy [1, 9], indications exist, that aggressive volume expansion for the treatment of severe vasospasm does not confer additional benefit [7] or may even be harmful because of the risk of vasogenic brain edema [8]. In our opinion, the most important and straightforward factor of the "Triple-H" approach is hypertension. The concept, that catecholamine-induced hypertension results in an improvement of cerebral blood flow (CBF) in ischemic regions is supported by the findings of Darby *et al.* [2], who demonstrated a significant increase of CBF in ischemic brain regions after dopamine administration. The fact that already in clinically asymptomatic patients, sites of increased Doppler velocities correlated to abnormalities of perfusion (hypoperfusion, perfusion deficits) in SPECT [3] speaks for its prophylactic initiation based on TCD results.

Our hypertensive therapy regimen led to a significantly decreased occurrence of delayed neurological deficits and proved to have a favorable effect on the number of patients discharged vegetative (GOS = IV). However, favorable effects of this pharmacological measure on the later quality of life of the surviving patients were not observed. Two reasons may account for this effect: First, the sample size of 71 patients might still be to small to uncover differential effects of one treatment modality on such a complex construct as quality of life which is predicted in SAH patients most of all by the severity of the initial bleeding [4]. Second, the results might be influenced by a selection bias, since those patients who remained vegetative were neither able to fill out the questionnaire nor did the questions of the proxy-rating version apply to this clinical subgroup.

An interesting effect was the observed negative influence of the covariate "maximally increased mean blood flow velocities" on some areas of the patients' quality of life as rated by their life-companions. When attributing the significantly higher mean blood flow velocities to catecholamine treatment, this finding invites to speculate that the positive effect of induced hypertension on neurological outcome may be over-compensated for in the long run by adverse effects of this treatment on the patients' later quality of life.

Conclusion

Although TCD-guided hypertensive therapy as a pharmacological treatment of severe vasospasm after aneurysmal SAH has a positive effect on neurological outcome, beneficial late effects on HQOL were not observed in the present study. This result may be explained by the fact that improvements of HQOL due to the therapeutical effect of this measure may remain marginal in comparison to the severe consequences of the hemorrhage itself.

References

1. Awad I, Carter LP, Spetzler RF, Medina M, Williams FC Jr (1987) Clinical vasospasm after subarachnoid hemorrhage: Response to hypervolemic hemodilution and arterial hypertension. Stroke 18: 365–372
2. Darby JM, Yonas H, Marks EC, Durham S, Snyder RW, Nemoto EM (1994) Acute cerebral blood flow response to dopamine-induced hypertension after subarachnoid hemorrhage. J Neurosurg 80: 857–864
3. Grosset DG, Straiton J, du Trevou M, Bullock R (1992) Prediction of symptomatic vasospasm after subarachnoid hemorrhage by rapidly increasing transcranial Doppler velocity and cerebral blood flow changes. Stroke 23: 674–679
4. Hütter BO, Kreitschmann-Andermahr I, Mayfrank L, Rohde V, Spetzger U, Giesbach JM (1999) Functional outcome after aneurysmal subarachnoid hemorrhage. Acta Neurochir [Suppl] (Wien) 72: 157–74
5. Hütter BO (2000) Neuropsychological sequelae of subarachnoid hemorrhage and its treatment. Springer, Wien New York, pp 67–72
6. Kreitschmann-Andermahr I, Hütter BO, Gilsbach JM (1996) Prävention und Therapie des Vasospasmus. In: Böker DK (ed) Neue Aspekte zu Pathogenese und Therapie des zerebralen Vasospasmus. Biermann, Zülpich, pp 74–86
7. Lennihan L, Mayer SA, Fink ME, Beckford A, Paick MC, Zhang H, Wu Yc, Klebanoff LM, Raps EC, Solomon RA (2000) Effect of hypervolemic therapy on cerebral blood flow after subarachnoid hemorrhage – a randomized controlled trial. Stroke 31: 383–391
8. Shimoda M, Oda S, Tsugane R, Sato O (1993) Intracranial complications of hypervolemic therapy in patients with a delayed ischemic deficit attributed to vasospasm. J Neurosurg 78: 423–429
9. Solomon RA, Fink ME, Lennihan L (1988) Prophylactic volume expansion therapy for the prevention of delayed cerebral ischemia after early aneurysm surgery. Arch Neurol 45: 325–332
10. Edginton ES (1995) Randomization tests, 3rd edn. Marcel Dekker, New York

Correspondence: Ilonka Kreitschmann-Andermahr, M.D., Department of Neurosurgery, University Hospital, University of Technology (RWTH) Aachen, Pauwelsstrasse 30, D-52074 Aachen, FRG.

Acta Neurochir (2001) [Suppl] 77: 255–258

Hypothermia Reduces Acute Vasospasm Following SAH in Rats

C. Thomé[1], **G. Schubert**[1], **A. Piepgras**[1], **V. Elste**[2], **L. Schilling**[1], and **P. Schmiedek**[1]

[1] Department of Neurosurgery, Fac. Clin. Med. Mannheim, Germany
[2] Department of Neuroradiology, University of Heidelberg, Germany

Introduction

Subarachnoid hemorrhage (SAH) due to rupture of an aneurysm results in acute brain injury manifesting itself clinically as an acute neurologic deficit. Depending on the severity of the bleeding, the patients are classified according to clinical grading scales. This classification allows estimation of individual prognosis, as the extent of acute injury constitutes the crucial parameter for outcome following SAH. This statement has only recently been confirmed by Proust *et al.* [8], who reported a favorable outcome after Hunt and Hess grades IV and V in only 10% of cases.

Cerebral blood flow (CBF) studies within the first 48 hours after SAH have demonstrated, that the higher the patients' clinical grade, the more reduced the cerebral perfusion [6]. This reduction in CBF may result in acute global ischemia due to decreased cerebral perfusion pressure (CPP) caused by the dramatic rise in intracranial pressure (ICP) at the time of bleeding. However, hypoperfusion lasting for many hours [6] cannot be sufficiently explained by intracranial hypertension. Acute vasospasm has been experimentally shown to cause early posthemorrhagic ischemia independently of changes in ICP and CPP [2]. In addition, the brain parenchyma is endangered by edema formation with consecutive increase in ICP and resulting hypoperfusion [6]. In view of this pathophysiological scenario, the course of SAH may be influenced favorably in particular during the acute stage of the disease by neuroprotective, antivasospastic and/or antiedematous measures.

The efficacy of cranial hypothermia to confer neuroprotection in ischemia has been established in several experimental studies. The effect of hypothermia on acute subarachnoid hemorrhage, however, is unclear. Therefore, the objective of this study was to examine the effects of moderate hypothermia on CBF and edema formation in the acute phase of experimental SAH.

Keywords: Acute vasospasm; hypothermia; laser doppler flowmetry; diffusion weighted magnetic resonance imaging.

Materials and Methods

Male Sprague-Dawley rats weighing 250 to 350 g were divided into two groups: rats were either used for measurement of CBF, ICP and CPP for 2 h following experimental SAH or for quantification of edema formation. Animals in both groups were allocated to normothermia (37 °C) or moderate hypothermia (32 °C). Cooling was performed prior to induction of SAH to study intra- and posthemorrhagic hypothermia.

Surgical Preparation

The animals were anesthetized with barbiturates, tracheotomized and artificially ventilated. The right femoral artery was cannulated for monitoring of arterial blood pressure (ABP) and blood gases, and ventilation was adjusted to maintain arterial blood gases within the normal range (arterial $PaCO_2$ of 35 mmHg).

Measurement of ICP and CBF

Rats were placed in a stereotactic frame with their heads in a slight forward flexion. A midline scalp incision was made over the parieto-occipital bone descending to the neck and the posterior cervical muscles were separated. The atlanto-occipital membrane was bluntly exposed to pass a 27-gauge saline-filled needle into the cisterna magna for ICP measurements.

For monitoring of cortical blood flow, a closed cranial window over the parietal cortex was prepared and a laser-Doppler flowmetry (LDF) probe (Moor Instruments Inc., Wilmington, De., USA) was advanced under stereotactic control avoiding large pial vessels.

Quantification of Edema

Having prepared the animals for induction of SAH (see below), they were placed in a 2.35 T Bruker Biospec 24/40 NMR scanner. Diffusion-weighted blipp epi spin echo sequences were used to cal-

Springer-Verlag and the Environment